Integrated Electronic Health Records:
A Worktext for
Greenway Medical Technologies'
PrimeSUITE®

M. Beth Shanholtzer, MAEd, RHIA

Lord Fairfax Community College,
Middletown, VA;
Blue Ridge Community & Technical College,
Martinsburg, WV;
and Carroll County Community College,
Westminster, MD

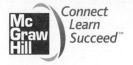

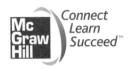

The McGraw·Hill Companies

Connect
Learn
Succeed™

INTEGRATED ELECTRONIC HEALTH RECORDS: A WORKTEXT FOR GREENWAY MEDICAL
TECHNOLOGIES' PrimeSUITE®

Published by McGraw-Hill, a business unit of The McGraw-Hill Companies, Inc., 1221 Avenue of
the Americas, New York, NY, 10020. Copyright © 2012 by The McGraw-Hill Companies, Inc. All
rights reserved. No part of this publication may be reproduced or distributed in any form or by
any means, or stored in a database or retrieval system, without the prior written consent of The
McGraw-Hill Companies, Inc., including, but not limited to, in any network or other electronic
storage or transmission, or broadcast for distance learning. Some ancillaries, including electronic
and print components, may not be available to customers outside the United States.
This book is printed on acid-free paper.

Printed in U.S.A.

6 7 8 9 0 QVS/LEH 1 0 9 8 7 6 5 4 3

ISBN   978-0-07-750872-2
MHID   0-07-750872-6

Vice president/Director of marketing: *Alice Harra*
Editorial director: *Michael S. Ledbetter*
Senior sponsoring editor: *Natalie J. Ruffatto*
Director, digital products: *Crystal Szewczyk*
Managing development editor: *Michelle L. Flomenhoft*
Executive marketing manager: *Roxan Kinsey*
Digital development editor: *Katherine Ward*
Digital product manager: *Thuan Vinh*
Director, Editing/Design/Production: *Jess Ann Kosic*
Lead project manager: *Rick Hecker*
Buyer II: *Sherry L. Kane*
Senior designer: *Marianna Kinigakis*
Senior photo research coordinator: *Jeremy Cheshareck*
Media project manager: *Brent dela Cruz*
Media project manager: *Cathy L. Tepper*
Cover design: *Cody Wallis and Nathan Kirkman*
Interior design: *Laurie Entringer*
Typeface: *11/13.5 Palatino*
Compositor: *Laserwords Private Limited*
Printer: *Quad/Graphics*

PrimeSUITE® is a Registered Trademark of Greenway Medical Technologies, Inc. Screenshots
and Material pertaining to PrimeSUITE® Software used with permission of Greenway Medical
Technologies, Inc. © 2011 Greenway Medical Technologies, Inc. All rights reserved.
All brand or product names are trademarks or registered trademarks of their respective companies.
CPT five-digit codes, nomenclature, and other data are © 2010 American Medical Association. All
rights reserved. No fee schedules, basic unit, relative values, or related listings are included in the
CPT. The AMA assumes no liability for the data contained herein.
CPT codes are based on CPT 2011.
ICD-9-CM codes are based on ICD-9-CM 2011.
All names, situations, and anecdotes are fictitious. They do not represent any person, event, or
medical record.

The Internet addresses listed in the text were accurate at the time of publication. The inclusion of a
Web site does not indicate an endorsement by the authors or McGraw-Hill, and McGraw-Hill does
not guarantee the accuracy of the information presented at these sites.

www.mhhe.com

brief contents

contents

EHR Matters!

Welcome to Integrated Electronic Health Records: An Online Course and Worktext for Greenway Medical Technologies' PrimeSUITE®!

Electronic Health Records implementation in the United States is creating great opportunities for people who want to work in the health professions. From front office staff to nurses, doctors, and every worker in between, understanding how health information is transferred and how that information can improve the quality of healthcare is a valuable skill. Everyone working in a healthcare setting will be impacted by electronic health records as they complete their daily tasks.

Developed as a comprehensive learning resource, this hands-on course for *Integrated Electronic Health Records* is offered through McGraw-Hill's *Connect Plus. Connect Plus* uses the latest technology and learning techniques to better connect professors to their students, and students to the information and customized resources they need to master a subject. It includes a variety of digital learning tools that enable instructors to easily customize courses and allow students to master content and succeed in the course.

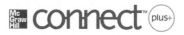

Integrated Electronic Health Records: A Worktext for Greenway Medical Technologies's PrimeSUITE complements the online *Connect Plus* course, and is written by an author with an extensive Health Information Management/Health Information Technology background—Beth Shanholtzer, MAEd, RHIA. Both the worktext and online course include coverage of Greenway Medical Technologies' PrimeSUITE, an ONC-ATCB-Certified, fully integrated, online Electronic Health Records, Practice Management, and interoperable physician-based solution. The book is not meant to be an extensive user manual for PrimeSUITE, but rather it covers the key topics for Electronic Health Records, with PrimeSUITE as the vehicle to demonstrate those topics. Attention is paid to providing the "why" behind each task so that the reader can accumulate transferable skills.

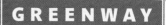

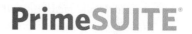

Electronic Health Records impact a variety of programs in the health professions; as such, this content will be relevant to Health Information Management, Health Information Technology, Medical Insurance, Billing, & Coding, Medical Assisting, and even Nursing programs! To help you determine with exercises would most benefit your students, all exercises are designated with PM (Practice Management), EHR (Electronic Health Records), HIM (Health Information Management) tags, or some combination of those three.

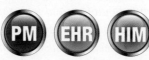

Instructors can access a correlation of the worktext's Learning Outcomes to key accrediting bodies such as CAHIIM, ABHES and CAAHEP via the book's website, **www.mhhe.com/greenway**.

Here are the advantages you will gain using this Online Course and Worktext:

- The opportunity to work hands-on with simulated content of real software—PrimeSUITE is used in physician practices across the country by more than 8,000 providers, impacting more than 29 million patient charts. The course contains 45 simulated PrimeSUITE exercises in the areas of Practice Management, Electronic Health Records, and Health Information Management.
- Having the same content for each mode of an exercise (Demo, Practice, Test, and Assessment) gives the student an opportunity to master the tasks.
- Simulating the software means the students' work can be assessed.
- *Connect Plus* is completely online—no software to install!

Here's How Instructors Have Described *Integrated EHR*:

This course is an excellent introduction for a student looking to become a part of the health information administration team! Multiple levels of knowledge and application are utilized in hands-on exercises to help you feel more comfortable in the challenging health dynamics of today.

—**Jill Ferrari, MA, MT, MLT (ASCP), Sullivan University**

I would list the following strengths for this product: it provides hands-on exposure to software that is compatible with those in current use in medical offices across the country; it provides exposure to day-to-day and administrator functions; and it introduces the use of the term 'meaningful use' as well as demonstrating examples of meaningful use.

—**Kathleen G. Bailey, CPA, MBA, CPC, CPC-I, Ultimate Medical Academy**

This product has the following strengths: it develops key concepts in understanding the function of an Electronic Health Record; it has a very methodical approach; and it uses a very hands-on skill development method allowing for as much review and practice as needed.

—**Kathy Jo Ellison, RN, DSN, Auburn University**

I like the approach of the book. It helps set the stage and prepare the student for a more in-depth approach later, after they have mastered the basics. Many of my textbooks jump right into the middle of a concept without laying the groundwork. This means the instructor has to set the stage. This book already has done that, and that allows the instructor to present more in-depth material, if desired, in the lectures.

—**Marsha Dolan, MBA, RHIA, FAHIMA, Missouri Western State University**

I would describe the book as . . . [one] that allows students to complete an entire EHR from registration to discharge of the patient. It allows the students to understand how reports are utilized and the importance of understanding the material to successfully run a medical office. In terms of the approach, hands-on experience can never be replaced with lecture. Most students become bored with lecture so using a hands-on approach brings the lecture 'to life' and provides a more thorough understanding of the topic.

—**Laura Michelsen, MS, RHIA, Joliet Junior College**

Content Highlights of *Integrated EHR* by Chapter

Chapter	Coverage
1	Introduces students to the applications used for administrative purposes (practice management) and electronic health records (EHR)—EHR's pros and cons, as well as EHR's purpose and how EHR can improve patient care. Also included is an overview of the flow of patient information—from registration to a complete health record and complete billing process.
2	Covers the transformation of data into information and the professionals who play key roles in the collection, maintenance, storage, and use of electronic information. The various tools used to collect data and the individual computerized applications used in healthcare are explored. Finally, the laws and standards that govern health information are introduced.
3	Administrative data—that which is collected to conduct the business side of healthcare—is addressed. The individual data elements that make up administrative data and the uses of that data are covered. The steps necessary to make an appointment and register a patient, collect administrative, including demographic data, and capture insurance information are all practiced through the exercises.
4	Data collection and maintenance from a clinical perspective is the focus. The past medical, surgical, family and social histories are collected through simulations. The importance of data accuracy, and proper handling of inconsistent, unclear, or incorrect data is covered in detail and practiced in PrimeSUITE.
5	Emphasizes the care provider's collection and use of healthcare data including the documentation of a patient's History of Present Illness, Review of Systems, and Physical Exam. Documentation methods, past and present, are discussed. Meaningful use of electronic health information is introduced in this chapter in relation to maintaining a Problem List, ePrescribing, and computerized order entry.
6	Returning to the administrative functions, this chapter addresses the claims management process including the use of a computer-generated Superbill, ICD-9-CM, CPT, and HCPCS coding using the practice management functionality of PrimeSUITE. The student will come away with a basic knowledge of billing and coding procedures through theory and practice. An introductory comparison of ICD-9-CM to ICD-10-CM/PCS coding is also addressed. Finally, the importance of billing and coding policies and standards to ensure compliance with regulations and agency requirements rounds out this chapter.
7	Regulations such as HIPAA and HITECH as well as legal concerns related to privacy and security are the emphasis. The HIPAA privacy and security standards are covered in depth. Through completion of PrimeSUITE simulated exercises, students learn methods to maintain security, safeguard data integrity, and audit compliance with access and release of information. Exercises also include Meaningful Use of electronic data for continuity of care and accounting for data disclosures.
8	Communication and managing information stored in an electronic environment is the focus. Storing all of this information and doing nothing with it is not the intent of an electronic health record. Improving the efficiency and effectiveness of communication is a goal of most offices; the electronic environment facilitates that. Documents do not always originate in an electronic format; thus, scanning of paper to a digital format is necessary and easily achieved through an electronic record. The use of templates allows for standardized data collection (and therefore more accurate and thorough information about a patient). An alert system prevents necessary screenings and testing from "slipping through the cracks," thus improving patient outcomes. Customization of screens permits flexibility and personal preferences of care providers and healthcare professionals to be taken into consideration, thus improving satisfaction with the electronic tools.
9	Explores the database—its use in decision support not only for clinical reasons but also for administrative reasons. In this chapter students will have the chance to write custom reports as well as system-generated reports. The differences between an index and a registry are covered as well. The credentialing process is covered in this chapter—not because the process utilizes the database, but because data is collected on care providers and healthcare professionals, which results in information that is supplied for a myriad of reasons.
10	Takes a look at where an electronic environment is taking healthcare—barriers that still exist though are diminishing; mobile access that makes caring for patients more efficient for care providers, for instance, the emergence of telemedicine, telehealth, and patient medical homes. And it includes an introduction to security methods currently used to ensure the sharing of electronic health information does not get into the wrong hands.

(Information about the worktext's pedagogical elements appears in the Walkthrough starting on page xiii.)

What You Can Expect from the Online Course in *Connect Plus*

Questions from the Worktext:

- Check Your Understanding (CYU) Questions only appear in Chapters 1, 2, and 10. There are two to four questions at the end of each section. These are conceptual chapters.
- End-of-Chapter (EOC) Questions include:
  - *Matching Questions for Key Terms*
  - *Multiple Choice Questions*
  - *Short Answer Questions*
  - *Applying Your Knowledge Questions [Critical Thinking]*
- The CYU and EOC Questions are all tagged with the following in *Connect Plus*:
  - *Learning Outcome*
  - *Level of Difficulty*
  - *Level of Bloom's Taxonomy*
  - *Correct Response Feedback*
- All of the Learning Outcomes are correlated to the key accrediting bodies: CAHIIM, ABHES, and CAAHEP for instructors at **www.mhhe.com/greenway**.

Forty-Five Hands-On Simulated PrimeSUITE Exercises:

- PrimeSUITE Exercises appear in Chapters 3 through 9. All are correlated to Learning Outcomes.
- PrimeSUITE Exercises include the following modes:
  - **Demo Mode**—*watch a demonstration of the exercise.*
  - **Practice Mode**—*try the exercise yourself with guidance.*
  - **Test Mode**—*complete the exercise on your own.*
  - **Assessment Mode**—*answer three to four conceptual questions about the exercise you just completed.*
- For each PrimeSUITE Exercise, the same data is used for all of the modes in order to reinforce the skill being taught in that exercise. This is a proven learning methodology.

- Each PrimeSUITE Exercise is labeled with:
  - *HIM (Health Information Management)*
  - *PM (Practice Management)*
  - *EHR (Electronic Health Records)*
  - *Or some combination of the above three.*
- The tagging for the PrimeSUITE Assessments is provided in the Instructor's Manual at the book's website. The tags are the same as the ones for the CYU and EOC questions.

Much more information on how to complete the exercises in *Connect Plus*, including detailed screenshots, can be found in the *McGraw-Hill Guide to Success for The Greenway/Shanholtzer Integrated EHR Online Course* at **www.mhhe.com/greenway**! The guide is divided into the following sections: Welcome, *Connect Plus* Functionality, Demo Mode, Practice Mode, Test Mode, Assessment Mode, Tips for Working with the Content, Instructor Resources, and Technical Support.

To the Instructor

McGraw-Hill knows how much effort it takes to prepare for a new course. Through focus groups, symposia, reviews, and conversations with instructors like you, we have gathered information about what materials you need in order to facilitate successful courses. We are committed to providing you with high-quality, accurate instructor support.

You can rely on the following materials to help you and your students work through the material in the book, all of which are available on the book's website, **www.mhhe.com/greenway** (instructors can request a password through their sales representative):

Supplement	Features
Instructor's Manual (organized by Learning Outcomes)	- Sample Syllabi and Lesson Plans - Answer Keys for Check Your Understanding Exercises, End-of-Chapter Exercises, and PrimeSUITE Exercises—including tagging for Learning Outcomes, Level of Difficulty, and Level of Bloom's Taxonomy - Documentation of Steps and Screenshots for PrimeSUITE Exercises
PowerPoint Presentations (organized by Learning Outcomes)	- Key Terms - Key Concepts - Teaching Notes

Electronic Testbank	- EZ Test Online (computerized)
	- Word Version
	- Questions are tagged with:
	  • Learning Outcome
	  • Level of Difficulty
	  • Level of Bloom's Taxonomy
	  • Feedback

Tools to Plan Course	- Correlations of the Learning Outcomes to Accrediting Bodies such as CAHIIM, ABHES, and CAAHEP - Sample Syllabi and Lesson Plans - Certificate of Completion - Asset Map—clickable PDF with links to all key supplements, broken down by Learning Outcomes, as well as information on the content available through *Connect Plus*
McGraw-Hill Guide to Success for the Greenway/Shanholtzer *Integrated EHR Online Course*	- Welcome - *Connect Plus* Functionality - Demo Mode - Practice Mode - Test Mode - Assessment Mode - Tips for Working with the Content - Instructor Resources - Technical Support

Need help with the book or online course? Contact McGraw-Hill Higher Education's Customer Experience Team.

Visit our Customer Experience Team Support website at **www.mhhe.com/support**. Browse our FAQs (Frequently Asked Questions) and product documentation, and/or contact a Customer Experience Team representative. The Customer Experience Team is available Sunday through Friday.

Want to learn more about this product? Attend one of our online webinars. To learn more about the webinars, please contact your McGraw-Hill sales representative. To find your McGraw-Hill representative, go to www.mhhe.com and click Find My Sales Rep.

About the Author

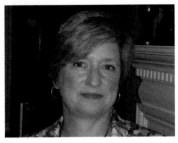

M. Beth Shanholtzer

M. Beth Shanholtzer, MAEd, RHIA

Beth Shanholtzer has been in the Health Information Management field for over 30 years. Her experience has included HIM department management positions within hospitals in New Jersey, Pennsylvania, West Virginia, and Maryland. Seventeen years ago she moved to academics, holding positions as program director/chair and instructor of associate degree programs, including online programs with Kaplan University. Most recently, she has been teaching at the community college level, currently with Blue Ridge Community and Technical College in West Virginia, Lord Fairfax Community College in Virginia, and Carroll County Community College in Maryland. She is active in the West Virginia Health Information Management Association, previously serving as Education Chair, and as President for the 2011-2012 year. Beth lives in Martinsburg, WV with her husband, and has three children.

Walkthrough

Many pedagogical tools have been incorporated throughout the book to help students learn.

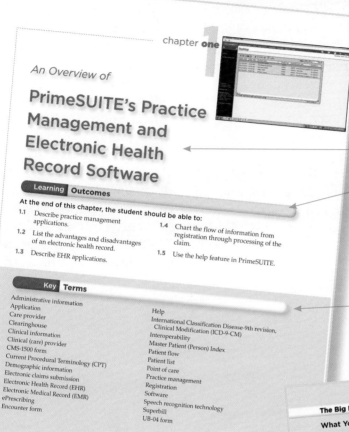

Chapter Opener

- Learning Outcomes—written to reflect Bloom's Taxonomy and to establish the key points the student should focus on in the chapter. The major chapter heads are structured to reflect the LOs and are numbered accordingly.

- Key Terms—will be defined in the chapter and in the end-of-book glossary.

The Big Picture starts off the content for each chapter and sets the stage for what students need to know and *why* they need to know it.

Marginal Tips

- **FYI Tips** highlight information that may be of interest to the reader, not related to the software.

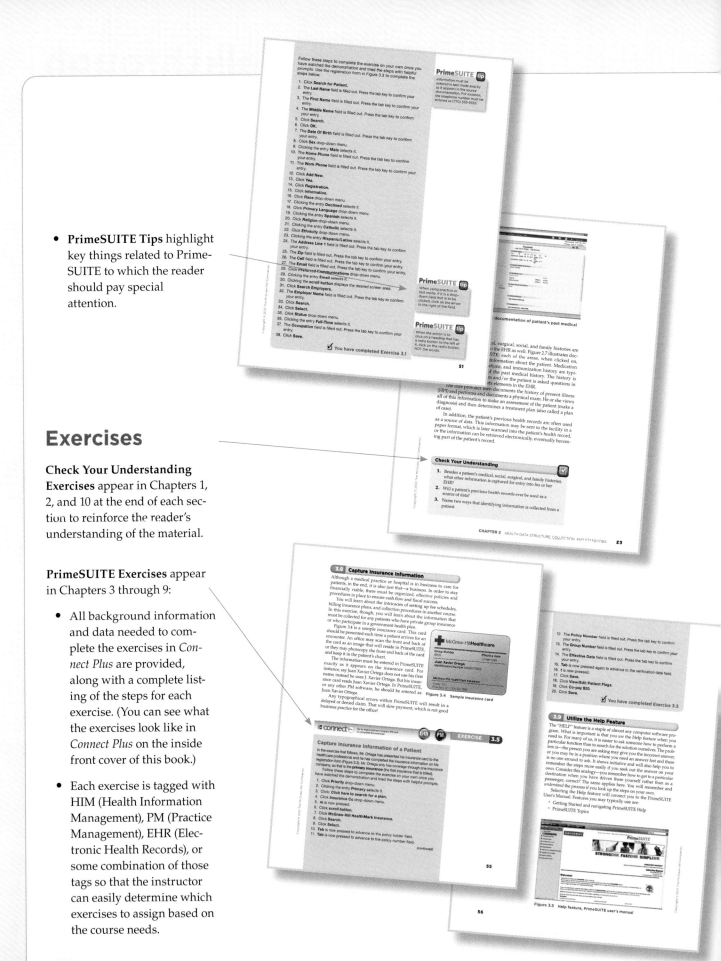

- **PrimeSUITE Tips** highlight key things related to Prime-SUITE to which the reader should pay special attention.

Exercises

Check Your Understanding Exercises appear in Chapters 1, 2, and 10 at the end of each section to reinforce the reader's understanding of the material.

PrimeSUITE Exercises appear in Chapters 3 through 9:

- All background information and data needed to complete the exercises in *Connect Plus* are provided, along with a complete listing of the steps for each exercise. (You can see what the exercises look like in *Connect Plus* on the inside front cover of this book.)

- Each exercise is tagged with HIM (Health Information Management), PM (Practice Management), EHR (Electronic Health Records), or some combination of those tags so that the instructor can easily determine which exercises to assign based on the course needs.

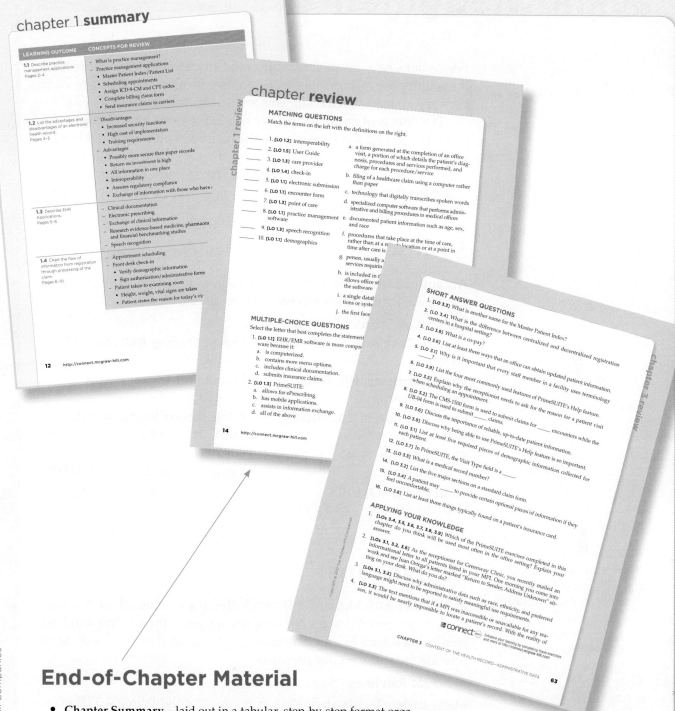

End-of-Chapter Material

- **Chapter Summary**—laid out in a tabular, step-by-step format organized by learning outcomes, with page references to help the reader review the material.

- **Chapter Review**—all questions are tagged with Learning Outcomes:

  - Matching Questions

  - Multiple-Choice Questions

  - Short Answer Questions

  - Applying Your Knowledge

acknowledgments

Suggestions have been received from faculty and students throughout the country. We rely on this vital feedback with all of our products. Each person who has offered comments and suggestions has our thanks.

The efforts of many people are needed to develop and improve a product. Among these people are the reviewers and consultants who point out areas of concern, cite areas of strength, and make recommendations for change. In this regard, the following instructors provided feedback that was enormously helpful in preparing the first edition of *Integrated EHR*.

Symposia

An enthusiastic group of trusted faculty members active in this course area attended symposia to provide crucial feedback.

Tucson, Arizona

Yvonne Beth Alles, MBA, DHA
Davenport University

Vanda Crossley, MS, RHIA
DeVry University

Patricia Elliot, M.Ed., RHIT
Concorde Career Colleges

Sharon Owen, MAC
Heald College

Lauri Perry, MJ, RHIA
Medical Careers Institute, ECPI University

Sheryl Starkey Bulloch, MMIS
Columbia Southern University

Emmanuel Touze, MHSA
Keiser University

Alice Jacobs Vestergaard, Ed.D., MS, CHES
Ashford University

Kathy H. Wood, Ph.D., FHFMA
Colorado Technical University

Workshops

In 2010 and 2011, McGraw-Hill conducted thirteen health professions workshops, providing an opportunity for more than seven hundred faculty members to gain continuing education credits as well as to provide feedback on our products.

Product Reviews

Many instructors participated in reviews of the PrimeSUITE exercises in *Connect Plus* and for the Worktext.

Kathleen G. Bailey, CPA, MBA, CPC, CPC-I
Ultimate Medical Academy

Amy Bledsoe, RHIA
Community Colleges of Spokane

Teresa Buglione, MBA, LPN, CPC
American Intercontinental University

Patricia DeiTos, MSN, RN, BC
Inova Health System-Military to Medicine Program

Marsha Dolan, MBA, RHIA, FAHIMA
Missouri Western State University

Patricia Elliot, M.Ed., RHIT
Concorde Career Colleges

Kathy Jo Ellison, RN, DSN
Auburn University

Jill Ferrari, MA, MT, MLT (ASCP)
Sullivan University

Lynette Garetz, MS
Heald College

Savanna Garrity, MPA
Madisonville Community College

Misty Hamilton, MBA, RHIT
Zane State College

Michelle Kistner, MBA, RHIA
Herzing University Online

Laura J. Michelsen, MS, RHIA
Joliet Junior College

Jenny Patton
West Virginia School of
Osteopathic Medicine

Lauri Perry, MJ, RHIA
Medical Careers Institute, ECPI
University

Libba Reed McMillan, Ph.D., RN
Auburn University

Tina Reynoso, RHIA
Rasmusssen College

Emmanuel Touze, MHSA
Keiser University

**Stacey Wilson, CMA (AAMA),
MT/PBT (ASCP), MHA**
Cabarrus College of Health Sciences

Kathy H. Wood, Ph.D., FHFMA
Colorado Technical University

Acknowledgments from the Author

I am grateful to my husband, Neil, for his support, patience, and encouragement throughout this process and in life. And, to my children, Alison, J.P., and Alex who are my constant inspiration to appreciate every moment and are always a reminder of what is important in life.

To my colleagues along the way—in the hospitals where I have worked, and the colleges where I have taught—I have learned so much from you over these many years.

To all of my students—you've challenged me, impressed me, enlightened me, and made me realize what a wonderful gift they have given me—the chance to *teach and to learn!*

To my editorial staff at McGraw-Hill—Michelle Flomenhoft and Natalie Ruffatto who gave support, excellent ideas, and were above all—patient! Ashley Dobbyn, who provided behind-the-scenes support, including finding photos and figures. And to Roxan Kinsey who planted the idea of someday being an author back in 2002 in Roswell, Georgia.

To my digital staff at McGraw-Hill—Crystal Szewczyk and Thuan Vinh who helped ensure that the simulations would work in *Connect,* as well as Katie Ward, Brent dela Cruz, and Cathy Tepper. Special thanks to Karen Jozefowicz and the QA team for their attention to the project. To my production staff at McGraw-Hill—Rick Hecker, Anna Kinigakis, Sherry Kane, and Jeremy Cheshareck—thank you for helping make this Worktext a reality!

And, to those who have made this project possible and contributed in countless ways:

The Greenway Medical Technologies team, particularly Kevin Kornegay for being our PrimeSUITE expert, as well as Matt Pierce and Diane Nivens for facilitating our partnership at every turn; W Hayden Childs, MD of Childs Medical Clinic, Samson, AL, who let us take a screen-shot of his practice's successful meaningful use dashboard for one of the exercises; the staff of datango, including Vince Lucey and Jim Brussard, but especially consultant Timothy Goodell who helped shepherd the simulations through every stage; Diana Gaviria, M.D., M.P.H., who wrote many of the patient scenarios, used in the PrimeSUITE exercises; Kathryn A. Booth, MS, RN, RMA (AMT), RPT, CPhT, who provided much of the initial patient data for the scenarios; Danielle Mbadu, MA, MEd, who helped write the assessments, reviewed the material throughout, and helped craft the instructor ancillaries; and Melinda Bilecki, who lent her copyediting and reviewing skills to the project.

And finally, thank you to the reviewers who helped write this book through their ideas, constructive criticism, and encouraging words.

1st Round: Author's Manuscript
Multiple Rounds of Review by Health Professions Instructors
2nd Round: Typeset Pages
Accuracy Checks by: • Author • Peer Instructors • 1st Proofread
3rd Round: Typeset Pages
Accuracy Checks by: • Author • 2nd Proofread
Final Round: Printing
Accuracy Check by 3rd Proofread
Supplements: • Proofreading • Accuracy Checks

A Commitment to Accuracy

You have a right to expect an accurate textbook, and McGraw-Hill invests considerable time and effort to make sure that we deliver one. Listed below are the many steps we take to make sure this happens.

Our Accuracy Verification Process

First Round—Development Reviews

STEP 1: Numerous **health professions instructors** review the draft manuscript and report on any errors that they may find. The authors make these corrections in her final manuscript.

Second Round—Page Proofs

STEP 2: Once the manuscript has been typeset, the **author** checks her manuscript against the first page proofs to ensure that all illustrations, graphs, examples, and exercises have been correctly laid out on the pages.

STEP 3: An outside panel of **peer instructors** completes a review of content in the page proofs to verify its accuracy. The author adds these corrections to her review of the pages.

STEP 4: A proofreader adds a triple layer of accuracy assurance in the pages by looking for errors; then a confirming, corrected round of page proofs is produced.

Third Round—Confirming Page Proofs

STEP 5: The **author** reviews the confirming round of page proofs to make certain that any previous corrections were properly made and to look for any errors she might have missed in the first round.

STEP 6: The **project manager,** who has overseen the book from the beginning, performs **another proofread** to make sure that no new errors have been introduced dutring the production process.

Final Round—Printer's Proofs

STEP 7: The **project manager** performs a final proofread of the book during the printing process, providing a final accuracy review. In concert with the main text, all supplements undergo a proofreading and technical editing stage to ensure their accuracy.

Results

What results is a textbook that is as accurate and error-free as is humanly possible. Our author and publishing staff are confdent that the many layers of quality assurance have produced books that are leaders in the industry for their integrity and correctness. *Please view the Acknowledgments for more details on the many people involved in this process.*

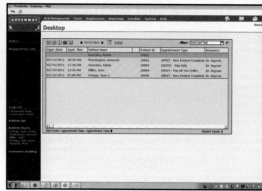

An Overview of

PrimeSUITE's Practice Management and Electronic Health Record Software

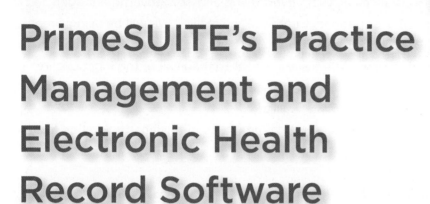

Learning Outcomes

At the end of this chapter, the student should be able to:

1.1 Describe practice management applications.

1.2 List the advantages and disadvantages of an electronic health record.

1.3 Describe EHR applications.

1.4 Chart the flow of information from registration through processing of the claim.

1.5 Use the help feature in PrimeSUITE.

Key Terms

Administrative information
Application
Care provider
Clearinghouse
Clinical information
Clinical (care) provider
CMS-1500 form
Current Procedural Terminology (CPT)
Demographic information
Electronic claims submission
Electronic Health Record (EHR)
Electronic Medical Record (EMR)
ePrescribing
Encounter form

Help
International Classification Disease-9th revision, Clinical Modification (ICD-9-CM)
Interoperability
Master Patient (Person) Index
Patient flow
Patient list
Point of care
Practice management
Registration
Software
Speech recognition technology
Superbill
UB-04 form

The Big Picture

What You Need to Know and Why You Need to Know It

The purpose of this worktext is to introduce students to **software** used to gather, track, and store the **clinical** and **administrative** (including **demographic**) **information** of patients seen in the medical facility. This information is used for patient care; to file claims for reimbursement; for reporting practice information to insurance carriers, government, and non-government agencies; and to gather statistics about the types of patients treated at the facility. We will be using Greenway Medical Technologies' PrimeSUITE **practice management (PM)** and **electronic health record (EHR)** software throughout the text. This worktext is not meant to teach all of the functionality of PrimeSUITE; instead it is meant to demonstrate the most common electronic functions carried out in a medical office, hospital, or other healthcare facility.

This first chapter is an introduction and overview. The concepts in this chapter will be further explained throughout the text.

1.1 Practice Management Applications

Typically, software (computer programs that carry out functions or operations) used in a medical office is known as **practice management (PM)** software. Through the use of PM software, data is gathered on every patient from the time an appointment is made through the time the bill for each visit is paid. **Electronic Health (Medical) Record (EHR/ EMR)** software includes the clinical documentation of patient care.

Greenway Medical Technologies' PrimeSUITE is both a PM and EHR solution using a single database. The use of this single database to document the administrative and clinical aspects of patient care allows the provider to concentrate on the care of the patient, improve quality of the documentation collected, and share that documentation with other healthcare providers as appropriate, with the result of better coordination of the patient's overall care.

We will first look at the applications typically found in practice management software, including PrimeSUITE. Practice management is a term used in physicians' offices. In other healthcare facilities, including hospitals, these functions will also be computerized, but are referred to as Admission, Discharge, Transfer (ADT) and billing systems.

The main applications include:

Entering Each Patient Seen into a Master List

Each patient seen, whether in a physician's office or a hospital, is only entered once into what is known as the **Patient List** or **Master Patient (Person) Index** (listings of all patients seen in an office or hospital). These will be further discussed in Chapter 2.

Scheduling Appointments

To maintain efficiency in an office, it is important that appointments be accurate. Think of it this way—if a patient were told to come to the office for an appointment at a particular date and time, but the appointment book showed another date and time for that patient to

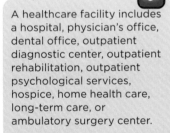

for your information **fyi**

A healthcare facility includes a hospital, physician's office, dental office, outpatient diagnostic center, outpatient rehabilitation, outpatient psychological services, hospice, home health care, long-term care, or ambulatory surgery center.

be seen, the end result would be disorganization as well as unhappy patients and staff. Computerizing this function allows sufficient time to be allotted to that patient based on the reason for his or her visit, and also allows for more efficient scheduling of the provider's time.

Assign ICD-9-CM Diagnosis and CPT Procedure Codes

You may have noticed on your own visits to your physician's office that you are given a piece of paper when you leave the examining room. This is referred to as a **Superbill** or **Encounter Form.** There are many numbers or codes found on this paper. Every diagnosis made by a care provider is written in narrative form on a patient's chart and then carried over to the Superbill. These narrative diagnoses are converted into numeric form with a coding system known as **International Classification of Diseases, 9th revision, Clinical Modification (ICD-9-CM)**. The same occurs for each procedure performed, but the coding system used is **Current Procedural Terminology (CPT)**. The Superbill and coding functions will be covered in detail in Chapter 6. Most likely, you will have a separate course or courses in billing and coding as well.

Complete a Billing Claim Form for Each Visit

In order to submit bills to health insurance carriers, a claim form must be generated for each visit. This is done by compiling the patient's identifying information, insurance information, and the ICD-9-CM and CPT codes into a form called the CMS-1500, which is used by physicians' offices, or the UB-04, which is used to bill hospital claims.

Send the Insurance Claims to Insurance Carriers

Once the claim form is generated, it is submitted to the insurance carrier for payment. Some hard-copy claim forms are still mailed to the insurance carrier, but the majority of forms are sent by **electronic claims submission.** Filing a claim electronically means that the information is sent by wire to a **clearinghouse** (service that processes insurance claims) or directly to the insurance carrier. Filing claims electronically cuts down on billing errors and cuts down on processing time, which results in faster payment. A clearinghouse is a service that processes data into a standardized billing format and checks for inconsistencies or other errors in the data.

The information collected as explained above is considered administrative information. The patient's **demographic** (identifying) information is collected as part of the administrative information, as well as information needed for the business processes that take place in a healthcare facility, for instance gathering of insurance information, completing a claim form, submitting a claim, and so on.

Administrative information includes the insurance information, authorization to bill the insurance company, correspondence related to billing matters, etc. Demographic information identifies the patient—name, address, phone numbers, etc. The demographic information is specific administrative information that helps differentiate one patient from another with the same name.

Check Your Understanding

1. Is PrimeSUITE a practice management tool or an electronic health record?
2. List the types of information that insurance companies need to be provided with on a billing claim form.

1.2 Why Adopt Electronic Health Record Applications?

The widespread acceptance of an electronic health record has been slow compared to other industries such as banking or retail. There are several reasons for this, including security concerns, cost, and the time involved in learning how to implement, maintain, and use an electronic system. These have been seen as disadvantages. It has long been thought that paper records were more secure from tampering, loss, unauthorized access, or theft. Overall, the advantages far outweigh the disadvantages as far as security is concerned. With today's technology, and with proper policies and procedures in place, although no system (including manual) is 100 percent secure, security need not prevent the use of an electronic record-keeping system. Paper records can more easily be stolen, lost, or tampered with. We will discuss in Chapter 7 the proper use of security measures.

The initial purchase and implementation costs are high. Writing in a chart or dictating into a microphone has been considered easier than pointing, clicking, and navigating within the screens of an electronic record. However, cost is an issue with any system—manual or electronic. Though it is true that the initial costs are high, the savings in supplies, space, archiving, greater staff and provider efficiency, and positive impact on patient care all increase the return on investment of an electronic system.

There is a high learning curve when implementing an electronic system, and it does require time-consuming hands-on training for all users. Care providers have been resistant to adopting an EHR due in part to this reason. But, once learned, the benefits of having all information in one place, quickly and readily retrievable by more than one person at a time, outweigh the disadvantages and will ultimately improve patient care. Informed decision-making regarding patient care or to manage a business can only be done through health information technology.

Interoperability is an advantage that really is not possible in a manual system. Interoperability means that through a single database, many different functions can take place and information can be shared. This is also known as an integrated database. An example is prescribing of medications. With a manual system, a separate piece of paper (the prescription pad) is used to write orders for the pharmacist to dispense a particular medication, at a particular dosage, and with particular instructions to a patient. Many times the writing is barely legible. This piece of paper has to be copied for inclusion in the patient's record, and the original is sent with the patient (or it is called in to the pharmacy). Hopefully all of that takes place, and the patient's record accurately reflects the medication ordered. With functionality called electronic prescribing, or ePrescribing, nothing is separate. The physician types the prescription into the EHR for that patient, it is electronically transmitted to the pharmacy chosen by the patient, a permanent, accurate record is maintained, and the prescription is filled and ready for pickup at the pharmacy.

Assuring regulatory compliance is also made easier and more efficient through use of an electronic health record. Report-writing capabilities available in electronic systems allow for fast, reliable data submission and retrieval.

From a more global perspective, the use of electronic medical records will allow for the collection and use of incredible amounts of clinical data for use in medical research and epidemiology, which will have a profound effect on healthcare worldwide.

Check Your Understanding

1. Is a paper-based system of records more secure than an electronic one? Explain your answer.
2. When transitioning to EHRs, which costs are higher: initial costs or long-term costs? Explain your answer.

1.3 Electronic Health Record Applications

Now, let us take a look at the electronic record using PrimeSUITE.

It is through the EHR functionality that clinical information is collected and includes the patient's medical history, current condition(s), treatment rendered, results of treatment, prognosis, plan of care, diagnosis, and any instructions given by the provider.

PrimeSUITE's EHR **applications** (functionality) include:

- Clinical documentation of a patient's visit (the progress note) by the **care provider**
- Prescribing medications electronically to the patient's pharmacy of choice through use of the ePrescribing solution.
- Exchange of clinical information between medical providers or other entities with a need to know, through the PrimeEXCHANGE solution.
- The ability to access clinical trials, evidence-based medicine, and pharmaceutical research to improve patient care, and access to clinical and financial benchmarking services to enhance financial management by using the PrimeRESEARCH solution.
- Mobile EHR applications available on personal digital assistants (PDAs) or SmartPhones to allow providers instant access anytime and anywhere through PrimeMOBILE.

- **Point of care** dictation of progress notes by the provider through PrimeSPEECH, which is a form of **speech recognition** technology. Speech recognition technology allows documentation to occur on the computer screen as the care provider dictates his notes. Point of care refers to the dictation occurring at the very time the patient is being seen.

Check Your Understanding

1. What does PrimeSUITE's PrimeEXCHANGE function do?
2. What is PrimeSPEECH?
3. Take a look at all of the functionality of PrimeSUITE. Open your Internet browser and access the following link, and then answer the following questions:

   http://www.greenwaymedical.com/specialties/family-practice/

   a. Where would you look to determine if a patient has had a polio vaccine?
   b. Where would you go to write a letter to a specialist to whom a patient is being referred?
   c. Where would you go to send tasks or make requests of physicians or other practice staff?

4. Take a look at the functionality and a demonstration of Greenway Medical Technologies' PrimeSUITE. Pay particular attention to the Web demonstration of PrimeSUITE applications to become familiar with it. Then answer the following questions:

   http://www.greenwaymedical.com/web-demo/

   a. PrimeSUITE uses a _____database, allowing for interoperability.
   b. The electronic Superbill is automatically generated from the _____.
   c. The Superbill includes charges, diagnosis, and _____ for the patient.
   d. PrimeSUITE is _____in meaningful use standards.

1.4 **The Flow of Information from Registration through Processing of the Claim**

If you think about your past experiences visiting a physician's office, you will recognize many of these steps and how similar they are to your experience. Of course, not every step is exactly the same in every office, but the basic premise is the same.

Step one (Figure 1.1) is that an appointment is made. Of course, if you are going to an urgent care center or an emergency room, this step would be skipped. Once the appointment is made, you go to the

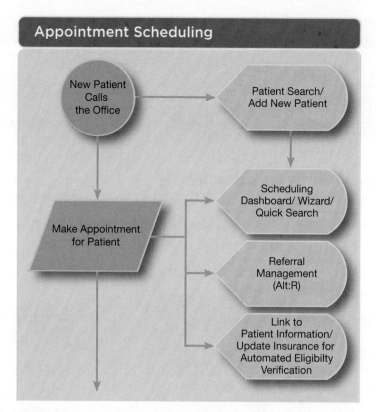

Appointment Scheduling

New Patient Calls the Office → Patient Search/ Add New Patient

Make Appointment for Patient

Scheduling Dashboard/ Wizard/ Quick Search

Referral Management (Alt:R)

Link to Patient Information/ Update Insurance for Automated Eligibilty Verification

Figure 1.1   Appointment scheduling flowchart

office on the day and time of the appointment and you are "checked in." This is known as registration, i.e., the patient's administrative information is taken either on the phone or when the patient appears for the appointment. It is during this time that any demographic information that is incorrect or that has not been collected is done. Also, if new authorization forms or other administrative forms need to be signed, that is done at this point.

After you are checked in, you wait to be seen by the care providers (Figure 1.2). First, you are called back to the exam room by a healthcare provider (Figure 1.3), your height, weight, and vital signs (temperature, pulse, blood pressure) are taken, and you are asked questions about why you are being seen today as well as questions about your medical history. Once those are complete, the care provider steps in for the actual exam (Figure 1.4).

Once the care provider has completed the exam, assessed the patient's condition, and given the patient a plan of care including instructions, the business functions begin (Figure 1.5 and Figure 1.6). These include the check-out and billing procedures. Some of these procedures are repeated or continue for several weeks or months until the claim is paid and the patient's account is at a zero balance.

In cases where the care provider ordered diagnostic procedures such as x-rays or laboratory tests, then the clinical documentation steps would be repeated (Figure 1.7).

for your information

The medical assistant, nurse, receptionist, health information technician, medical biller/coder, and office administrative personnel will be referred to as *healthcare professional* throughout the text.

for your information

The term *care provider* will be used to refer to any physician, physician's assistant, dentist, psychologist, nurse practitioner or midwife.

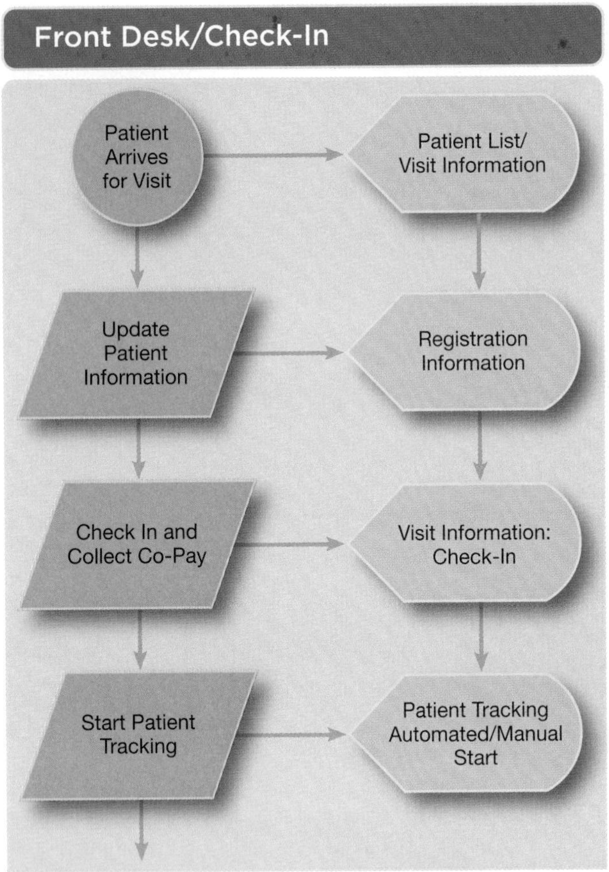

Front Desk/Check-In

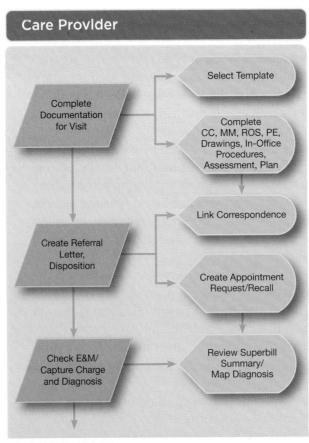

Figure 1.2 Front desk check-in flowchart

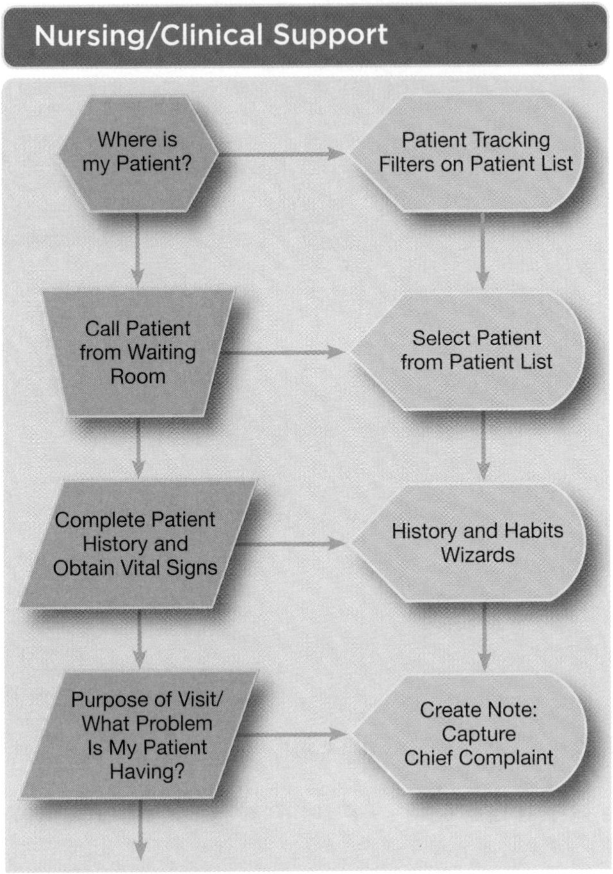

Nursing/Clinical Support

Figure 1.3 Nursing/clinical support flowchart

Care Provider

Figure 1.4 Care provider flowchart

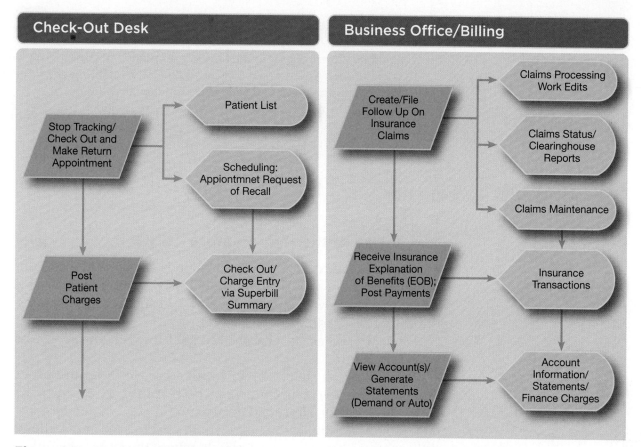

Check-Out Desk

Stop Tracking/ Check Out and Make Return Appointment

Patient List

Scheduling: Appiontmnet Request of Recall

Post Patient Charges

Check Out/ Charge Entry via Superbill Summary

Figure 1.5   Check-out desk flowchart

Business Office/Billing

Create/File Follow Up On Insurance Claims

Claims Processing Work Edits

Claims Status/ Clearinghouse Reports

Claims Maintenance

Receive Insurance Explanation of Benefits (EOB); Post Payments

Insurance Transactions

View Account(s)/ Generate Statements (Demand or Auto)

Account Information/ Statements/ Finance Charges

Figure 1.6   Business office/billing flowchart

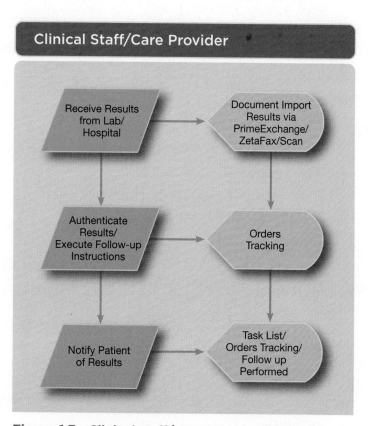

Clinical Staff/Care Provider

Receive Results from Lab/ Hospital

Document Import Results via PrimeExchange/ ZetaFax/Scan

Authenticate Results/ Execute Follow-up Instructions

Orders Tracking

Notify Patient of Results

Task List/ Orders Tracking/ Follow up Performed

Figure 1.7   Clinical staff/care provider flowchart

Check Your Understanding

1. Put the following steps in the flow of information into the correct order: Care Provider; Front Desk/Check-In; Business Office/Billing; Check-Out Desk; Appointment Scheduling; Nursing/Clinical Support; Clinical Staff/Care Provider.

2. Under what circumstances would the clinical documentation steps need to be repeated?

1.5 Use of the Help Feature

The use of help text or of a help function is standard in most software applications. You have no doubt used it from time to time when preparing word processing or spreadsheet applications. PrimeSUITE is no different.

PrimeSUITE help text can be accessed through any screen, as you see in Figure 1.8.

By clicking on Help, you will gain access to the entire user's guide (Figure 1.9). The guide can be searched by topic, or by using the index or glossary. For instance, if you wanted to know more about vocabulary reconciliation, clicking on index allows the user to access a keyword search, where the system begins to

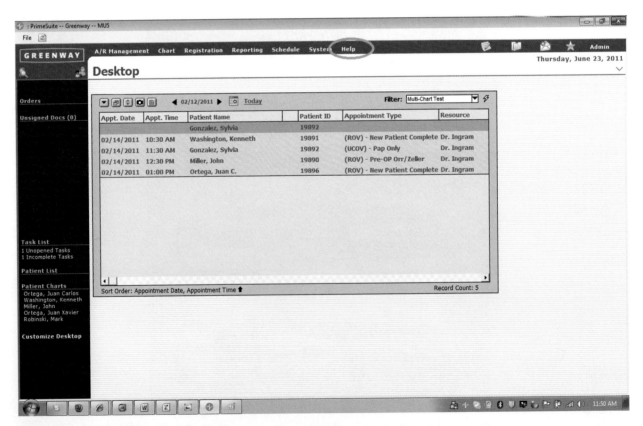

Figure 1.8 Location of Help feature on any screen

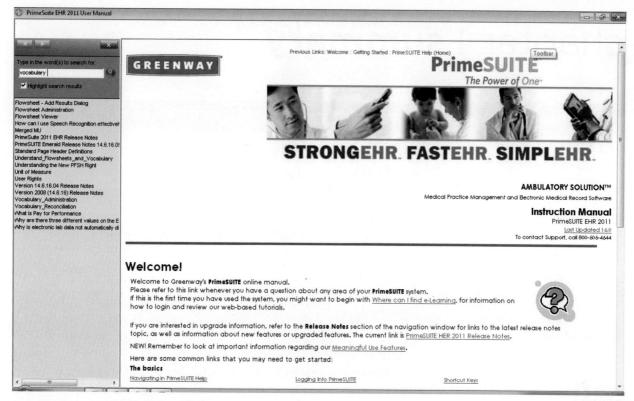

Figure 1.9   PrimeSUITE EHR 2011 user manual

predict what the user is searching for based on the first few characters typed or by typing the entire word in the search field (Figure 1.9).

The important thing about Help is that it is there for just that—to help you learn PrimeSUITE, assist you when you are unsure of the steps you need to complete, and to help you keep up to date with changes or new functionality added to the software.

Check Your Understanding

1. How do you access the Help feature in PrimeSUITE?
2. How many ways are there to locate information?
3. Using the Help feature, describe how to add a new allergy to a patient's chart.

chapter 1 **summary**

LEARNING OUTCOME	CONCEPTS FOR REVIEW

1.1 Describe practice management applications. Pages 2–4	– What is practice management?
	– Practice management applications
	  • Master Patient Index/Patient List
	  • Scheduling appointments
	  • Assign ICD-9-CM and CPT codes
	  • Complete billing claim form
	  • Send insurance claims to carriers

1.2 List the advantages and disadvantages of an electronic health record. Pages 4–5	– Disadvantages
	  • Increased security functions
	  • High cost of implementation
	  • Training requirements
	– Advantages
	  • Possibly more secure than paper records
	  • Return on investment is high
	  • All information in one place
	  • Interoperability
	  • Assures regulatory compliance
	  • Exchange of information with those who have a need to know

1.3 Describe EHR Applications. Pages 5–6	– Clinical documentation – Electronic prescribing – Exchange of clinical information – Research evidence-based medicine, pharmaceutical research, clinical and financial benchmarking studies – Speech recognition

1.4 Chart the flow of information from registration through processing of the claim. Pages 6–10	– Appointment scheduling
	– Front desk check-in
	  • Verify demographic information
	  • Sign authorization/administrative forms, if necessary
	– Patient taken to examining room
	  • Height, weight, vital signs are taken
	  • Patient states the reason for today's visit (chief complaint)

| --- | --- |
| | – Care provider meets with the patient
  • Provider verifies reason for visit; updates history
  • Provider examines of patient
  • Provider makes referrals, if necessary
  • Prescriptions are electronically sent to pharmacy, if necessary
  • Provider completes the chart, which then starts the coding and claims process
  • Provider completes the visit and provides patient with a Superbill or encounter form
– Patient stops at the check-out desk
  • Superbill is given to staff member at the check-out desk
  • Patient pays co-pay, if not done during check-in process
  • Patient leaves the office
– Business Office/Billing
  • Insurance claim form is completed electronically
  • Insurance claim is submitted electronically
  • Insurance payment (or notice of denial) is received
  • Payment is entered in the system
  • Patient's account is updated
  • Statement is sent, if necessary
– Follow-up
  • Results of diagnostic tests received, if applicable
  • Record is updated with results
  • Provider reviews results
  • Patient is contacted, if necessary |
| **1.5** Use the help feature in PrimeSUITE.
Pages 10–11 | – Use of Help from menu bar
– Other means of accessing help feature
– User's Guide |

chapter **review**

MATCHING QUESTIONS

Match the terms on the left with the definitions on the right.

_____ 1. **[LO 1.2]** interoperability

_____ 2. **[LO 1.5]** User Guide

_____ 3. **[LO 1.3]** care provider

_____ 4. **[LO 1.4]** check-in

_____ 5. **[LO 1.1]** electronic submission

_____ 6. **[LO 1.1]** encounter form

_____ 7. **[LO 1.3]** point of care

_____ 8. **[LO 1.1]** practice management software

_____ 9. **[LO 1.3]** speech recognition

_____ 10. **[LO 1.1]** demographics

a. a form generated at the completion of an office visit, a portion of which details the patient's diagnosis, procedures and services performed, and charge for each procedure/service

b. filing of a healthcare claim using a computer rather than paper

c. technology that digitally transcribes spoken words

d. specialized computer software that performs administrative and billing procedures in medical offices

e. documented patient information such as age, sex, and race

f. procedures that take place at the time of care, rather than at a remote location or at a point in time after care is complete

g. person, usually a physician, who performs healthcare services requiring specialized education and training

h. is included in the Help feature of PrimeSUITE and allows office staff to search for assistance in using the software

i. a single database to sync multiple unrelated functions or systems

j. the first face-to-face step in the patient encounter

MULTIPLE-CHOICE QUESTIONS

Select the letter that best completes the statement or answers the question:

1. **[LO 1.1]** EHR/EMR software is more comprehensive than practice management software because it:
   a. is computerized.
   b. contains more menu options.
   c. includes clinical documentation.
   d. submits insurance claims.

2. **[LO 1.3]** PrimeSUITE:
   a. allows for ePrescribing.
   b. has mobile applications.
   c. assists in information exchange.
   d. all of the above

3. **[LO 1.1]** A patient is entered into the patient list:
   a. once.
   b. twice.
   c. after a procedure.
   d. each time he or she is seen.

4. **[LO 1.2]** In the long term, costs will _____ when transitioning to an electronic health record system.
   a. increase
   b. decrease
   c. stay the same
   d. disappear

5. **[LO 1.4]** The process of moving a patient from appointment making through check-out is called:
   a. patient cycle.
   b. patient process.
   c. patient flow.
   d. patient records.

6. **[LO 1.3]** Clinical documentation of a patient's visit is known as the:
   a. Superbill.
   b. progress note.
   c. medical claim.
   d. point of care.

7. **[LO 1.1]** An encounter form is also known as a/an:
   a. EHR.
   b. history.
   c. claim form.
   d. Superbill.

8. **[LO 1.1]** The _____ is a form used to bill inpatient claims.
   a. CMS-1500
   b. ICD-9
   c. CPT
   d. UB-04

9. **[LO 1.2]** One factor that might contribute to slow acceptance of EHRs is:
   a. security fears.
   b. laziness.
   c. fear of change.
   d. space concerns.

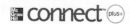 Enhance your learning by completing these exercises and more at http://**connect.mcgraw-hill.com**!

10. **[LO 1.5]** PrimeSUITE's User Guide is accessed through the _____ feature.
    a. Help
    b. Information
    c. Lookup
    d. Query

11. **[LO 1.3]** The _____ is an example of clinical information that is collected through an EHR.
    a. insurance policy
    b. plan of care
    c. research effects
    d. regulatory guidelines

12. **[LO 1.2]** _____ is not easily attained when using a manual record system.
    a. Communication
    b. Data capture
    c. Interoperability
    d. Maintenance

SHORT ANSWER QUESTIONS

1. **[LO 1.4]** List the steps included in patient flow of information.

2. **[LO 1.2]** Discuss three advantages to electronic health records as discussed in the text.

3. **[LO 1.1]** What is practice management software?

4. **[LO 1.3]** What feature of PrimeSUITE allows practitioners to access clinical trials and other research?

5. **[LO 1.5]** If you needed to use PrimeSUITE's Help feature to look up how to register a patient, how would you do it?

6. **[LO 1.4]** What is the first step in the patient flow of information?

7. **[LO 1.1]** What is the CMS-1500 form?

8. **[LO 1.3]** Mobile EHR applications are currently available on what mobile devices?

9. **[LO 1.2]** Define interoperability and give an example of how it might be used in the healthcare field.

10. **[LO 1.2]** List three advantages of ePrescribing.

11. **[LO 1.1]** What is electronic claims submission? Why is this the preferred method of claims submission?

12. **[LO 1.1]** List at least three main applications found in a typical practice management program.

13. **[LO 1.4]** What is the final step in the Front Desk/Check-In process?

APPLYING YOUR KNOWLEDGE

1. **[LO 1.2]** Your medical office is preparing to transition from a paper-based office to an electronic one; you are really excited about this change. One day you receive an email from one of your colleagues negatively discussing the change and wondering why things cannot stay how they are now. Your colleague is looking to you and asking your opinion. What would you say to convince the person that this transition is a good thing?

2. **[LOs 1.1, 1.3, 1.5]** Which of PrimeSUITE's many EHR applications do you feel is the most beneficial or useful? Explain your answer.

3. **[LO 1.4]** Denisse Cruz arrives at your office for her annual check-up appointment with Dr. Smith. Discuss what will happen with Denisse as she moves through each step of patient flow.

4. **[LOs 1.2, 1.3]** A patient is admitted to the hospital with a constant, severe migraine headache. After numerous tests, no cause for the headache can be determined. Discuss how EHRs might help diagnose this patient.

5. **[LOs 1.1, 1.2, 1.3]** Contrast a typical day in a paper-based office with a day at an office that uses practice management software.

6. **[LOs 1.1, 1.2, 1.3, 1.4, 1.5]** The medical office you work in recently transitioned into an electronic office and is implementing practice management software. You are excited about this change and are learning all you can about the new technology. However, some of your coworkers are having trouble grasping the basics, and are now saying they don't want to use the software at all. What steps could you take to assist your struggling coworkers?

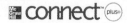 Enhance your learning by completing these exercises and more at http://connect.mcgraw-hill.com!

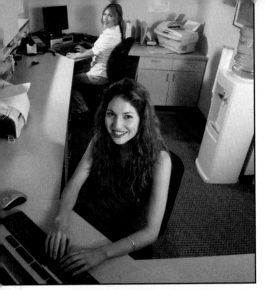

chapter **two**

Health Data Structure, Collection, and Standards

Learning Outcomes

At the end of this chapter, the student should be able to:

2.1 Describe the role of six healthcare professionals who maintain or use practice management and electronic health record applications.

2.2 Explain the difference between data and information.

2.3 Identify computer-based health information media.

2.4 Relate how screen-based data collection tools are used in healthcare.

2.5 Demonstrate how individual data elements are collected.

2.6 Describe electronic health record applications.

2.7 Identify laws, regulations, and standards that govern electronic health information.

2.8 Distinguish between practice management software and hospital health information software.

Key Terms

American Recovery and Reinvestment Act of 2009 (ARRA)

Clinical decision support

Certification Commission for Health Information Technology (CCHIT)

Clearinghouse

Data

Decision support

Electronic health record (EHR)

Electronic medical record (EMR)

Federal Register

Healthcare administrator

Healthcare manager

Health Information Exchange (HIE)

Health systems administrator

Health Insurance Portability and Accountability Act (HIPAA)

Health Information Technology for Economic and Clinical Health (HITECH) Act

Information

Institute of Medicine (IOM)

Master Patient (Person) Index

Meaningful use (MU)

Medical assistant (MA)

National Health Information Network (NHIN)

National Provider Identifier (NPI)

Office administrator (manager)

Office of the National Coordinator for Health Information Technology (ONC)

Patient list

Personal health record (PHR)

Protected Health Information (PHI)

Regional Extension Center (REC)

Regional Health Information Organization

Registered Health Information Administrator (RHIA)

Registered Health Information Technician (RHIT)

Voice Recognition

What You Need to Know and Why You Need to Know It

As a healthcare professional you will be one of many who will be selecting, maintaining, and using electronic health record and management software. Knowing who within the organization is using the software and how they are using it is important to selecting a system that meets the needs of the organization. The collection of **data** must be done efficiently while meeting the documentation requirements of licensing and accrediting agencies, as well as insurance carriers (including Medicare), and conforming to the legal definition of an electronic health record. We will begin this chapter by reviewing the professionals involved and the positions they may hold within the organization. Then, the concepts of data structure, collection, and standards will be introduced in preparation for a more detailed level of instruction found in the remaining chapters of the text. We will also cover how data is collected, the tools used to collect the data, how data is transformed into **information,** and the regulations and standards that dictate the collection, maintenance, use, and storage of health information in an electronic form.

Health Information Management spans a wide range of functions and processes within a healthcare organization. Just about every decision that is made is based on statistics that are largely collected from the health records of a facility. The data that is captured will result in information that is used by care providers to make decisions regarding patient care and to justify reimbursement. In addition, various levels of administrators will use information in risk management activities, budgeting, strategic planning, quality assessment, and financial reporting. Report writing will be discussed in greater detail in Chapter 9.

Table 2.1 depicts a few of the medical professions within healthcare, the education or certifications they may hold, and the responsibilities they may have as pertains to the collection and use of information. This is not an exhaustive list, as there are myriad other positions such as therapists, laboratory technicians, and radiology technicians, just to name a few. Those listed are the positions held by individuals who will most likely be involved in selecting, implementing, maintaining, and using the electronic systems in a healthcare facility.

During the selection process, it is imperative that people with knowledge of health information standards, structure, and content be involved. The health information professional fulfills this role, particularly in hospitals. In addition, administrative staff who are responsible for the effective operation of the entire organization, including facility- or enterprise-wide information systems, are key to the process as well. That is not to say that individual department managers (laboratory, nursing, radiology, etc.) do not have a say—but the administrator(s) responsible for those departments may be the key players in the early stages of system selection.

| Table 2.1 | Medical Professions within Healthcare |

Profession	Certifications	Description
Health Information and Informatics	• Registered Health Information Administrator (RHIA) • Registered Health Information Technician (RHIT) • Certified Health Data Analyst (CHDA) • Certified in Healthcare Privacy and Security (CHPS)	• Work in any healthcare setting, but most often in acute care or specialty hospitals • Work in healthcare-related professions such as consultants, software trainers and installers, government agencies, insurance companies, and law offices • Associate's, bachelor's and master's degrees available • Many healthcare facilities, particularly hospitals, require certification Positions held in the following areas: • Health Information Department managers • Information Technology and Systems • Project management • Software analyst • Implementation support • Information system design • EHR implementation and management • Data analyst • Documentation management • Privacy/security • Release of healthcare information • Risk management • Compliance • Utilization management • Quality Assessment/Assurance • Cancer Registrar • Medical staff coordinator
Health Information Specialty Areas (HITPro™)	Require completion of non-degree educational programs that prepare students to sit for competency exams in: • Clinician/Practitioner Consultant • Implementation Manager • Implementation Support Specialist • Practice Workflow & Information Management Redesign Specialist • Technical/Software Support Staff • Trainer	• The most recent health information/informatics roles • May work in any healthcare facility, inpatient or outpatient • Each competency exam is specific to a particular role that plays a part in meaningful use of the electronic health record (EHR)
Coding professionals	• Certified Coding Associate (CCA) • Certified Coding Specialist (CCS) • Certified Coding Specialist-Physician (CCS-P) • Certified Professional Coder (CPC) • Certified Professional Coder-Hospital (CPC-H) • Certified Interventional Radiology Cardiovascular Coder (CIRCC®)	• Work in all healthcare settings • Work in healthcare-related settings such as consulting firms, software vendors, insurance companies • Certificate or associate's degree Positions held in the following areas: • Medical Coder • Reimbursement specialist • Insurance biller • Chargemaster specialist • Insurance claims specialist

Medical Assistants	• Certified Medical Assistant (CMA) • Registered Medical Assistant (RMA)	• Typically employed in physicians' office or other outpatient setting • Requires associate's degree or certificate • Perform clinical duties such as prepping patients, taking vital signs, taking medical histories, assisting physician during exams, explaining minor procedures and giving instructions based on physician's orders, and collecting specimens • Perform administrative duties such as answering phone, making appointments, registering patients, maintaining health records, handing correspondence, filing health insurance claims, scheduling outpatient services, arranging referrals, and managing the office in general • May hold positions as office managers or business managers within a medical practice
Healthcare Administrators	• Certified Health Care Facility Manager (CHFM) • Fellow of the American College of Healthcare Executives (FACHE) • American College of Medical Practice Executives (ACMPE) Certification	• Work in all healthcare organizations • Bachelor's or master's degree typically required • Plan, organize, coordinate, and direct facility or department operations Positions held with the following titles: • Hospital administrator • Chief Information Officer/Manager • Project manager • Department manager • Office manager • Office administrator
Care Providers	• Physicians (Doctor of Medicine [MD]), Doctor of Osteopathy (DO) • Physicians' Assistants (PA, PA-C) • Certified Nurse Practitioners (CNP) • Certified Registered Nurse Midwives (CRNM)	• Work in any healthcare setting • Requires advanced education, licensure, and possibly certification • The only medical professionals who can diagnose a patient, order diagnostic testing and therapeutic (including medications) measures
Nursing	• Registered Nurse (RN) • Licensed Practical Nurse (LPN)	• Provide direct care to patients • May also hold non-direct care positions in Utilization Management, Risk Management, Quality Assessment, and general management positions within a healthcare facility • Nursing Informatics • Requires associate's or bachelor's degree at a minimum; management positions and informatics positions may require a master's degree

2.1 The Professionals Who Maintain and Use Health Information

In the inpatient setting, the **healthcare administrator** may be a chief executive officer (CEO), chief operating officer (COO), chief financial officer (CFO), or chief information officer (CIO). These individuals typically have a bachelor's or master's degree (preferred) in healthcare administration and are responsible for overseeing several departments (or the entire organization). Their degree is most likely in healthcare administration, healthcare management, or health systems administration. These individuals, who may also be called a **healthcare manager** or **health systems administrator**, concentrate on the big picture—the operation of the organization as a whole, and in regard to health information they are concerned with how an automated systems affects individual departments—will it meet the needs of the board of directors and administration to supply adequate, easily obtainable decision support data—will the clinicians have easily accessible, fast information—is the system secure and does it meet all standards and regulations? The health systems administrator may be known as the chief information officer and will typically have a great deal of knowledge and experience related to the technical aspects of automated systems.

In a hospital setting, the Director of the Health Information Department and the Chief Information Officer work closely. Each plays a key role in the selection of the product. Health Information Professionals have basic clinical knowledge, technical knowledge of automated systems, and expertise in record-keeping practice, putting them in a position to lead automation of health information efforts. Depending on the level and content of his or her education, a health information management professional may hold the position of chief information officer. Traditionally, the data itself has been the health information manager's main concern, and the use of the actual technology has been scope of the chief information officer's domain. The staff of the health information department will need to enter, maintain, and retrieve data from electronic health records and may be certified by the American Health Information Management Association (AHIMA). Various certifications are listed in Table 2.1, as well as other certifications for health information professional. The most recent development in health information careers and competencies is the recognition of competency exams in specialty areas which are also explained in Table 2.1.

In a medical office or other outpatient setting, healthcare administrators may have the same titles as are used in the inpatient setting, or they may be called Office Manager, Office Administrator, Business Manager, and the like. These individuals are keenly aware that electronic systems can greatly enhance the efficiency of an office, or can just as easily be a negative force that causes inefficiencies; therefore, they are at the forefront of selecting and maintaining electronic systems that meet the needs of the practice and its practitioners. Certification of professionals in the outpatient setting is just as important as in the inpatient setting.

Healthcare professionals such as medical assistants, nurses, medical coders and billers, and other administrative professionals will be using the software in a medical practice and will want it to be "user friendly," since they will be required to enter and retrieve data quickly yet accurately. The office administrator (manager**)** will be gathering information from the **practice management** and **EHR** systems to ensure claims are filed and paid accurately and in a timely manner, to ensure requirements of managed care organizations are met, and to ensure compliance with **meaningful use (MU)** requirements. Meaningful use will be discussed throughout this worktext.

The American Health Information Management Association (AHIMA), the American Association of Medical Assistants (AAMA), and the American Medical Technologists (AMT) are professional associations that offer certifying exams, and provide members with up-to-date, relevant information about their respective fields, continuing education opportunities, networking opportunities, publications, and career assistance. The websites for each are www.ahima.org, www.aama-ntl.org, and www.americanmedtech.org, respectively.

Check Your Understanding

1. What roles might be held by a Healthcare Administrator?
2. What does AHIMA do?
3. What is the difference between a medical assistant and an office administrator?

2.2 Data versus Information

Throughout this worktext you will see the terms *data* and *information*. They are often used interchangeably, but they are not entirely the same. Look up each term in a dictionary, and you will see within the definitions that the terms are almost interchangeable or synonymous. Think of it this way, though—data is a single fact, such as the patient is *60 years old,* or that the *patient is female,* or the *patient is African American.* Single facts come together to form information. For example, the fact that Elena Jones is allergic to penicillin is a piece of data. But, add to that piece of data the fact that she breaks out in hives, has difficulty breathing, and required an emergency room visit for her last allergic reaction and we have information about Elena and her allergy to penicillin. It is vitally important that each piece of data is accurate, valid, and timely to ensure that the information resulting from the data is also accurate, valid, timely, and in a usable format to ensure quality medical care.

Data may be unstructured or structured. Examples of unstructured data are a dictated report, a written progress note, voice files, or scanned images of original documents. In this unstructured format, it is difficult, if not impossible, to track or trend statistics, or to share information with healthcare agencies, public health agencies, or insurance carriers. Structured data—such as standard templates that are used to collect the elements of the dictated report or progress note, bar codes to identify types of reports or individual files, or numeric codes that equate to a written diagnosis or procedure—allow computers to process the data into usable information.

Check Your Understanding

1. Define data.
2. _____ makes up _____.

Prior to there being an electronic health record system, clinicians relied on one medium to collect and access information about patients—paper. Many pieces of paper make up the health record, and records of patients are often several inches thick. Paper records are contained in a folder that is filed numerically by a medical record number or alphabetically by the patient's last name. It is not that paper is no longer in use, but electronic media is gaining acceptance in the healthcare community. And in the coming years, the electronic health record will be a requirement rather than a choice thanks to the **Health Information Technology for Economic and Clinical Health Act (HITECH)**, which will be addressed later in this chapter. Many health insurance plans are making electronic **personal health records (PHR)** available to their subscribers. A PHR contains a person's health history, immunization status, current and past medications, allergies, and instructions given by a care provider; it often includes patient education materials as well. Though insurance carriers may provide the means to keep a PHR online, this does not replace the legal health record kept by the patient's care provider.

Electronic health records provide physicians with **decision support** software, which is used to access current information about a disease or condition. This technology alerts the care provider to possible medication interactions, gives treatment options based on results of clinical trials or research, and alerts the provider that a patient may have a particular diagnosis based on the data found in his or her electronic record. Not so long ago, physicians were opposed to this technology, thinking it was "cookbook medicine"; this is no longer the case, since great advances in the diagnosis and treatment of illnesses occur so quickly, making it very difficult or impossible to keep up with the most recent studies, findings, and recommended treatments. Thus, decision support applications within an EHR software package help to keep physicians up to date as well as improve the quality of care given to patients.

Physicians can use computerized models within the EHR to show where a patient's rash is located, for example, rather than placing an "X" on a crudely drawn picture of a patient's back (Figures 2.1 and 2.2).

The use of videos or DVDs is not new technology, although they are now used more often to educate patients about the procedure they are about to undergo than are handouts or educational booklets. The care provider may choose to show patients a video while they are in the office, or provide a link to a video for patients to view from their home computer. Using this type of media ensures that the information used to educate patients is consistent.

Most EHRs now provide educational materials for patients, and the educational materials can be specific to a particular patient's conditions, including treatment options, medications, etc. The educational materials may be printed out for the patient, or they

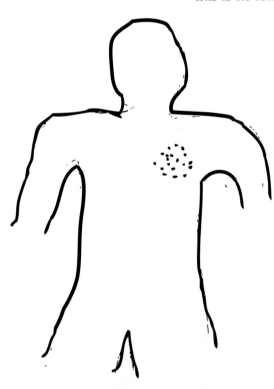

Figure 2.1 Drawing of placement of rash on patient's back as it would have appeared in a paper health record

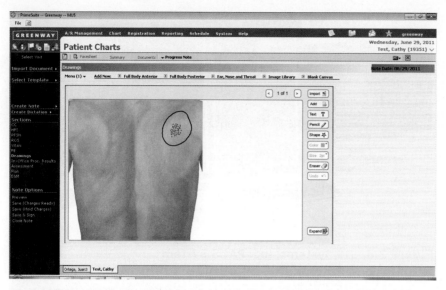

Figure 2.2 **Computer-generated drawing of placement of rash on patient's back**

can be provided through a secure portal that the patient accesses from home.

Physicians and administrators may want to visually present findings of a study or to consult with another physician and show a patient's disease progression. This can be done through use of software that has been available for years—presentation software such as Microsoft Power-Point® or Open Office IMPRESS. Spreadsheets are often useful in making a point as well. EHR software provides the ability to visually chart changes in a patient's vital signs, for example, and show trends or statistical changes. Patient care and treatment is greatly enhanced with the ability to track vital signs over time, thus alerting the care provider to changes in a patient's condition.

Let us look at a particular scenario. Patti Wolfe has been seeing Dr. Raszkowski for the past five years. She has been faithful about having a yearly physical exam. For the past four years, her blood pressure has increased on each visit. In 2008, her blood pressure was 130/80; in 2009, it was 135/82; in 2010, it was 130/83; and in 2011, it was 140/88. Seeing this steady climb, Dr. Raszkowski explained the situation to Mrs. Wolfe, and began her on a treatment regimen. Without this quick visual of her blood pressures, the subtle changes may not have been picked up by the physician, and her high blood pressure could have gone untreated.

Voice recognition technology is a medium that has been available for many years and has steadily gained in popularity. This software translates what a provider is saying and types those words into text. Whereas physicians used to dictate into a microphone and a medical transcriptionist would type the words, using word processing software, with voice recognition software the physician still dictates, but the software captures his or her words, then converts speech into text. With speech recognition, the medical transcriptionist's role has changed from transcriber to editor. The software is not 100 percent accurate, however, and in the world of medicine, it needs to be. Thus, a human being must still review the final document for accuracy.

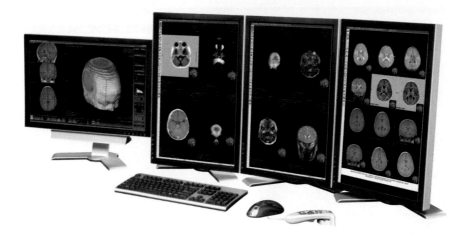

Figure 2.3   DS Systems, Inc. PACS System

Picture Archiving and Communication Systems (PACS) allow providers to view images such as x-rays, scans, ultrasounds, and the like. Originally used as a means to store x-ray film, PACS systems make it possible for providers to remotely view x-ray film to aid in **clinical decision support.** The improved image quality using PACS systems as well as the ability to add alerts or reminders based on the findings noted in PACS greatly improves patient care. Figure 2.3 illustrates a typical PACS system used to view radiologic images.

Check Your Understanding

1. In the past, physicians marked the location of a patient's pain by drawing an "X" on a picture of a body. With the advantage of EHRs, what are they now able to do?
2. What does PACS stand for?
3. What do PACS allow providers to do?

2.4   Screen-Based Data Collection Tools

Those who are entering (also known as capturing) data typically do so on a computer screen. It may be done on a desktop computer, a laptop, a notebook computer, or a personal digital assistant (PDA). Each of these pieces of hardware will be discussed in Chapter 10, but the commonality between them is that data can be entered and then retrieved by using a computer screen. Think of the screen as the replacement for paper. Advantages include the portability of the hand-held devices, the ability to have multiple monitors showing different images at the same time, and the ability to customize a screen based on user preference. With paper records, there is typically an order in which the individual papers are filed within the folder, but not all care providers prefer that same order. Take a look at the two screens showing a patient's history in Figures 2.4 and 2.5—you see that the same information is collected but that the information is in different places on the screen.

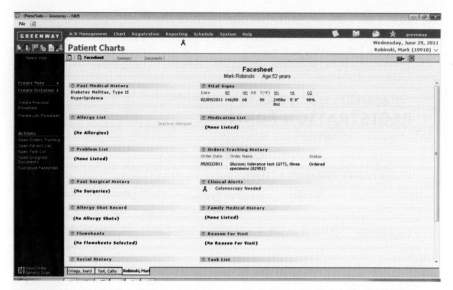

Figure 2.4 Facesheet format as preferred by one care provider

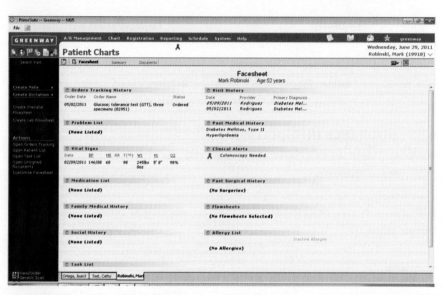

Figure 2.5 Facesheet format as preferred by a different care provider

Check Your Understanding

1. What types of computers are used for data capture?
2. In this digital era, the computer screen is considered the replacement for _____.

2.5 Collecting Data Elements

So, we have this data, but how did we get it in the first place? It all starts when the patient makes an appointment with a physician's office or comes to the hospital for an emergency department visit, outpatient laboratory, outpatient surgery, or inpatient admission.

We collect identifying information verbally from the patient (or representative), or we ask the patient to complete a form (or a combination of both). See Figure 2.6 for an example of a registration form.

Greensburg Medical Center
REGISTRATION FORM
(Please Print)

Today's date:	Care Provider:

PATIENT INFORMATION

Patient's last name:	First:	Middle:	❏ Mr. ❏ Mrs.	❏ Miss ❏ Ms.	Marital status (circle one) Single / Mar / Div / Sep / Wid

Is this your legal name? ❏ Yes ❏ No	If not, what is your legal name?	(Former name):	Birth date:	Age:	Sex: ❏ M ❏ F

Street address:	Social Security no.:	Home phone no.:

P. O. Box:	City:	State:	ZIP Code:

Occupation:	Employer:	Employer phone no.:

E-mail address:	Cell phone:	

Race:	Ethnicity:	Primary language:	Religion:

Other family members seen here:

INSURANCE INFORMATION
(Presentation of Insurance Card is required at time of each visit)

Person responsible for bill:	Birth date: / /	Address (if different):	Home phone no.: ( )

Is this person a patient here?   ❏ Yes   ❏ No

Occupation:	Employer:	Employer address:	Employer phone no.: ( )

Is this patient covered by insurance?   ❏ Yes   ❏ No

Please indicate primary insurance	❏ McGraw-Hill Healthmark Insurance	❏ BlueCross/Shield	❏ [Insurance]	❏ [Insurance]	❏ [Insurance]
❏ [Insurance]	❏ Workers' Compensation	❏ Medicare	❏ Medicaid *(Please provide card)*	❏ Other	

Subscriber's name:	Subscriber's S.S. no.:	Birth date: / /	Group no.:	Policy no.:	Co-payment: $

Patient's relationship to subscriber:	❏ Self	❏ Spouse	❏ Child	❏ Other	Effective Date:

Name of secondary insurance (if applicable):	Subscriber's name:	Group no.:	Policy no.:

Patient's relationship to subscriber:	❏ Self	❏ Spouse	❏ Child	❏ Other

IN CASE OF EMERGENCY

Name of local friend or relative (not living at same address):	Relationship to patient:	Home phone no.: ( )	Work phone no.: ( )

The above information is true to the best of my knowledge. I authorize my insurance benefits be paid directly to the physician. I understand that I am financially responsible for any balance. I also authorize [Name of Practice] or insurance company to release any information required to process my claims.

_____   _____
Patient/Guardian signature   *Date*

Figure 2.6   Patient registration form

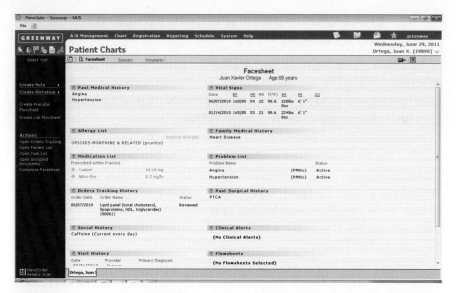

Figure 2.7   PrimeSUITE documentation of patient's past medical history

The patient's past medical, surgical, social, and family histories are collected and entered into the EHR as well. Figure 2.7 illustrates documentation in PrimeSUITE; each of the areas, when clicked on, includes more detailed information about the patient. Medication allergies, current medications, and immunization history are typically captured as part of the past medical history. The history is taken from a history form and/or the patient is asked questions in order to capture those data elements in the EHR.

The care provider then documents the history of present illness (HPI) and performs and documents a physical exam. He or she views all of this information to make an assessment of the patient (make a diagnosis) and then determines a treatment plan (also called a plan of care).

In addition, the patient's previous health records are often used as a source of data. This information may be sent to the facility in a paper format, which is later scanned into the patient's health record, or the information can be retrieved electronically, eventually becoming part of the patient's record.

Check Your Understanding

1. Besides a patient's medical, social, surgical, and family histories, what other information is captured for entry into his or her EHR?

2. Will a patient's previous health records ever be used as a source of data?

3. Name two ways that identifying information is collected from a patient.

2.6 Electronic Health (Medical) Records (EHR) (EMR)

A health record that is in electronic form is referred to as an **electronic health record (EHR)** and sometimes an **electronic medical record (EMR)**. The **Office of the National Coordinator for Health Information Technology (ONC)**, however, differentiates between the two, based on a white paper by Garets and Davis. According to Garets and Davis, the EMR is the legal patient record that is created within any healthcare facility (hospital, nursing home, ambulatory surgery facility, physician's office, etc.). The information in that EMR relates solely to that episode of care, and the EMR is the data source for the EHR. The individual records feed into the EHR so that healthcare providers, patients, employers, and insurance carriers can access a patient's health records as appropriate and in accordance with **Health Insurance Portability and Accountability Act (HIPAA)** regulations. Only those who have a need to know should access the information found in a patient's record.

Let us look at an example. Alison Holt is seen in the emergency room of Memorial Hospital on July 15, 2009. An EMR is compiled for that visit. She also has an EMR for an inpatient stay in Memorial Hospital from October 5 to October 10, 2009. There are additional EMRs for Alison Holt that pertain to various physician office visits and outpatient diagnostic testing. Then, in April, 2010, Ms. Holt sees a pulmonary specialist who needs to review her previous health records. Her providers and the hospitals she has been admitted to are able to share information through a **Regional Health Information Organization (RHIO)**, which includes healthcare organizations in her area that exchange patient information in order to improve care. This **health information exchange (HIE)** resulted in the quick and easy sharing of her medical history with the pulmonary specialist. Her individual records thus became part of an EHR. In effect, an EHR allows for the exchange of information among caregivers and others (insurance, employers, etc.) who have a need to know, but in a secure environment and according to certain standards.

In 2003, the **Institute of Medicine** defined the functions of an EHR. The eight core functions are:

- health information and data
- result management
- order management
- decision support
- electronic communication and connectivity
- patient support
- administrative processes and reporting
- reporting and population health

We will no doubt continue to use the terms EMR and EHR interchangeably, but it is important to remember that in order for the benefits of the EMR to be realized, an EHR must exist. Without the EMR, the EHR, by definition, would not exist.

Check Your Understanding

1. The legal patient record created for one episode of care is known as the _____.

2. Who is allowed to access the information contained in a patient's record?

2.7 Laws, Regulations, and Standards

Health Insurance Portability and Accountability Act (HIPAA)

As a healthcare professional, you will get used to the fact that there are many outside influences that affect how and why we do our jobs. We will start our journey through the agencies, regulations, and laws that govern the keeping and exchange of health information with HIPAA, although many laws and standards have come before it. HIPAA stands for Health Insurance Portability and Accountability Act. HIPAA was passed on August 21, 1996, with a multifaceted purpose. It included regulations that afforded people who left their employment the ability to keep their insurance or obtain new health insurance even if they had a pre-existing medical condition. It also set standards for several aspects of storing, maintaining, and sharing electronic health information while ensuring the privacy and security of health information.

There are several rules that are addressed in HIPAA. With an effective compliance date of April 14, 2003, is the Privacy Rule. Its intent was to ensure the privacy of health information, and the use of **Protected Health Information (PHI)**, which is information that identifies the patient. The Office of Civil Rights that enforces compliance with the Privacy Rule. The specifics of the Privacy Rule will be covered in more detail in Chapter 7, Privacy, Security, Confidentiality, and Legal Issues; however, it is important to know that electronic data collection, maintenance, use, and storage are all governed by standards, and many of these come from HIPAA. Health records are legal documents and must be compliant with state and federal regulations as well as standards set forth by accrediting agencies and insurance carriers.

In February 2003, the Security Rules were published. The deadline for facilities to implement the security rules was April 20, 2005. The security standards require health care organizations to include safeguards (administrative, physical, and technological) that ensure health information is protected, that it is kept private, and that it is retrievable in the event that the integrity of the electronic system is compromised. As noted above, Chapter 7 includes more specific information regarding the security requirements.

The Electronic Healthcare Transactions, Code Sets, and National Identifiers Rules required that medical providers who submit claims electronically be compliant with regulations requiring standardization of electronic collection and exchange of health information.

for your information

To learn fast facts about HIPAA privacy, go to http://www.hhs.gov/ocr/privacy/hipaa/understanding/coveredentities/cefastfacts.html or http://www.hhs.gov/ocr/privacy/index.html

for your information

The final Security Standards, as published in **The Federal Register**, which is published daily and includes all actions taken by the federal government, may be found at http://aspe.hhs.gov/admnsimp/FINAL/FR03-8334.pdf

Hospitals, physicians' offices, and **clearinghouses** (entities that process medical claims prior to payment) were required not only to submit claims (and diagnosis and procedure codes) electronically, but also to receive information, such as remittance advices, from insurance companies electronically. Compliance was required by October 23, 2003. However, yet another change is coming, and on January 1, 2012, version 5010 of the Code Set Rule will go into effect. The version 5010 HIPAA transaction upgrade is being made in part because the previous version, 4010, is several years old and has its share of problems, the use of ICD-10-PCS codes beginning in 2013 required significant revision, and version 5010 includes improved instructions for use of the **National Provider Identifier (NPI)** number, which is a unique identifier that must be used on insurance claims to identify the care provider and/or group practice that rendered care to the patient. The NPI implementation was the last of the original HIPAA regulations to take effect.

HITECH Act

The **Health Information Technology for Economic and Clinical Health (HITECH) Act** is part of the **American Recovery and Reinvestment Act of 2009 (ARRA)**, which was signed into law by President Obama on February 17, 2009. The HITECH portion of ARRA is meant to increase the use of an EHR by hospitals and physicians. The incentive program, made possible through HITECH, includes $18 billion in funding for this purpose. Physicians and hospitals that show **meaningful use** of the information collected through use of an EHR will benefit from HITECH. The incentives can be used for implementation of new EHR systems, or upgrades to those that are already in place. Later in this text, we will demonstrate the meaningful use of data. There are three stages of meaningful use; the first is the collection and use of data, the second is the secure exchange of information, and the third is use of patient data to improve patient outcomes. Figure 2.8 depicts the HITECH interim final rule from the Health and Human Services (HHS) website.

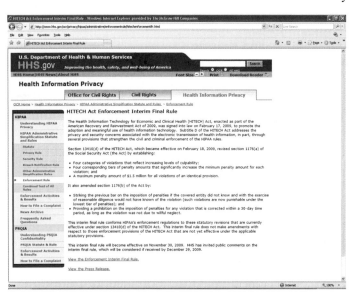

Figure 2.8   HITECH Act enforcement interim final rule

Office of the National Coordinator (ONC)

From ARRA also came the **Office of the National Coordinator**, or **ONC.** The ONC was created in 2004 through a presidential order, but was later mandated by legislation (HITECH). According to the ONC website "ONC is the principal Federal entity charged with coordination of nationwide efforts to implement and use the most advanced health information technology and the electronic exchange of health information"; its mission includes:

- promoting development of a nationwide Health IT infrastructure that allows for electronic use and exchange of information that:
  - ensures secure and protected patient health information
  - improves healthcare quality
  - reduces healthcare costs
  - informs medical decisions at the time/place of care
  - includes meaningful public input in infrastructure development
  - improves coordination of care and information among hospitals, labs, physicians, etc.
  - improves public health activities and facilitates early identification/rapid response to public health emergencies
  - facilitates health and clinical research
  - promotes early detection, prevention, and management of chronic diseases
  - promotes a more effective marketplace
  - improves efforts to reduce health disparities
- providing leadership in the development, recognition, and implementation of standards and the certification of Health IT products
- health IT policy coordination
- strategic planning for Health IT adoption and health information exchange
- establishing governance for the Nationwide Health Information Network"

NATIONAL HEALTH INFORMATION NETWORK (NHIN)

The ultimate goal of using EHR technology is to improve patient care—sharing information to improve diagnosis, treatment, and prognosis—while doing so in an economically efficient manner. In order to share health information electronically, though, standards must be set, and policies must be adhered to. According to the ONC website, the **National Health Information Network (NHIN)** is "a set of standards, services, and policies that enable the secure exchange of health information over the Internet." (National Health Information Network: Overview)

Three activities are currently available through NHIN:

National Health Information Network Exchange—a group of federal agencies and private organizations that are developing NHIN standards, services, and policies; they are also demonstrating live, a health information exchange.

Direct Project—a project aimed at developing standards and services that will enable secure exchange of information on a local level among trusted providers to support stage 1 of the meaningful use incentives, which went into effect on January 1, 2011.

CONNECT—free, open source software that supports health information exchange.

CERTIFICATION COMMISSION FOR HEALTH INFORMATION TECHNOLOGY (CCHIT) AND OTHER CERTIFYING AGENCIES

To ensure that health information is indeed shared securely, and that the shared information is being used for its intended purpose, the **Certification Commission for Health Information Technology (CCHIT)** was founded in 2004. Its purpose is to certify EHRs for functionality, interoperability, and security and it is a non-government, non-profit organization. CCHIT began certifying EHR systems in 2004, and by 2009 over 200 systems had been certified. There is reference to the importance of certification within ARRA, specifically in the area of meaningful use of health information through the adoption of a certified EHR.

The Healthcare Information and Management Systems and Society (HIMSS), a non-profit organization that focuses on the use of information technology (IT) and management systems needed to improve heathcare, provides important information regarding the EHR on its website found at http://www.himss.org/ASP/topics_ehr.asp

The Medicare and Medicaid EHR Incentive Programs require the use of certified EHR technology; a listing of certified EHR technologies can be found at http://onc-chpl.force.com/ehrcert. When you access this list, you will see that there are other EHR certifying agencies; they will be discussed further in Chapter 7.

REGIONAL EXTENSION CENTERS

As part of HITECH, extension centers are funded by the federal government. The purpose of the extension centers is to lend technical assistance and guidance regarding best practices in the selection, implementation, and maintenance of an EHR that will satisfy the meaningful use requirements. Each **Regional Extension Center,** or REC (pronounced R-E-C), is responsible for a geographic region within the United States and is a non-profit entity. A map is available at http://www.hhs.gov/about/regionmap.html; click on your location to see what is happening in your area.

So you can see that there are many outside entities to ensure that health information is shared so that safe, effective, quality medical care is provided, yet in a manner that allows for the security and privacy of that information exchange.

Check Your Understanding

1. CCHIT is a _____ agency.
2. Name the four subcategories of HIPAA.
3. What does PHI stand for?
4. What office ensures compliance with the Privacy Rule?
5. What does the Office of the National Coordinator (ONC) do?
6. List the three activities currently available through the National Health Information Network.

2.8 Similarities and Differences between a Physician's Office and Hospital Information Systems

Regardless of the healthcare setting—inpatient or outpatient—every patient seen must have a health record that describes his or her history of present illness, past medical and surgical history, record of physical exam, record of treatment rendered, results of diagnostic tests, plan of care, and diagnoses. In a physician's office setting, the patient schedules an appointment, which is part of the registration process. In a hospital setting, a patient may arrive without an appointment for an emergency department visit, or to have outpatient lab work done, for example. In either case, appointments would typically be unnecessary or impossible. In other instances, such as for a CT scan, which requires a significant amount of time and specially trained staff, an appointment is necessary. And, in a hospital setting, a patient may be scheduled for an elective surgery such as cholecystectomy (removal of the gall bladder).

The steps taken to capture the fact that a patient was seen, no matter what the setting, are most easily (and accurately) done using computerization. In a physician's office, this is done using **Practice Management** (PM) software. In a hospital, this is called the **Master Patient (person) Index (MPI)** and it is part of the RADT (Registration, Admission, Discharge, Transfer) functions of the hospital's automated information system. Each patient is entered only once into the MPI or Patient List, although there may be several visits (encounters) for each patient as a subset of the main entry. This allows the documentation of each individual visit to be filed in one place within the MPI or Patient List.

Practice Management software is used to handle the administrative functions in an office such as listing all patients who have been seen in that practice; capturing insurance and demographic information; entering charges and diagnosis and procedure codes; filing, maintenance, and follow-up of medical claims and collections (billing procedures); running statistical reports about the practice; and scheduling patients' appointments.

The capturing of the identifying information and the clinical documentation discussed earlier in this chapter becomes part of the electronic health record in both the hospital and physicians' offices.

The various functions performed are called by different names in different settings, but the goals are the same—registration of the patient and then compilation a health record for every encounter the patient has in that facility or office.

Table 2.2 compares common jargon used in a hospital to that used in a physician's office.

The objective of an EHR is to capture timely, accurate, usable health information to ensure quality medical care; provide for coordination of care; support the medical necessity for diagnostic testing; protect the legal interests of the patient, provider, and hospital; collect data used in statistical reporting; and file insurance claims.

TABLE 2.2   Comparison of Outpatient to Inpatient Setting

Action	Physician's Office or Other Outpatient Setting	Hospital
Patient seeks care	Schedule patient or make an appointment	Register or admit a patient
Health record is compiled	End product is a SOAP note, progress note, or "chart"	End product is a health (medical) record
Listing of all patients seen by the facility	Once the patient is registered one time, he/she appears in the Patient List	Once the patient is registered one time, he/she appears in the Master Patient (person) Index (MPI)
Patient has outpatient care	Each is called an encounter or visit	Each is called an encounter
Patient stays over night	n/a	The patient is an admission or inpatient
Patient is finished with the encounter	Patient checks out	Patient is discharged

Check Your Understanding

1. SOAP notes are generally used in a/an _____ setting.
2. Could a patient ever have outpatient care in a hospital setting? If so, what is an episode of outpatient care called?
3. What term describes a hospital's historical list of patients?

In order to select, implement, maintain, and use practice management software or the electronic health record, it is necessary to include professionals who understand not only how to use the software, but also what to look for when selecting software that will meet the stiff regulations that govern the keeping of health information. It is vitally important that this health information be maintained in a way that is private, confidential, and secure, yet readily available when needed. In addition, the information needs to be accurate, reliable, and valid. Over the past several years, the federal government has affirmed that there is an urgent need for an electronic health record that will provide for more efficient, effective, and safe healthcare for Americans.

chapter 2 **summary**

LEARNING OUTCOME	CONCEPTS FOR REVIEW
2.1 Describe the role of six healthcare professionals who maintain or use practice management and electronic health record applications. Pages 21–23	– Healthcare professionals, their educational background, their certifications, and how they use health information: • Chief Information Officer • Health Information Professionals • Chief Financial Officer • Healthcare Administrators/Managers/Office Administrators • Care Providers • Nurses, Medical Assistants
2.2 Explain the difference between data and information. Page 23	– Often used interchangeably – Data is a single fact – Single facts come together to form information – Structured vs. unstructured data
2.3 Identify computer-based health information media. Pages 24–26	– Role of the health Information Technology for Economic and Clinical Health (HITCH) Act in the adoption of an electronic health record – Define Personal Health Record (PHR) – Electronic health record includes decision support technology – Electronic health record includes computerized models and images – Electronic health record includes presentation aids – Electronic health record includes voice recognition technology – Electronic health record includes Picture Archiving and Communication Systems (PACS)
2.4 Relate how screen-based data collection tools are used in healthcare. Pages 26–27	– Hardware used to collect health information includes: • Desktop computers • Laptop computers • Notebook computers • iPad • iPhone • Personal Digital Assistants (PDA) – Advantages include portability and customization

LEARNING OUTCOME	CONCEPTS FOR REVIEW
2.5 Demonstrate how individual data elements are collected. Pages 27–29	– Data collected through use of forms or in person – Registration forms used as method of collecting patient identifying and demographic information – Patient history form used as method of collecting past medical, surgical, family, and social histories; allergies; medication history
2.6 Describe electronic health record applications, Pages 30–31	– Differentiate between electronic medical record (EMR) and electronic health record (EHR) – Role of the Office of the National Coordinator (ONC) – Differentiate between Regional Health Information Organization (RHIO) and Health Information Exchange (HIE) – List the functions of the EHR as detailed by the Institute of Medicine (IOM)
2.7 Identify laws, regulations, and standards that govern electronic health information. Pages 31–34	– Identify the privacy, security, transactions, and code set rules of HIPAA – Define Protected Health Information (PHI) – Define National Provider Identifier (NPI) number – Describe the Health Information Technology for Economic and Clinical Health (HITECH) Act and its role in requiring electronic health records – Define meaningful use of data collected through use of an EHR – Describe the purpose of the Office of the National Coordinator (ONC) – Explain the National Health Information Network (NHIN) – Explain the Certification Commission for Health Information Technology (CCHIT) – Relate the purpose of Regional Extension Centers (REC)
2.8 Distinguish between practice management software and hospital health information software. Pages 35–36	– Describe the functions of Practice Management software – Differentiate between RADT systems and EHR systems within a hospital setting – Discuss the use of a Master Patient (Person) Index and Patient List – Articulate the purpose of an EHR

chapter **review**

MATCHING QUESTIONS

Match the terms on the left with the definitions on the right.

_____ 1. **[LO 2.2]** data

_____ 2. **[LO 2.5]** progress note

_____ 3. **[LO 2.6]** electronic medical record (EMR)

_____ 4. **[LO 2.1]** office administrator

_____ 5. **[LO 2.7]** meaningful use

_____ 6. **[LO 2.3]** clinical decision support

_____ 7. **[LO 2.8]** Master Patient Index

_____ 8. **[LO 2.1]** medical assistant

_____ 9. **[LO 2.5]** capture

_____ 10. **[LO 2.6]** electronic health record (EHR)

a. staff member who uses EHR software

b. entering or editing information about a patient

c. staff member whose responsibilities may include management of the EHR and other office systems to ensure efficient claims management and compliance with meaningful use requirements.

d. use of health information in an effective and efficient manner to improve patient care

e. a single fact often used interchangeably with information

f. comprehensive record of all health records for a patient which can be shared electronically with other healthcare providers as necessary

g. method of accessing current treatment options for a disease, through electronic or remote methods

h. documentation that usually contains the patient's chief complaint, history of present illness, results of physical exam, assessment, and plan.

i. record of the names of all patients seen in a hospital setting

j. legal patient record for a single instance of treatment

MULTIPLE-CHOICE QUESTIONS

Select the letter that best completes the statement or answers the question:

1. **[LO 2.7]** The acronym HIE stands for:
   a. health information exchange.
   b. hospital information exchange.
   c. health information electronically.
   d. hospital institutional exchange.

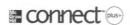 Enhance your learning by completing these exercises and more at http://connect.mcgraw-hill.com!

2. **[LO 2.4]** An advantage of using screen-based data collection tools is that the layout of the information can be:
   a. printed.
   b. deleted.
   c. shredded.
   d. customized.

3. **[LO 2.6]** The _____ defined the eight core functions of an EHR.
   a. National Institute of Health
   b. American Recovery and Reinvestment Act
   c. Institute of Medicine
   d. HITECH Act

4. **[LO 2.7]** Which of the following is a goal of HIPAA?
   a. establish standards for keeping of health care information
   b. ensure patients receive timely treatment
   c. allow a person's insurance to transfer from one job to another
   d. to guide how Picture Archiving and Communication Systems are used

5. **[LO 2.5, 2.8]** In a physician's office, patient data collection begins when:
   a. the patient exam begins.
   b. the patient calls to make an appointment.
   c. the medical assistant takes the patient's vital signs.
   d. the patient signs in at the front desk.

6. **[LO 2.3]** An advantage of EHRs is that patients are now able to _____ about procedures they are undergoing.
   a. hear lectures
   b. see diagrams
   c. ask questions
   d. view videos

7. **[LO 2.2]** Knowing that Jim Smith had a heart attack when he was 53 is an example of:
   a. data.
   b. information.
   c. support.
   d. technology.

8. **[LO 2.8]** When patients are finished with their encounter at a hospital, they:
   a. are admitted.
   b. check out.
   c. complete a SOAP note.
   d. are discharged.

9. **[LO 2.7]** If a hospital uses information gathered through their EHRs to justify the purchase of state-the-art equipment to improve patient care, they are:
   a. violating the Privacy Rule.
   b. engaging in meaningful use.
   c. abusing Protected Health Information.
   d. following CCHIT.

SHORT ANSWER QUESTIONS

1. **[LO 2.1]** List and define the roles of the six healthcare professionals involved in EMR use.

2. **[LO 2.7]** What is the purpose of CCHIT?

3. **[LO 2.1]** Explain the differences between a healthcare administrator, healthcare manager, and health systems administrator.

4. **[LO 2.3]** What does PACS stand for?

5. **[LO 2.8]** List five objectives of an EHR.

6. **[LO 2.7]** HIPAA is an acronym for _____.

7. **[LO 2.6]** Contrast an EHR with an EMR.

8. **[LO 2.6]** List the eight core functions of an EHR as defined by the Institute of Medicine.

9. **[LO 2.2]** Explain the difference between data and information, and give an example of each.

10. **[LO 2.3]** Why were so many physicians opposed to clinical decision support in the past?

11. **[LO 2.5]** List the four types of histories entered into a patient's electronic record.

12. **[LO 2.4]** Name two advantages of using screen-based data collection tools.

13. **[LO 2.1]** If someone has the letters "RHIA" after his or her name, what does that mean?

14. **[LO 2.8]** What does the ADT acronym mean in a hospital setting?

15. **[LO 2.7]** Explain the purpose of a Regional Extension Center (REC).

16. **[LO 2.3]** List one way that voice recognition technology can be used in a medical setting.

APPLYING YOUR KNOWLEDGE

1. **[LOs 2.3, 2.4, 2.6, 2.7]** Discuss any potential drawbacks to the full-scale use of EHRs, and explain what precautions or regulations have been put in place to deal with each drawback.

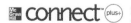 Enhance your learning by completing these exercises and more at http://connect.mcgraw-hill.com!

2. **[LO 2.7]** Incentives are a significant part of the HITECH Act. Discuss the advantages and potential disadvantages associated with using incentives as a tool for implementing EHRs.

3. **[LOs 2.2, 2.5]** In the following case study, determine what would be considered data and what would be considered information: New patient Alice Jones is a 32-year-old female who presents with chest pains. She tells you that, in the past, she has been diagnosed with rosacea and is allergic to latex. In addition, she has had surgery for a broken arm. She does not smoke; is a social drinker; and has no family history of heart problems.

4. **[LO 2.8]** A physician's office and a hospital employ different terminology and process flow when maintaining records and monitoring patient flow. Why is there no set protocol that is used by all health-care settings?

5. **[LO 2.4]** Describe a scenario where presentation software might be used in a physician's office practice.

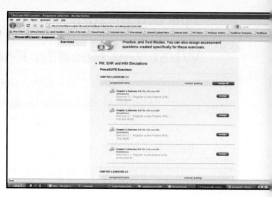

Content of the Health Record— Administrative Data

Learning Outcomes

At the end of this chapter, the student should be able to:

3.1 Identify administrative data elements.

3.2 Explain the administrative uses of data.

3.3 Explain the use of the Master Patient (person) Index (MPI).

3.4 Apply procedures to register a new patient in PrimeSUITE.

3.5 Apply procedures to schedule a patient's appointment in PrimeSUITE.

3.6 Apply procedures to edit demographic information in PrimeSUITE.

3.7 Follow the steps performed upon patient check-in.

3.8 Apply procedures to capture insurance information in PrimeSUITE.

3.9 Locate the Help feature in PrimeSUITE.

Key Terms

Administrative data
Chief complaint
CMS-1500
Current Procedural Terminology (CPT) codes
Data dictionary
Demographic data
Health Level Seven (HL7)
International Classification of Diseases, 9th revision, Clinical Modification (ICD-9-CM) codes
Library

Master Patient (person) Index (MPI)
Master Patient List
Meaningful use (MU)
Medical record number
Patient List
Policyholder
Primary insurance
Shortcut key
UB-04

What You Need to Know and Why You Need to Know It

In Chapters 1 and 2 we talked about the importance of each patient having only one record in the EHR of that facility. Remember though, that one record may have many individual encounters attached to it, one for each visit to the facility as a patient. In this chapter we will discuss the administrative data, including demographic (identifying) data that is collected about each patient, thus forming the master record or master patient index for each patient.

3.1 Administrative Data Elements

Administrative data is non-clinical data; it does not include data relative to the diagnosis, prognosis, treatment, or plan of care. **Demographic data** is a subset of administrative data and includes data collected to identify a particular patient. It includes the patient's full name, date of birth, gender, social security number, marital status, address, and phone number. Additional information that may be collected includes employer/student status, employer name and address, next of kin, race, ethnicity, and insurance policy name, policy number, and group number. In addition to identifying patients, many administrative data elements are required to complete insurance claim forms such as the **CMS-1500** and the **UB-04,** as required by HIPAA. The CMS-1500 form is used to bill outpatient encounters, and the UB-04 is used to bill hospital admissions/ encounters. Both the CMS-1500 and the UB-04 are available on the Online Learning Center at http://www.mhhe.com/greenway.

Identifying information for inpatients and outpatients, as included in the core health data elements recommended by the National Center for Vital and Health Statistics in 1996, should include the data elements listed below.

- Full Name
- Personal/Unique Identifier – this is also referred to as medical record number or chart number
- Account or billing number
- Date of Birth
- Gender
- Race and Ethnicity
- Residence (address)
- Marital Status
- Current or Most Recent Occupation (employer)
- Type of Encounter (inpatient, emergency room visit, physician's office visit, etc.)
- Admission Date (inpatient) or date of encounter (outpatient)
- Discharge Date (inpatient)
- Facility Identification (unique identifier of the medical office, hospital, outpatient surgery center, etc.)

- Type of Facility/Place of Encounter (hospital, physician's office, surgi-center, etc.)
- Healthcare Practitioner Identification (outpatient)
- Provider Location or Address of Encounter (outpatient)
- Attending Physician Identification (inpatient)
- Patient's Expected Sources of Payment (Medicare, Medicaid, insurance, self-pay, etc.)
- Injury Related to Employment
- Total Billed Charges

These data elements are also included in the **Health Level Seven (HL7)** standards. HL7 allows different software packages to interface with one another, i.e., it allows them to share data. There are many different companies that develop healthcare applications and systems, and by writing the software according to HL7 standards, the applications "talk to each other;" otherwise the data would have to be entered separately for each. Hospitals or medical practices may have different vendors for different systems. For instance, there may be one vendor for the laboratory system, one for the pharmacy system, one for tracking incomplete records, etc. Through use of HL7 standards, if something is changed in one system, say the patient's telephone number, the change would be reflected in all three. This is a very important requirement, because without this standard language the interoperability that was discussed in Chapter 1 would not be possible. More explanation of the protocol itself is not necessary in this text, but will be covered in more advanced health information technology courses.

One data element that is not included above, but that should be collected is a patient's previous name, if applicable. This could be a maiden name or previous married name. Collecting this data element allows for cross-referencing of files. If a woman was previously seen at that facility under her maiden name, but is being seen for the first time using her married name, she is still one and the same person and should be listed only one time in the master list of patients.

In an outpatient setting, the data elements listed above are collected on a patient registration form, which is completed at the time care is established with that facility or office. The information should be verified with the patient each time he or she is seen to assure that there has been no change in information, and that there have been no additions or deletions to the information. Examples would be change in address, telephone number, or marital status. In a hospital setting, the information may be required prior to a patient undergoing an elective admission, or would be collected face-to-face in the registration department when the patient presents for care.

Equally important for collecting sufficient identifying information is that each data element is consistently defined in the facility. Use of a **data dictionary** will ensure that each member of the registration staff has defined the data element correctly, and that only valid entries are made in a particular data element.

Let us look at a few examples. First, consider the possible data dictionary choices for marital status. The typical choices are single, married, separated, widowed, divorced, or unknown. If that is the definition of marital status in your facility, then those are the *only* choices available in the practice management system. Data dictionaries should be very specific. Each choice could be further defined. An example is the definition of "separated." Some facilities may consider a patient to be separated only if she presents a legal document stating such, and if she cannot do that, she is considered married for data collection purposes even though she considers herself to be separated in the legal sense. Another example is the patient's full name. In the facility's data dictionary the full name may be defined as the patient's last name, first name, middle name. Or, it may be defined as the last name, first name, middle initial. Thus, when a patient is registered, the name should be collected exactly as defined in that facility's data dictionary. Failure to follow the data dictionary definitions will result in unreliable data.

For consistency of wording and to save time, many fields in Prime-SUITE have a **library** of possibilities from which to choose. These are called drop-down menus. Examples of libraries would be: employers, common medications, religions, ethnicities, medical conditions, and elements of a physical exam, just to name a few.

3.2 Administrative Uses of Data

In addition to identifying a particular patient, administrative data is also used to satisfy HIPAA data requirements, which in turn are used to file electronic health claims for reimbursement. The **CMS-1500** form is used to submit claims electronically for outpatient encounters, and the **UB-04** is used to submit hospital claims. There are five major sections or levels on the claim form:

1. Provider information

The name, address, national provider identifier (NPI) number, and telephone number of the provider.

2. Subscriber and patient information

This section includes information about the person who is the **policyholder** (subscriber) of the insurance and the patient identifying information. These may be one and the same, if the patient is the policyholder (the primary insured). Below is a partial list of information collected but it is not limited to:

- Policyholder's (subscriber's) name
- Group or insurance plan name
- Identification (policy) number
- Patient's relationship to the policyholder

3. Payer information

- Group or insurance plan name
- Plan identification
- Address
- Assignment of benefits authorization (allows payment to be made directly to the provider)

- Release of information authorization (allows clinical information to be released to the insurance company)
- Referral number (if patient was referred by another provider)
- Prior authorization number (obtained when insurance plan requires procedures to be approved for payment in advance)

4. Claim details. A partial list of data includes:
- Individual account number or identification for that particular encounter
- Total charges submitted
- Place of service code
- Provider signature
- Details about the onset of the illness/accident
- Date(s) of service
- Amount collected from the patient
- Unique identifier (medical record number or chart number)
- **International Classification of Diseases, 9th edition, Clinical Modification (ICD-9-CM)** diagnosis codes. ICD-9-CM is a classification system that converts diagnoses and procedures into numeric form. It is published by the World Health Organization (WHO) and is the required code set for documenting diagnoses and procedures for inpatients. An example of an ICD-9-CM code is 250.01, which is type I diabetes mellitus.
- Whether the encounter was due to an auto or other accident or was a work-related injury

5. Services
- Procedures performed as indicated by **Current Procedural Terminology (CPT)** codes. CPT codes convert written procedures and services into numeric form. It is published by the American Medical Association (AMA) and is the required code set for submitting procedures and services for outpatients. An example of a CPT code is 82247, which is the code for a total bilirubin test.
- Date(s) of service

Information collected in each of these major sections may overlap. For instance, the place of service code or dates of service code would be collected only once, but satisfies the claim details as well as the services section requirements.

Administrative data, as well as clinical data which describes the patient's diagnosis and procedures, may also be used to satisfy reporting requirements. **Meaningful use** of data was discussed in Chapter 2—reporting that the race and ethnicity of all patients is collected would be an example of the administrative use of data to satisfy meaningful use regulations. Other administrative data elements that are required to satisfy meaningful use are the patient's preferred language, gender, and date of birth. An example of a clinical data element that is collected from within the provider's documentation or in the health history would be the patient's smoking status (if the patient is 13 years of age or older). A report that includes the total number of patients living in a particular ZIP code with a diagnosis of COPD is an example of a report that uses both administrative and clinical data. Another would be the total number of patients between the ages of 13 and 50 years of age who are smokers and have a diagnosis of asthma. Either of these reports may be used by public health agencies or in educational materials used in a smoking cessation class.

3.3 The Master Patient (Person) Index (MPI)

All of the administrative data elements discussed above are included in a **Master Patient Index,** also known as the Master Person Index, and referred to as the MPI. The acronym MPI is used more in the hospital setting than in the outpatient setting, although the objective is the same: one file of all the patients seen in the facility, with each patient listed in the index only *once.* In a medical practice, this may be referred to as the **Patient List or Master Patient list.** Each patient then has a second level of information that reflects individual visits to the facility. For instance James Philips has been a patient at Memorial Hospital. He was admitted as an inpatient in January 2010 for appendicitis. He was then seen in the emergency department of the hospital in June of 2010 for a fracture of his right radius. In September he underwent outpatient blood work ordered by his primary care physician. In this instance, James will have one entry in the MPI, but will have three individual encounters attached to his record (one inpatient, two outpatient encounters).

The MPI should be kept permanently, since it is the master list of all patients seen at a particular facility. In the hospital setting, records are filed by **medical record number,** which is a unique number assigned to each individual patient. Should the MPI be destroyed or unavailable for some reason, it would be difficult if not impossible to locate the patient's health record, if using paper records. Though physician's offices typically file alphabetically by the patient's last name, best practice still dictates that a master index (list) of all patients be kept.

In some facilities or offices, the MPI is kept manually. With the move toward an electronic record, an electronic MPI is more the norm. Figure 3.1 is an example of a manual MPI card. Figure 3.2 is

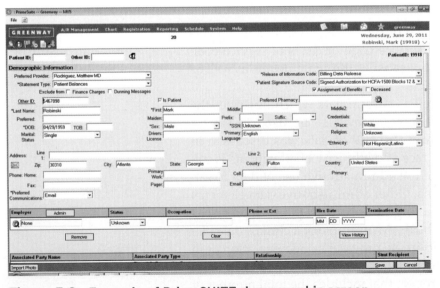

MEMORIAL HOSPITAL 7652 HORIZON WAY ANYWHERE, TX 44555			
Last Name, First Name, Middle Name	DOB	Gender Male Race Caucasian Medical Record Number	
Philips, James Bernard	07/31/1990	07-45-85	
Home Address		Telephone Number	
1234 Oriole Way, Anywhere, TX 44555		555-555-3333	
Previous Name		Social Security Number	
n/a		123-45-6780	
ADM/ENCOUNTER DATE	DISCHARGE DATE	TYPE OF SERVICE	PROVIDER
1/15/2010	1/28/2010	IP	Howard Hinkins, MD
6/22/2010	6/22/2010	ED	Sylvia Crowell, MD
9/30/2010	9/30/2010	OP	Lloyd Wright, Md

Figure 3.1   Master Patient Index (MPI) card

Figure 3.2   Example of PrimeSUITE demographic screen

an example of the equivalent of an MPI entry in PrimeSUITE. Notice that in the electronic version, much more demographic information is collected and stored in this patient's master file than for the patient with the manual MPI card.

3.4 Registering a New Patient in PrimeSUITE

Before any information, administrative or clinical, is entered for a patient, he or she must be registered in the practice management software, which, in turn, populates basic information in the EHR as well. This function is carried out in every healthcare setting.

In a physician's office the registration process is completed by the reception staff. In the hospital setting this is part of the registration process. Some hospitals have a centralized registration department, meaning that regardless of the type of patient (inpatient or outpatient), all registration is done from a central location. Other hospitals have decentralized registration, meaning that there is an admissions department that registers inpatients, an emergency department registration area for emergency patients, a Radiology Department registration area for outpatient radiology patients, and so on. In Exercise 3.1 we will follow a patient through registration in a physician's office.

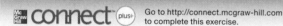

PM **EXERCISE 3.1**

Register a New Patient

In this exercise, we will be registering a new patient, Juan X. Ortega. He has called Greensburg Medical Center, asking if any of the providers were taking new patients. The healthcare professional tells him that Dr. Ingram, a Family Practice physician, is taking new patients and asks if he would like to establish care with Dr. Ingram. Since Mr. Ortega does want to do so, the following steps are completed to register him in the Practice Management and EHR system of Greensburg Medical Center.

From the initial phone call, basic information such as full name, date of birth, address, and telephone number(s) are taken. He tells the healthcare professional that his name is Juan Xavier Ortega. He was born on 07/31/1945. His address is 117 Greenway Blvd., Carrollton, GA 30117, and his phone number is (770) 555-5555.

The healthcare professional will mail Mr. Ortega some paperwork to complete before he arrives for his appointment. Typically, the paperwork includes a form to collect administrative information, a past medical history form, and authorization forms. The administrative information includes information such as address, telephone number, next of kin, insurance information, ethnicity, race, etc. The insurance information is entered as soon as it is available so that verification of insurance can be done (more about insurance verification is in Chapter 6).

For our purposes, we will assume that Mr. Ortega completed the initial paperwork and brought it to the office before the day of his appointment with Dr. Ingram, as noted in Figure 3.3.

(continued)

Greensburg Medical Center
REGISTRATION FORM
(Please Print)

Today's date: *February 12, 2011*   **Care Provider: Dr. Ingram**

PATIENT INFORMATION

Patient's last name:	First:	Middle:	x Mr.	❏ Miss	Marital status (circle one)
Ortega	*Juan*	*Xavier*	❏ Mrs.	❏ Ms.	(Single) / Mar / Div / Sep / Wid

Is this your legal name?	If not, what is your legal name?	(Former name):		Birth date:	Age:	Sex:
☒ Yes ❏ No				*07 / 31 / 1945*	65	☒ M ❏ F

Street address:	Social Security no.:	Home phone no.:
117 Greenway Blvd.		(*770*) *555-5555*

P. O. Box:	City:	State:	ZIP Code:
	Carrollton	*GA*	*30117*

Occupation:	Employer:	Employer phone no.:
Project Manager	*Greenway Medical Tech*	(*770*) *555-6666*

E-mail address: *jxuanortega@greenwaymedical.com*   **Cell phone:** (770) 555-7777

Race: *declined*   **Ethnicity:** *Hispanic*   **Primary language:** *Spanish*   **Religion:** *Catholic*

Other family members seen here:

INSURANCE INFORMATION
(Presentation of Insurance Card is required at time of each visit)

Person responsible for bill:	Birth date:	Address (if different):	Home phone no.:
Juan Ortega	*07 / 31 / 1945*		( )

Is this person a patient here?   ☒ Yes   ❏ No

Occupation:	Employer:	Employer address:	Employer phone no.:
			( )

Is this patient covered by insurance?   ☒ Yes   ❏ No

Please indicate primary insurance	❏ McGraw-Hill Healthmark Insurance	❏ BlueCross/Shield	❏ [Insurance]	❏ [Insurance]	❏ [Insurance]

❏ [Insurance]	❏ Workers' Compensation	❏ Medicare	❏ Medicaid *(Please provide card)*	❏ Other

Subscriber's name:	Subscriber's S.S. no.:	Birth date:	Group no.:	Policy no.:	Co-payment:
Juan Xavier Ortega		*07 / 31 / 1945*	*6500*	*GAR5679009*	$ *20.00*

Patient's relationship to subscriber:	☒ Self	❏ Spouse	❏ Child	❏ Other	Effective Date: *01/06/1999*

Name of secondary insurance (if applicable):	Subscriber's name:	Group no.:	Policy no.:
None			

Patient's relationship to subscriber:	❏ Self	❏ Spouse	❏ Child	❏ Other

IN CASE OF EMERGENCY

Name of local friend or relative (not living at same address):	Relationship to patient:	Home phone no.:	Work phone no.:
		( )	( )

The above information is true to the best of my knowledge. I authorize my insurance benefits be paid directly to the physician. I understand that I am financially responsible for any balance. I also authorize [Name of Practice] or insurance company to release any information required to process my claims.

Patient/Guardian signature   *Date*

Figure 3.3   Juan Ortega registration form

Follow these steps to complete the exercise on your own once you have watched the demonstration and tried the steps with helpful prompts. Use the registration form in Figure 3.3 to complete the steps below.

1. Click **Search for Patient.**
2. The **Last Name** field is filled out. Press the tab key to confirm your entry.
3. The **First Name** field is filled out. Press the tab key to confirm your entry.
4. The **Middle Name** field is filled out. Press the tab key to confirm your entry.
5. Click **Search.**
6. Click **OK.**
7. The **Date Of Birth** field is filled out. Press the tab key to confirm your entry.
8. Click **Sex** drop-down menu.
9. Clicking the entry **Male** selects it.
10. The **Home Phone** field is filled out. Press the tab key to confirm your entry.
11. The **Work Phone** field is filled out. Press the tab key to confirm your entry.
12. Click **Add New.**
13. Click **Yes.**
14. Click **Registration.**
15. Click **Information.**
16. Click **Race** drop-down menu.
17. Clicking the entry **Declined** selects it.
18. Click **Primary Language** drop-down menu.
19. Clicking the entry **Spanish** selects it.
20. Click **Religion** drop-down menu.
21. Clicking the entry **Catholic** selects it.
22. Click **Ethnicity** drop-down menu.
23. Clicking the entry **Hispanic/Latino** selects it.
24. The **Address Line 1** field is filled out. Press the tab key to confirm your entry.
25. The **Zip** field is filled out. Press the tab key to confirm your entry.
26. The **Cell** field is filled out. Press the tab key to confirm your entry.
27. The **Email** field is filled out. Press the tab key to confirm your entry.
28. Click **Preferred Communications** drop-down menu.
29. Clicking the entry **Email** selects it.
30. Clicking the **scroll button** displays the desired screen area.
31. Click **Search Employers.**
32. The **Employer Name** field is filled out. Press the tab key to confirm your entry.
33. Click **Search.**
34. Click **Select.**
35. Click **Status** drop-down menu.
36. Clicking the entry **Full-Time** selects it.
37. The **Occupation** field is filled out. Press the tab key to confirm your entry.
38. Click **Save.**

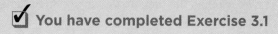 You have completed Exercise 3.1

PrimeSUITE **tip**

Information must be entered in test mode exactly as it appears in the source documentation. For instance, the telephone number must be entered as (770) 555-5555.

PrimeSUITE **tip**

When using practice or test mode, if it is a drop-down field that is to be clicked, click on the arrow to the right of the field.

PrimeSUITE **tip**

When the action is to click on a heading that has a radio button to the left of it, click on the radio button, NOT the words.

In PrimeSUITE, the "Appointment Scheduling" function is used to make the appointment with the provider who has been assigned to that patient. In Juan Ortega's example, he was a new patient, and was assigned to Dr. Ingram.

In an office setting, the healthcare professional will need to know the reason for the visit in order to allot enough time for the visit. For example, a follow-up visit for hypertension is going to take less time than a physical exam. She will also ask for convenient days and times before beginning the search for the appointment. In a hospital setting, outpatient procedures such as CT scans or MRIs are scheduled in advance, and the process is similar.

Appointment scheduling is a very involved process. The time allotted to a patient is dependent on the reason the patient is being seen. A follow-up appointment for a child's ears following an ear infection may be allotted only 15 minutes, whereas a patient who is going to have a complete medical exam may be allotted 30 minutes. Each care provider is set up in the PM system to show their typical schedule. For instance, Dr. Ingram may prefer to start the day at 9:00 a.m., break for lunch from noon to 1 p.m., and end his day at 5:30 p.m. Dr. Rodriguez, on the other hand, may prefer to start seeing patients at 8 a.m., break from seeing patients between 11 and 11:30 a.m. to return phone calls and perform administrative tasks, see patients from 11:30 a.m. until 1:00 p.m., and then break for lunch from 1:00 p.m. until 2:00 p.m. His last appointment of the day is scheduled for 4:30 p.m. In addition, some care providers prefer to do complete physical exams only in the morning. Many offices leave open appointment times for urgent visits. Patients who do not show up for an appointment, or who cancel at the last minute, can wreak havoc on a schedule!

EXERCISE **3.2**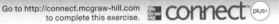

Go to http://connect.mcgraw-hill.com
to complete this exercise.

Schedule an Appointment

Recall that we registered Mr. Ortega in Exercise 3.1, so his name is located in PrimeSUITE's master patient list. The healthcare professional asked Mr. Ortega which day(s) of the week work best for him. He does not have a preference of day, but he would like to be seen soon, so she starts the search beginning with May 10. Since Mr. Ortega is establishing care with this office, the type of visit he will have is a Routine Office Visit (ROV). He will be having a complete exam. By selecting the correct type of visit, the amount of time allotted for that visit is automatically assigned by the system. In this case, it will be a 30-minute appointment. He then states that a morning visit on a Wednesday is best for him, so 9:30 a.m. on May 11th is selected by the healthcare professional. Mr. Ortega also stated that he was having shortness of breath, so that will be entered as his **chief complaint**, which is the reason (in the patient's own words) that he has made the appointment.

Now we will perform the process of scheduling an appointment for Juan Ortega.

Follow these steps to complete the exercise on your own once you have watched the demonstration and tried the steps with helpful prompts.

PrimeSUITE tip

In PrimeSUITE, when the search function is used, the first patient who meets the criteria entered (in this case, the last name Ortega) is highlighted. By clicking anywhere on the line of the patient you are actually looking for, then clicking Select, you will choose the correct person.

1. Click `Search for Patient.
2. Type Ortega in the **Last Name** field. Press the tab key to confirm your entry.
3. Click **Search**.
4. Click on the line with the patient record for Juan Xavier Ortega.
5. Click **Select**.
6. Click **Appointment Scheduling**.
7. Click the check box next to Dr. Ingram's name.
8. Click the check box next to Greensburg Medical Center.
9. The ***From Date** field is filled out. Press the tab key to confirm your entry.
10. Click **View Schedules** near the bottom left corner of the screen.
11. Click the Next Day blue arrow next to the date at the top of the screen.
12. Click the plus sign next to **Routine Office Visit** to open it.
13. Drag the **ROV** icon "New Patient Complete Exam" to the 9:30 a.m. time slot.
14. Click in the **Chief Complaint** field.
15. The **Chief Complaint** field is filled out. Press the tab key to confirm your entry.
16. Click **Save**.

✔ **You have completed Exercise 3.2**

3.6 Editing Demographic Data

People move, their last names change, their emergency contact information changes—just about anything except their first name and date of birth can change at one time or another. It is important that an office always have up-to-date information on a patient.

At the time of check-in, many offices will print out the identification page and have the patient review it either on a yearly basis or even every time a patient is seen. If changes need to be made, the patient communicates them to the office staff, and the information is edited appropriately. To save paper, some offices have a computer terminal where the patient can view the information on the screen, or the healthcare professional may just swivel her screen around for the patient to view and either verify that there are no changes necessary or tell her what information does need to be changed.

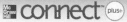 (plus+) Go to http://connect.mcgraw-hill.com to complete this exercise.   **EXERCISE 3.3**

Edit Demographic Information

In this exercise, Mr. Ortega realizes that he has moved since initially completing the registration paperwork; he calls in to the office to give his new address. He tells the healthcare professional that his address is now 2024 Peachtree Parkway, Carrollton, GA 30117

Follow these steps to complete the exercise on your own once you've watched the demonstration and tried the steps with helpful prompts.

(continued)

PrimeSUITE tip

A plus sign (+) next to a menu designates that there are more submenus available for that item. To find them, click on the plus sign.

1. Click **Search for Patient.**
2. The ***Last Name** field is filled out. Press the tab key to confirm your entry.
3. Click **Search.**
4. Click **Xavier.**
5. Click **Select.**
6. Click **Information.**
7. Click **Address Line 1.**
8. The **Space bar** key on the keyboard is now pressed.
9. The **Address Line 1** field is filled out. Press the tab key to confirm your entry.
10. Click **Save.**

✔ **You have completed Exercise 3.3**

PrimeSUITE tip

Default values are used throughout PrimeSUITE. This means that the most common entry in a particular field is already placed in a field when the screen appears. If that information is correct, nothing is done, and the healthcare professional tabs through the field. If the default information for that patient is not correct, then the drop-down menu of choices is searched for the appropriate information. Examples include the Visit Type and Service Location fields.

3.7 Checking in a Patient

One of the advantages of using PM software is the ability to track a patient's flow through the office. The flow starts when the patient checks in. As a patient, you are aware of this part of the process—it is when you either sign your name on a log sheet or verbally inform the healthcare professional that you have arrived. This process is used in a physician's office setting, but would not necessarily have a use in the hospital environment other than in the outpatient registration area.

The typical flow is the following:

Patient checks in at front desk > patient is seen by clinical support team (MA or nurse) > patient is seen by the care provider (physician or physician's assistant or nurse practitioner) > patient stops at the cashier or check-out desk > billing processes begin.

EXERCISE 3.4 **PM**

Go to http://connect.mcgraw-hill.com to complete this exercise.

Check in a Patient Who Has Arrived

In the following demonstration, Juan Ortega has arrived and he has just signed the log, which alerts the healthcare professional that she can check him in for his appointment.

Follow these steps to complete the exercise on your own once you have watched the demonstration and tried the steps with helpful prompts.

1. Click **Ortega, Juan X.**
2. Click **Close.**
3. **Click *Visit Type** drop-down button.
4. Clicking the entry **Routine Office Visit** selects it.
5. Click ***Service Location** drop-down button.
6. Clicking the entry **Greensburg Medical Center** selects it.
7. Click **Check-In.**

✔ **You have completed Exercise 3.4**

Although a medical practice or hospital is in business to care for patients, in the end, it is also just that—a business. In order to stay financially viable, there must be organized, effective policies and procedures in place to ensure cash flow and fiscal success.

You will learn about the intricacies of setting up fee schedules, billing insurance plans, and collection procedures in another course. In this exercise, though, you will learn about the information that must be collected for any patients who have private group insurance or who participate in a government health plan.

Figure 3.4 is a sample insurance card. This card should be presented each time a patient arrives for an encounter. An office may scan the front and back of the card as an image that will reside in PrimeSUITE, or they may photocopy the front and back of the card and keep it in the patient's chart.

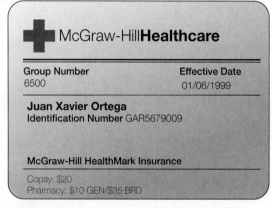

The information must be entered in PrimeSUITE exactly as it appears on the insurance card. For instance, say Juan Xavier Ortega does not use his first name; instead he uses J. Xavier Ortega. But his insurance card reads Juan Xavier Ortega. In PrimeSUITE, or any other PM software, he should be entered as Juan Xavier Ortega.

Figure 3.4 Sample insurance card

Any typographical errors within PrimeSUITE will result in a delayed or denied claim. That will slow payment, which is not good business practice for the office!

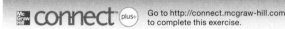 Go to http://connect.mcgraw-hill.com to complete this exercise.   **EXERCISE** **3.5**

Capture Insurance Information of a Patient

In the exercise that follows, Mr. Ortega has presented his insurance card to the healthcare professional and he has completed the insurance information on his registration form (Figure 3.3). Mr. Ortega only has coverage through one insurance company, so that is the **primary insurance** (the first insurance that is billed).

Follow these steps to complete the exercise on your own once you have watched the demonstration and tried the steps with helpful prompts.

1. Click **Priority** drop-down menu.
2. Clicking the entry **Primary** selects it.
3. Click: **Click here to search for a plan.**
4. Click **Insurance Co** drop-down menu.
5. **m** is now pressed.
6. Click **scroll button.**
7. Click **McGraw-Hill HealthMark Insurance.**
8. Click **Search.**
9. Click **Select.**
10. **Tab** is now pressed to advance to the policy holder field.
11. **Tab** is now pressed to advance to the policy number field.

(continued)

12. The **Policy Number** field is filled out. Press the tab key to confirm your entry.
13. The **Group Number** field is filled out. Press the tab key to confirm your entry.
14. The **Effective Date** field is filled out. Press the tab key to confirm your entry.
15. **Tab** is now pressed again to advance to the verification date field.
16. **t** is now pressed.
17. Click **Save.**
18. Click **View/Edit Patient Flags.**
19. Click **Co-pay $20.**
20. Click **Save.**

☑ **You have completed Exercise 3.5**

3.9 Utilize the Help Feature

The "HELP" feature is a staple of almost any computer software program. What is important is that you *use* the Help feature when you need to. For many of us, it is easier to ask someone how to perform a particular function than to search for the solution ourselves. The problem is—the person you are asking may give you the incorrect answer, or you may be in a position where you need an answer fast and there is no one around to ask. It shows initiative and will also help you to remember the steps more easily if you seek out the answer on your own. Consider this analogy—you remember how to get to a particular destination when you have driven there yourself rather than as a passenger, correct? The same applies here. You will remember and *understand* the process if you look up the steps on your own.

Selecting the Help feature will connect you to the PrimeSUITE User's Manual. Features you may typically use are:

- Getting Started and navigating PrimeSUITE Help
- PrimeSUITE Topics

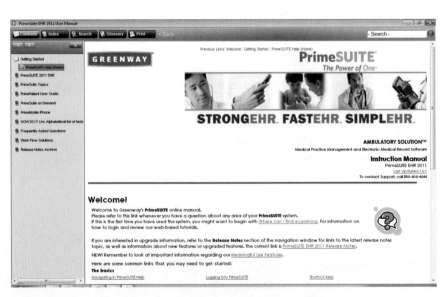

Figure 3.5 Help feature, PrimeSUITE user's manual

- Frequently Asked Questions
- Work Flow Solutions

Also readily available in PrimeSUITE Help is material that speaks to the newest upgrades in functionality, and also a listing of what Greenway has determined to be the most frequently asked questions about topics (see Figure 3.5).

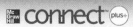 Go to http://connect.mcgraw-hill.com to complete this exercise.   **EXERCISE 3.6**

Use the Help Feature

In this scenario you are fairly new to Greensburg Medical Center, but you have been there for several weeks and you are comfortable using Prime-SUITE. You would like to make the process easier, and one of your coworkers has told you about using **Shortcut Keys** (keys that link directly to a function rather than choosing it from a menu). She has told you about some of the more common ones, but you would like to know more, so you go to PrimeSUITE Help for more guidance.

Follow these steps to complete the exercise on your own once you have watched the demonstration and tried the steps with helpful prompts.

1. Click **PrimeSUITE Help.**
2. Click **Shortcut Keys.**

 You have completed Exercise 3.6

chapter 3 **summary**

LEARNING OUTCOME	CONCEPTS FOR REVIEW
3.1 Identify administrative data elements. Pages 44–46	– Demographic data is identifying data – Administrative data includes demographic data as well as additional non-clinical data – A data dictionary is necessary to assure consistency and reliability of data – CMS-1500, UB-04, and HIPAA regulations dictate much of the administrative data captured

3.2 Explain the administrative uses of data. Pages 46–48	– Insurance purposes (file claims)
	– Satisfy regulatory requirements and meaningful use
	– Five sections of the claim form
	  • Provider
	  • Subscriber
	  • Payer
	  • Claim detail
	  • Services

3.3 Explain the use of the Master Patient (person) Index (MPI). Pages 48–49	– A means of tracking that a patient was seen in a healthcare facility – Only one entry per patient • Each encounter has its own entry, filed under the patient's master entry – Medical record (chart) number is unique to each patient—links the patient to his/her health record – Can be manual or electronic – Is kept permanently
3.4 Apply procedures to register a new patient in PrimeSUITE. Pages 49–51	– Patient must have an entry in the Master Patient Index or patient list before any other functions can occur (scheduling, patient's chart, etc.) – Registration process occurs in every healthcare setting – Registration process ultimately results in the patient being a part of the MPI – In the physician office setting this is done by a healthcare professional – In hospital setting this is done by a registration department
3.5 Apply procedures to schedule a patient's appointment in PrimeSUITE. Pages 52–53	– Before scheduling an appointment, a provider has to be assigned, if a new patient, or select the patient's usual provider – Must know the reason for the visit in order to allot sufficient time for the visit – Select a date and time that works for the patient
3.6 Apply procedures to edit demographic information in PrimeSUITE. Pages 53–54	– All information about a patient must be current and correct – Verification of demographic and administrative information is done by administrative personnel at the time a patient checks in – Information is edited, added, or deleted as appropriate

Copyright © 2012 The McGraw-Hill Companies

http://connect.mcgraw-hill.com

LEARNING OUTCOME	CONCEPTS FOR REVIEW
3.7 Follow the steps performed upon patient check in. Page 54	– Knowing where the patient is in the flow through the office is important to maintain efficiency – Typical flow: • Patient checks in at reception desk • Patient is called back to the exam room by the healthcare professional • Patient is seen and examined by the provider • Patient checks out • Claim process begins
3.8 Apply procedures to capture insurance information in PrimeSUITE. Pages 55–56	– Capturing complete, correct insurance information is vital to cash flow and financial success – Require patients to present their insurance card on every visit – Information in the practice management system must match what is on the insurance card
3.9 Locate the Help feature in PrimeSUITE. Pages 56–57	– Help feature is available in any software – User's Manual Includes: • Getting Started and navigating PrimeSUITE Help • PrimeSUITE Topics • Frequently Asked Questions • Work Flow Solutions

chapter **review**

MATCHING QUESTIONS

Match the terms on the left with the definitions on the right.

_____ 1. **[LO 3.5]** chief complaint

_____ 2. **[LO 3.2]** ICD-9-CM

_____ 3. **[LO 3.7]** check-in

_____ 4. **[LO 3.1]** administrative data

_____ 5. **[LO 3.4]** registration

_____ 6. **[LO 3.3]** medical record number

_____ 7. **[LO 3.8]** policy number

_____ 8. **[LO 3.9]** Frequently Asked Questions

_____ 9. **[LO 3.2]** policyholder

_____ 10. **[LO 3.1]** data dictionary

a. information, such as a patient's gender and date of birth, that is required to be collected under HIPAA

b. list of correct definitions for a facility's unique terms and jargon

c. administrative task that begins patient flow

d. primary person who is covered by an insurance policy and whose name is on an insurance card

e. found on a patient's insurance card,

f. unique identifier assigned to an individual patient

g. reason for a patient's appointment; may determine the length of an exam visit

h. process of entering a new patient into the Master Index

i. feature of the PrimeSUITE Help section that helps users locate information

j. comprehensive listing of national diagnosis codes

MULTIPLE-CHOICE QUESTIONS

Select the letter that best completes the statement or answers the question:

1. **[LO 3.1]** _____ data includes demographic data.
   a. Useful
   b. HIPAA
   c. Administrative
   d. Patient

2. **[LO 3.3]** Anna Jacobs presented to the ER of County Hospital three times in the past year. She will appear in County's MPI:
   a. once.
   b. twice.
   c. three times.
   d. four times.

3. **[LO 3.1]** Which of the following is NOT an example of demographic data?
   a. Full name
   b. Primary physician
   c. Social security number
   d. Date of birth

4. **[LO 3.2]** Administrative data is used to satisfy _____ requirements.
   a. CCHIP
   b. HITECH
   c. HIPAA
   d. ONC

5. **[LO 3.4]** Before a patient can be treated at a healthcare setting, she must be:
   a. prepped.
   b. registered.
   c. logged.
   d. admitted.

6. **[LO 3.3]** How many years should a facility's Master Patient Index be kept?
   a. three
   b. five
   c. seven
   d. permanently

7. **[LO 3.1]** Recording a patient's previous or married name might help with:
   a. cross-referencing data.
   b. compiling family history.
   c. legal proceedings.
   d. Privacy Rule compliance.

8. **[LO 3.9]** One of the common Help features is:
   a. Work Flow Help.
   b. Quick Start Guide.
   c. Frequently Asked Questions.
   d. Topical Outline.

9. **[LO 3.4]** _____ is part of a patient's administrative information found on a registration form.
   a. Occupation
   b. Chief complaint
   c. Provider number
   d. Co-pay amount

10. **[LO 3.1]** Patient demographic information should be verified:
    a. at initial visit.
    b. at each visit.
    c. once a year.
    d. when patient initiates a change.

connect (plus+) Enhance your learning by completing these exercises and more at http://connect.mcgraw-hill.com!

11. **[LO 3.8]** An insurance claim may be denied if the receptionist fails to:
    a. collect a patient's co-pay.
    b. make a copy of the patient's insurance card.
    c. enter all data correctly.
    d. have the patient sign the front-desk log.

12. **[LO 3.5]** _____ is part of the appointment scheduling feature of PrimeSUITE.
    a. Occupation
    b. Chief complaint
    c. Provider number
    d. Co-pay amount

13. **[LO 3.3]** A Master Patient Index can be kept:
    a. electronically.
    b. manually.
    c. both are acceptable
    d. neither are acceptable

14. **[LO 3.2]** A facility's collection of patient data might be used to satisfy _____ requirements.
    a. data dictionary
    b. meaningful use
    c. incentive
    d. interoperability

15. **[LO 3.6]** Editing a patient's mailing address is accomplished by using:
    a. drop-down menus.
    b. free-text fields.
    c. Help topics.
    d. patient flags.

16. **[LO 3.3]** In a hospital's health information department, patient records are most often filed by:
    a. patient's last name.
    b. number of patient encounters.
    c. provider identification number.
    d. medical record number.

17. **[LO 3.7]** Patient check-in is the _____ part of patient flow.
    a. first
    b. second
    c. last
    d. least important

18. **[LO 3.2]** Information such as a policyholder name and insurance plan name appear in the _____ section of a claim form.
    a. payer
    b. provider
    c. services
    d. subscriber

http://connect.mcgraw-hill.com

SHORT ANSWER QUESTIONS

1. **[LO 3.3]** What is another name for the Master Patient Index?

2. **[LO 3.4]** What is the difference between centralized and decentralized registration centers in a hospital setting?

3. **[LO 3.8]** What is a co-pay?

4. **[LO 3.6]** List at least three ways that an office can obtain updated patient information.

5. **[LO 3.1]** Why is it important that every staff member in a facility uses terminology _____?

6. **[LO 3.9]** List the four most commonly used features of PrimeSUITE's Help feature.

7. **[LO 3.5]** Explain why the receptionist needs to ask for the reason for a patient visit when scheduling an appointment.

8. **[LO 3.2]** The CMS-1500 form is used to submit claims for _____ encounters while the UB-04 form is used to submit _____ claims.

9. **[LO 3.6]** Discuss the importance of reliable, up-to-date patient information.

10. **[LO 3.9]** Discuss why being able to use PrimeSUITE's Help feature is so important.

11. **[LO 3.1]** List at least five required pieces of demographic information collected for each patient.

12. **[LO 3.7]** In PrimeSUITE, the Visit Type field is a _____.

13. **[LO 3.3]** What is a medical record number?

14. **[LO 3.2]** List the five major sections on a standard claim form.

15. **[LO 3.4]** A patient may _____ to provide certain optional pieces of information if they feel uncomfortable.

16. **[LO 3.8]** List at least three things typically found on a patient's insurance card.

APPLYING YOUR KNOWLEDGE

1. **[LOs 3.4, 3.5, 3.6, 3.7, 3.8, 3.9]** Which of the PrimeSUITE exercises completed in this chapter do you think will be used most often in the office setting? Explain your answer.

2. **[LOs 3.1, 3.2, 3.6]** As the receptionist for Greenway Clinic, you recently mailed an informational letter to all patients listed in your MPI. One morning you come into work and see Juan Ortega's letter marked "Return to Sender, Address Unknown" sitting on your desk. What do you do?

3. **[LOs 3.1, 3.2]** Discuss why administrative data such as race, ethnicity, and preferred language might need to be reported to satisfy meaningful use requirements.

4. **[LO 3.3]** The text mentions that if a MPI was inaccessible or unavailable for any reason, it would be nearly impossible to locate a patient's record. With the reality of

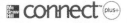 Enhance your learning by completing these exercises and more at http://connect.mcgraw-hill.com!

computer system freezes and crashes, would this not be an argument against maintaining an electronic MPI? Explain your answer.

5. **[LOs 3.1, 3.2, 3.3]** One of your colleagues has been asked to update the office's data dictionary. She remarks that she does not see why having the data dictionary is so important, because most terms are easily understood by most people in the office. How would you explain to her, with examples, the importance of a solid data dictionary for your practice?

6. **[LOs 3.4, 3.5, 3.6, 3.7]** Discuss the advantages of using a practice management tool such as PrimeSUITE to complete tasks such as patient registration and appointment scheduling.

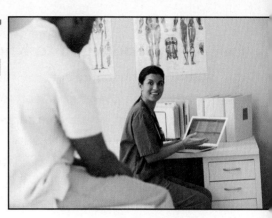

chapter **four**

Content of the Health Record—the Past Medical, Surgical, Family, and Social History

Learning Outcomes

At the end of this chapter, the student should be able to:

4.1 Outline the use of forms as data collection tools.

4.2 Execute a step-by-step procedure to document past medical, surgical, family, and social histories in PrimeSUITE.

4.3 Examine the necessity of properly documenting and correcting inconsistent or unclear information.

4.4 Apply procedures to document vital signs in PrimeSUITE.

Key Terms

Chief complaint
History of present illness
Past family history
Past medical history

Past surgical history
Review of systems
Social history
Vital signs

Copyright © 2012 The McGraw-Hill Companies

65

What You Need to Know and Why You Need to Know It

Before patients are seen by the care provider, they first meet with the healthcare professional to go over the reason for the visit and to capture historical information about their health status. In this chapter we will cover the types of history collected. We will also cover *why* knowing this information is so important in the care of the patient. As with all documentation in a health record, the history must be accurate because often the past history plays a part in the diagnosis and treatment of the current condition. The history generally begins with the **history of present illness (HPI)**, which is documented in the patient's (or legal representative's) own words. It is in the HPI that the patient relates what is wrong, how long it has been present, and whether he has been taking any medications to relieve the symptoms (and did the symptoms improve), etc. As mentioned earlier, either the history is taken from a form that the patient or legal representative completes or it is taken verbally. Most of the time, both the form and a conversation with the patient are needed to accurately capture the patient's history.

4.1 Forms as Data Collection Tools

Take a moment to think of forms that you have completed recently. Most likely they were on paper, and you can probably think immediately of one that was long, cumbersome, and took quite a bit of thought to complete. You can also think of one or two that were organized well, easy to complete, and seemed rather logical. The same goes for forms that are on screen rather than on paper. When we speak of paper forms, we refer to "boxes" that we are filling out. On screen, we often refer to each item of data as a field rather than a box. For our purposes, we will refer to each piece of data on a form as a field. In most healthcare settings, at this point in time, much of the information gathered from a patient will continue to be done through use of a paper form, and then that information will be transferred to the patient's EHR. Thus, it is important that the design of the paper forms be logical to minimize the amount of time it takes to transfer the information and to minimize the likelihood of having missing or incorrect information end up in the EHR. As the transition to an electronic record progresses, patients will increasingly complete the forms electronically, though paper forms will not disappear completely since there will always be patients who do not want to complete the forms electronically due to lack of a computer, lack of computer literacy, or privacy concerns.

When designing a form, keep in mind the following:

- Name the form—give it a title that correlates to the information gathered on the form.

- Each page of a multipage form should include the patient's name and the medical record number or chart number to guard against mixing up the records of patients with the same or similar names and to guard against documentation errors in general.

- The information collected should be relevant to the purpose of the form. Only information that is necessary should be collected—a medical history form in a dermatologist's office will probably not include the patient's menstrual history, for example. If that information were needed for some reason, it could still be added elsewhere in the patient's record.

- Related information should be adjacent—for instance the street address, city, and ZIP code of a patient's address would be located adjacent to one another on the form.

- Clearly mark the field names (also called labels) by use of bolding, colored font, or italics.

- Separate the form into sections, if it is a lengthy form.

- Completion of the form should be easy for the person completing it; in other words it should be obvious whether the answer to each field should be written on the same line as the field heading or needs to go in the line below.

- Each piece of information should be requested only once on a given form.

- Provide sufficient space for the answer to each field.

- Typically, do not duplicate questions that are answered on other forms; an exception to this would be medication allergies—this question is often asked on more than one form due to the importance of the information. It may slip a patient's mind when completing a form at home but he or she will recall the allergy later in the interview process.

Following the guidelines above will make it easy for the patient to fill out the form. A thoroughly completed form will benefit the care provider as well. Care providers need complete, accurate information quickly, and so proper development of data collection tools—whether on paper or on screen—should be an important task in any healthcare setting.

The registration form used in Chapter 3 is an example of a form that has individual fields in block format. The medical history form in Figure 4.1 is an example of one that has a more free-form format rather than individual fields.

As noted earlier, though forms do exist today, many "paperless" offices are requesting their patients to complete their history form online. Think of the last time you applied for a job or when you applied to the college you are attending. Most likely you did so online rather than with a paper application. The rules noted above about ease of completion apply to online forms as well as paper forms. You have no doubt experienced the frustration of completing a confusing, lengthy form online! In Chapter 10, when we discuss coming trends, we will discuss this subject in more detail.

for your information **fyi**

In some offices, the registration form and the history form are one document rather than individual documents.

Page 1

GREENSBURG MEDICAL CENTER   MEDICAL HISTORY FORM

PATIENT NAME	DOB	MEDICAL RECORD NUMBER

PLEASE ANSWER THE FOLLOWING QUESTIONS THOROUGHLY. IF A QUESTION DOESN'T APPLY, PLEASE ENTER N/A OR PLACE A LINE IN THAT AREA.

PRESENT MEDICAL CONDITION (*why are you being seen today*)

_____

_____

_____

ALLERGIES/REACTIONS TO MEDICINES/FOODS:

NAME OF MEDICATION/AGENT		TYPE OF REACTION

MEDICATIONS: Enter all prescription _and_ non-prescription medicines, herbal remedies, vitamins, or birth control medications here:

MEDICATION	DOSE	HOW OFTEN?	TAKEN FOR?

PERSONAL MEDICAL HISTORY: Please check all conditions you have had (with approximate date or year)

Heart Disease ____ _____   Cancer ____ _____   Type _____

Heart Attack ____ _____   Diabetes ____ _____   Type _____

Hypertension ____ _____   Thyroid ____ _____   Type _____

Stroke ____ _____   Bleeding Disorder ___ _____   Type _____

High cholesterol _____ _____   Other ___ _____

Depression/Suicide Attempt ___ _____   Other ___ _____

Alcoholism _____   Other _____

1

Page 2

Patient Name _____ DOB _____ Med. Record Number _____

SURGICAL HISTORY: Please indicate all procedures or surgeries you have had (with approximate date or year)

Type of surgery	Date (year)	Name of surgeon

FAMILY HISTORY: Please place a check under the family member who has had any of the conditions:

CONDITION	Mo	Dad	Sib.	Child	Other	CONDITION	Mom	Dad	Sibling	Child	Other
Alcoholism						Environmental allergies					
Anemia						Loss of hearing					
Anesthesia problem						Heart problems (heart attack, coronary artery disease, congestive heart failure)					
Arthritis						Hypertension					
Asthma						High cholesterol					
Bleeding problem						Mitral valve disorders					
Cancer, breast						Lupus					
Cancer, colon						HIV/AIDS					
Cancer, melanoma/basal cell						Kidney disease					
Cancer, ovarian						Mental health disorders					
Cancer, prostate						Migraine headaches					
Cancer, other						Osteoarthritis					
Depression						Rheumatoid arthritis					
Type I Diabetes						CVA (stroke)					
Type II Diabetes						Cerebral hemorrhage					
Eczema						Thyroid disorder					
Seizure disorder or epilepsy						Other					
Glaucoma						Other					

IMMUNIZATION HISTORY: Please indicate date (or best guess) of last immunization for:

Hepatitis A _____ Hepatitis B _____ Measles _____ Mumps _____ Rubella _____ Pneumovax (pneumonia) _____

Tetanus (Td) _____ MMR _____ Chicken pox _____ Flu _____ Other _____

SOCIAL HISTORY

Tobacco Use

Cigarettes (current use) ☐ yes ☐ no If yes, packs per day _____ for _____ years

Cigarettes (past use) ☐ yes ☐ no If yes, no. of years _____; quit when? _____

2

Page 3

Other current tobacco use: ☐ snuff/chew ☐ pipe ☐ cigar

Other past tobacco use: ☐ snuff/chew ☐ pipe ☐ cigar

Alcohol Use

Do you drink alcohol? ☐ yes ☐ no If yes, no. of drinks per week _____

Recreational Drug Use

Do you use any recreational drugs? ☐ yes ☐ no If yes, what and how often? _____

_____

Physical Activity

How often do you exercise? _____ times/week

Are you relatively active (engage in recreational sports, take stairs daily, job involves standing, walking often, etc). ☐ yes ☐ no

SOCIOECONOMIC HISTORY

Occupation _____ Student status ☐ Full time ☐ Part time

Education Completed : ☐ High School graduate ☐ College graduate ☐ Graduate School

Marital Status ☐ Single ☐ Married ☐ Separated ☐ Divorced ☐ Widowed

REVIEW OF SYSTEMS Answer the following questions for any _current_ problems you are experiencing:

Constitutional: Are you experiencing?

___ Fever/chills/nigh-sweats   ___ Tiredness/weakness

___ Unexpected weight gain/loss   ___ Excessive thirst or urination

___ Tiredness/weakness   ___ Difficulty falling or staying asleep

Eyes, Ears, Nose, Throat and Mouth   *Skin*

____ Change in vision   ___ Rash

____ Difficulty hearing/ringing in ears   ___ Change in moles

____ Teeth/gum problems

____ Hay fever or allergies

Cardiovascular   *Respiratory*

___ Chest pain or discomfort   ___ Cough/wheeze

3

Page 4

___ Leg pain during exercise   ___ Difficulty breathing/shortness of breath

___ Palpitations (racing heart)

Gastrointestinal   *Genitourinary*

___ Abdominal pain   ___ Frequent urination during night

___ Blood in stool   ___ Leaking urine

___ Nausea/vomiting/diarrhea   ___ Vaginal bleeding (not related to period)

Musculoskeletal   ___ Discharge from penis

___ Muscle/joint pain   *Breasts*

Neurological   ___ lump or discharge

___ Headaches   *Psychiatric*

___ Dizziness/light-headed   ___ Anxiety/stress

___ Numbness   ___ Depression

___ Memory Loss   *Blood/Lymphatic*

___ Lumps

___ Easily bruises/bleeding

Is there anything you want the doctor to address with you today? _____

_____

WOMEN'S HEALTH HISTORY

No. pregnancies _____ No. deliveries _____ No. abortions _____ No. miscarriages _____

Date of last menstrual period _____ Frequency of periods _____ Length _____

_____   _____

Patient's Signature   Date

FOR INTERNAL USE ONLY (ENTER DATE REVIEWED AND INITIALS) ANY CHANGES, ADDITIONS, DELETIONS SHOULD BE DOCUMENTED ABOVE, DATED AND INITIALED.

4

Figure 4.1   Medical history form

A patient's **past medical history** often contains information that is pertinent to his current health status. It is important that the care provider be aware of the patient's past medical history, which includes:

- Medical conditions (past and current) for which the patient has been treated or which he or she is experiencing
- Date of onset and date resolved for each
- Known allergies (particularly to medications) as well as the actual reaction
- Immunization status, particularly in children
- Current list of medications, including name, dosage, frequency, and reason it is being taken
- A **review of systems (ROS)**, that is, a body system inventory of symptoms he or she may be having

Many offices include the patient's current condition on the history form, or the particulars of the current condition may be documented in the progress note for the visit. The information about the current condition includes:

- **Chief complaint** (the reason the patient is being seen that day; generally speaking, the reason he made the appointment)
- History of present illness: location of the condition (for example, pain in the right shoulder); type of pain (ache, sharp pain, etc.); severity (mild, severe); duration (how long the complaint has been present); and any associated signs and symptoms (for example, difficult to raise arm above head when pain is present)

The **past surgical history** includes information about procedures the patient has undergone. If a patient, Carolyn Wright, is experiencing right lower quadrant pain, yet her history shows she had an appendectomy 14 years ago, the care provider will concentrate diagnostic testing for other possibilities. Past surgical history includes:

- Name of operation or procedure
- Date that the procedure was performed (may be approximate)
- Name of surgeon who performed the procedure
- Anesthesia reactions or complications, if any

The **past family history** includes information that will alert the care provider to any conditions that may affect the patient's overall health now or in the future. For example, Neil Alexander is a 45-year-old patient who has been experiencing chest pains and shortness of breath. He notes that his father and paternal grandfather both had a myocardial infarction (heart attack) before the age of 50. In this case, that information is important to the care provider in order to make diagnostic and treatment decisions for the patient. Past family history includes:

- Name of condition(s)
- Family member(s) who had the condition(s)

- Sometimes, whether immediate family members (parent, sibling) are still alive and, if not, the date/cause of death

The **social history** is important because the care provider needs to know the patient's habits in order to assess possible causes of conditions or potential health concerns that could arise as a result of the habits or the lifestyle of a patient. An example would be a patient who is overweight, works in a sedentary job, and has noted that she does not exercise or participate in any other strenuous activity. That patient would be at risk for heart disease, stroke, and other serious medical conditions. Elements of a social history include:

- Smoking history – past or current use
- Other tobacco use (snuff, pipe, cigar, for example)
- Alcohol use – current or past
- Recreational drug use
- Socioeconomic data – occupation, education, marital status
- Sexual activity and use of protection
- Exercise and physical activity

 EXERCISE 4.1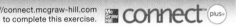

Go to http://connect.mcgraw-hill.com to complete this exercise.

Enter a Patient's Past Medical History

In this exercise, we will be following the past medical history of a patient, Nancy Evans. She has arrived and checked in for her appointment with Dr. Rodriguez at Greensburg Medical Center. The healthcare professional has called Mrs. Evans back to the exam room for the initial portion of the visit. Mr. Evans has accompanied the patient to the appointment, and is in the exam room as well. The healthcare professional begins by accessing Nancy Evans' Facesheet screen in PrimeSUITE as noted in Figure 4.2.

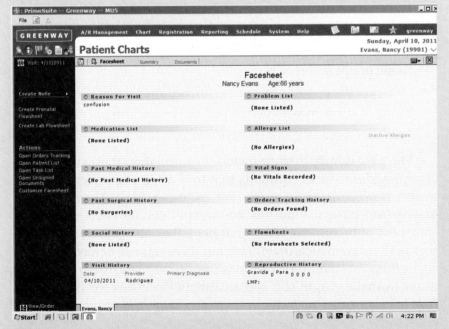

Figure 4.2 Nancy Evans' Facesheet

The reason for the visit, confusion, already appears on the screen because that information was collected at the time the appointment was made. The healthcare professional will verify that information, and change it if necessary before going on to the Past Medical History. In our scenario, that information is correct. The reason for the visit is also known as the chief complaint and it is the reason, as noted by the patient, that an appointment was made with the care provider.

The healthcare professional clicks on the Past Medical History screen from the Facesheet.

Though a medical history form had been completed last year, the healthcare professional asks Mrs. Evans about any other conditions she has. Mrs. Evans and her husband confirm that she has osteoporosis and osteoarthritis, but no other medical conditions. The healthcare professional asks about any previous surgeries. Mr. Evans responds that she had an appendectomy back in 1971 and she had a cataract removed from her right eye in 2007. They are the only surgical procedures Mrs. Evans has had, but she does have one child, so the healthcare professional asks Mrs. Evans about her reproductive history. Mrs. Evans says that she was pregnant once and has one child. The pregnancy was a full-term pregnancy.

Follow these steps to complete the exercise on your own once you have watched the demonstration and tried the steps with helpful prompts. Use the information provided in the scenario above to complete the information.

1. Click **Past Medical History.**
2. Click **Osteoarthritis.**
3. Click **Osteoporosis.**
4. Click **PSHx.**
5. Click **Appendectomy.**
6. Click **details.**
7. The **Procedure Date** field is filled out. Press the tab key to confirm your entry.
8. Click **OK.**
9. Click **Cataract removal.**
10. Click **details.**
11. The **Procedure Date** field is filled out. Press the tab key to confirm your entry.
12. Click **Notes.**
13. The **Notes** field is filled out. Press the tab key to confirm your entry.
14. Click **OK.**
15. Click **RHx.**
16. Click **Total Preg.**
17. The **space bar** is now pressed on the keyboard.
18. **1** is now pressed.
19. Click **Full Term 0.**
20. The **space bar** is now pressed on the keyboard.
21. **1** is now pressed.
22. Click the x in the upper right corner of the reproductive history screen to close it.

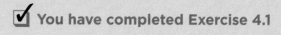 **You have completed Exercise 4.1**

Go to http://connect.mcgraw-hill.com
to complete this exercise.

Enter a Patient's List of Current Medications

In this exercise the patient's current medications are entered. Part of the functionality of PrimeSUITE is the differentiation between those medications prescribed by Greensburg Medical Center and to those that were prescribed by another provider or are bought over the counter.

This process begins by accessing Mrs. Evans' Facesheet in PrimeSUITE and then selecting **Medication List** (see Figure 4.2, on page 70). Mrs. Evans shares with the healthcare professional that she takes ibuprofen for her osteoarthritis. She takes 800 mg tablets, 3 times a day. She also takes glucosamine chondroitin every day. These are tablets as well, and she takes the 750-600 mg tablets. She is also taking alendronate, which is a drug for post-menopausal osteoporosis prevention. These are taken in tablet form as well, 35 mg one time a week.

Follow these steps to complete the exercise on your own once you have watched the demonstration and tried the steps with helpful prompts. Use the information provided in the scenario above to complete the information.

1. Click **Medication List.**
2. Click **Record Medication** in the *Outside Prescribed Medication* section.
3. The **Medication Name** field is filled out. Press the tab key to confirm your entry.
4. Click **ibuprofen.**
5. Click **Osteoarthritis.**
6. Click **Oral.**
7. Click **800 mg Oral Tablet.**
8. Click **OK.**
9. Click **Sig** and select the appropriate option.
10. Click **OK.**
11. Click **Record Medication** in the *Outside Prescribed Medication* section.
12. The **Medication Name** field is filled out. Press the tab key to confirm your entry.
13. Click **glucosamine-chondroitin.**
14. Click **750-600 mg Oral Tablet.**
15. **2** is now pressed.
16. Click on the line to the left of the yellow sticky note to **Modify the frequency.**
17. Click **QD.**
18. Click **Done.**
19. Click **Add Another.**
20. The **Medication Name** field is filled out. Press the tab key to confirm your entry.
21. Click **alendronate.**
22. Click **Post-Menopausal Osteoporosis Prevention.**
23. Click **35 mg Oral Tablet.**
24. Click **OK.**
25. Click **Save.**

✓ **You have completed Exercise 4.2**

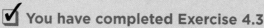

Enter a Patient's Known Drug Allergies

Mrs. Evans has an allergy to amoxicillin. Knowing the patient's medication allergies is a very important piece of information. Not knowing her allergies, and prescribing a drug that she is allergic to could cause a very serious reaction. Her allergy to amoxicillin will be documented in the Allergies List section of the Facesheet (see Figure 4.2).

Follow these steps to complete the exercise on your own once you have watched the demonstration and tried the steps with helpful prompts. Use the information provided in the scenario above to complete the information.

1. Click **Allergy List.**
2. Click **Add.**
3. The **Allergen** field is filled out with **amox.** Press the tab key to confirm your entry.
4. Clicking the entry **amoxicillin** selects it.
5. Click **OK.**
6. Click **amoxicillin.**
7. Click the small "x" in the top right corner to close the allergy list screen.

☑ **You have completed Exercise 4.3**

4.3 Handling Inconsistent or Unclear Information

As we discussed earlier, a patient's history is gathered by use of a form as well as through an interview with the patient. Sometimes, what a patient has documented on the history form is contradictory to what comes out during the interview. When entering any information about a patient, for instance if you are reviewing a past medical history with the patient, and you see on the past medical history form that the patient had an appendectomy in 1997 yet she tells you verbally that she has never had any surgeries, you need to question the patient to determine the correct answer. Though the patient completed the form, she could have checked the wrong box on the form, or she may have forgotten that she had the surgery. Sometimes, patients choose not to tell the healthcare professional or care provider all of the facts. Often, the healthcare professional senses the fact that the patient is being evasive or is only partly answering questions. It is part of the healthcare professional's role to act in such a way that instills trust; communicating *why* these questions are being asked is often all that is needed for a patient to become more comfortable. The fact that there is a discrepancy (or that there is information missing) should never be ignored, and should be documented. The medical practice or hospital must have written policies on how to handle such situations.

An example of a policy statement regarding inconsistent information is: *In the event that an error or inconsistency is found in a health record or in the information given verbally by a patient/legal representative,* an attempt should be made to verify the information and document same. The circumstances surrounding the discrepancy should be documented sufficiently in the health record to explain the situation thoroughly.

PrimeSUITE, as in other EHR software, has built-in mechanisms to amend, delete, or add documentation. Though a change to documentation may occur, the original version of the documentation is always retrievable. In the example given above regarding the discrepancy about the patient's surgery, the explanation of the discrepancy can be documented in a details box that is found in the past surgical history section of the record. Later in this worktext, we will further examine correcting and amending entries and will test your knowledge through PrimeSUITE exercises.

4.4 Documenting Vital Signs

The patient's **vital signs** are taken by the healthcare professional—some offices take them before completing the history and others take them after. PrimeSUITE software includes a very helpful feature—the ability to see a patient's vital signs over time The tracking of the vital signs can be seen in graph form or chronologically. This will help the provider assess such conditions as hypertension or significant weight gain (or loss).

Like the history documentation, entering the vital signs is done from the vital signs section of the Facesheet.

The vital signs include the patient's blood pressure, heart rate, respiratory rate, temperature, height, weight, body mass index (BMI), and oxygen saturation. Technically, height and weight are not vital signs, but both are taken around the same time as the vital signs and are therefore included in that section of the record.

 EXERCISE 4.4 (EHR)

Go to http://connect.mcgraw-hill.com to complete this exercise.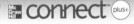

Enter a Patient's Vital Signs

PrimeSUITE allows documentation of the position the patient is in when the blood pressure is taken. The positions include sitting, standing, or lying down.

In our example, the healthcare professional is in the process of taking Nancy Evans' vital signs. She asks Nancy to sit on the exam table and takes her blood pressure. The reading is 110/65. Her heart rate is 68 beats per minute (bpm) and regular, with a respiratory rate of 22. Mrs. Evans' temperature is 97.6 F. Her weight was taken before coming into the exam room, and she weighed 135 pounds. She is 5 feet 2 inches (62 inches) tall. Her oxygen saturation today is 99%.

Follow these steps to complete the exercise on your own once you have watched the demonstration and tried the steps with helpful prompts. Use the information provided in the scenario above to complete the information.

1. Click **Vital Signs.**
2. Click **Add New Vitals.**

 for your information

The body mass index (BMI) is now a standard entry in most health records. BMI is a formula showing body weight adjusted for a patient's height. A healthy BMI is between 18.5 and 24.9. EHR software will automatically compute the BMI once the patient's height and weight are entered in the vital signs.

3. The **Systolic** field is filled out. Press the tab key to confirm your entry.

4. The **Diastolic** field is filled out. Press the tab key to confirm your entry.

5. **Tab** is now pressed to advance to the next field.

6. The **Heart Rate** field is filled out. Press the tab key to confirm your entry.

7. **Tab** is now pressed to advance to the next field.

8. The **Respiratory Rate** field is filled out. Press the tab key to confirm your entry.

9. The **Temperature** field is filled out. Press the tab key to confirm your entry.

10. The **Weight** field is filled out. Press the tab key to confirm your entry.

11. Press **tab** to advance through the oz. field.

12. Press **tab** again to advance through the height (in feet) field.

13. The **Height (inches)** field is filled out. Press the tab key to confirm your entry.

14. The **O2 Saturation** field is filled out. Press the tab key to confirm your entry.

15. Click **Add Vitals.**

16. Click the small **"x"** in the top right corner of the vitals history screen to close it.

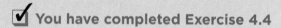 **You have completed Exercise 4.4**

At this point in the process, the patient has been taken to the exam room, vital signs have been taken, and she is ready to be seen by the care provider, which we will cover in Chapter 5.

chapter 4 **summary**

LEARNING OUTCOME	CONCEPTS FOR REVIEW

4.1 Outline the use of forms as data collection tools. pp. 66–68	– Paper form versus computer screen
	– When designing a form, keep the following in mind:
	  • name the form
	  • patient's name on every page
	  • purpose of the form
	– Keep related information close together on the form
	– Clearly mark field headings
	– Lengthy forms should be separated into sections
	– Ease of completion and of reading
	– Don't duplicate information on the form
	– Sufficient space for answers on paper forms

4.2 Execute a step-by-step procedure to document past medical, surgical, family, and social histories in PrimeSUITE. pp. 69–73	– All histories are important in the assessment of patients – Past medical history includes: current and past medical conditions; allergies; medications; immunization status; chief complaint; history of present illness; review of systems – Surgical history includes all surgeries or procedures the patient has had and the dates (approximate) – Past family history is collected to assess whether the patient is predisposed to certain conditions – Social history is collected to determine if patient may be at a greater risk for certain conditions
4.3 Examine the necessity of properly documenting and correcting inconsistent or unclear information. pp. 73–74	– Office or facility must have clear policies to deal with inconsistent information – When a discrepancy is found and the patient is present, ask which is correct; amend the record according to policy – If the correct information is not certain, document that as well

4.4 Apply procedures to document vital signs in PrimeSUITE. pp. 74–75	– Vital signs include:
	  • blood pressure
	  • temperature
	  • heart rate
	  • respiratory rate
	  • height
	  • weight
	  • body mass index
	  • blood oxygen
	– PrimeSUITE will show vital signs over time, which may alert the provider to certain risk factors such as high blood pressure or significant weight loss or gain

chapter review

MATCHING QUESTIONS

Match the terms on the left with the definitions on the right.

_____ 1. **[LO 4.2]** review of systems

_____ 2. **[LO 4.2]** surgical history

_____ 3. **[LO 4.2]** past medical history

_____ 4. **[LO 4.2]** social history

_____ 5. **[LO 4.2]** past family history

_____ 6. **[LO 4.2]** history of present illness

_____ 7. **[LO 4.2]** chief complaint

_____ 8. **[LO 4.4]** vital signs

a. reason for a patient's visit

b. patient information such as blood pressure and respiratory rate

c. patient information that includes immunizations and allergies

d. patient information that includes frequency of drinking and smoking

e. patient information that includes duration of the complaint, associated symptoms, and presence of pain

f. comprehensive inventory of patient symptoms such as headaches, vision, heart palpitations, swelling of joints, etc.

g. patient information that includes past procedures and who performed the procedures

h. patient information that includes possibly inherited conditions

MULTIPLE-CHOICE QUESTIONS

Select the letter that best completes the statement or answers the question:

1. **[LO 4.1]** An on-screen item of data is known as a:
   a. box.
   b. crate.
   c. carton.
   d. field.

2. **[LO 4.3]** PrimeSUITE allows you to note discrepancies in the _____ box.
   a. details
   b. discrepancies
   c. information
   d. registration

3. **[LO 4.1]** It is important to keep the design of paper forms:
   a. cumbersome.
   b. detailed.
   c. logical.
   d. short.

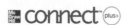 Enhance your learning by completing these exercises and more at http://connect.mcgraw-hill.com!

4. **[LO 4.4]** A patient's vital signs are taken _____ the patient history interviews.
   a. before
   b. after
   c. during
   d. A and B are correct

5. **[LO 4.2]** Which of the following is **not** a required patient history?
   a. Family
   b. Birth
   c. Social
   d. Surgical

6. **[LO 4.1]** Of the following, who will benefit from thoroughly completed paper forms?
   a. Care providers
   b. Patients
   c. Receptionists
   d. All of the above

7. **[LO 4.2]** The patient's _____ history could possibly help predict a future health condition.
   a. family
   b. medical
   c. social
   d. surgical

8. **[LO 4.4]** A patient's vital signs are entered via PrimeSUITE's _____ screen.
   a. Facesheet
   b. History
   c. Patient
   d. Registration

9. **[LO 4.3]** Which of the following is an acceptable way of gathering a patient's history?
   a. Assessment
   b. Critique
   c. Discussion
   d. Interview

10. **[LO 4.1]** Which piece of information might be included multiple times on a form?
    a. Address
    b. Allergies
    c. Marital status
    d. Patient history

11. **[LO 4.1]** What information should you see on all forms in a patient chart?
    a. Name
    b. DOB
    c. Medical record number
    d. All of the above

12. **[LO 4.2]** A patient's past surgical history includes the:
    a. approximate date of the procedure.
    b. name of the attending physician.
    c. patient's recovery time.
    d. type of sutures used.

13. **[LO 4.1]** For ease of completion, related information should be _____ on a form.
    a. adjacent
    b. duplicated
    c. labeled
    d. separate

14. **[LO 4.4]** What does BMI stand for?
    a. Basic Medical Information
    b. Body Mass Index
    c. Body Matter Indicator
    d. Base Measurement Index

15. **[LO 4.2]** Which of the following would include a patient's exercise regimen?
    a. Family history
    b. Medical history
    c. Social history
    d. Surgical history

16. **[LO 4.3]** Any discrepancies in patient information need to be:
    a. detailed.
    b. documented.
    c. filed.
    d. transcribed.

SHORT ANSWER QUESTIONS

1. **[LO 4.1]** Explain why it is important to keep the design of paper forms logical and orderly.

2. **[LO 4.1]** List at least eight things to keep in mind when designing a form as explained in the text.

3. **[LO 4.2]** Explain why a patient's social history is important.

4. **[LO 4.1]** Why might it be recommended that a patient's name and chart number/medical record number appear on each page of a multi-page form?

5. **[LO 4.4]** List the vital signs that are typically taken at each patient visit.

6. **[LO 4.1]** Why, in the age of EHRs, is patient information still gathered mainly through the use of paper forms?

7. **[LO 4.2]** Differentiate between the social and family histories.

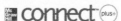 Enhance your learning by completing these exercises and more at http://connect.mcgraw-hill.com!

8. **[LO 4.3]** Why does a medical office need to have clear policies in place for dealing with discrepancies in patient information?

9. **[LO 4.4]** PrimeSUITE asks you to record what position—sitting, standing, or lying down—a patient was in when his or her blood pressure was taken. Why does this matter?

10. **[LO 4.2]** Why might so many patient histories need to be taken?

APPLYING YOUR KNOWLEDGE

1. **[LO 4.2]** Amy Lewis comes to your office for her annual wellness check-up. As the healthcare professional who will be doing her initial interview, create a list of questions you might ask Amy to obtain her social history.

2. **[LO 4.4]** How can the PrimeSUITE tracking feature assist you in analyzing a patient's vital signs over time? Give a specific example.

3. **[LO 4.1]** As an office manager for a large healthcare practice, you have been asked to design a new patient intake form. In the space below, sketch out your form's layout, keeping in mind the best practices discussed in the chapter.

4. **[LO 4.3]** Bob Larks is a new patient in your practice, and he brought his informational form with him on his first visit. During the patient history portion of his exam, he says that he does not drink, but while entering that information in Bob's chart you notice that his initial history stated that he was a "social drinker." What should you do?

5. **[LOs 4.2, 4.3]** As a healthcare professional, you are attempting to obtain the medical histories of your patient, Lisa Sanchez. However, you are having difficulty because Lisa is evading your questions and is refusing to respond. What could you do?

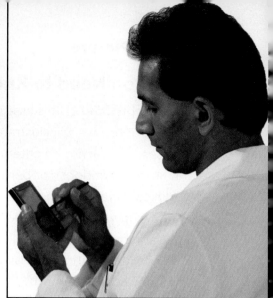

Content of the Health Record—the Care Provider's Responsibility

Learning Outcomes

At the end of this chapter, the student should be able to:

5.1 Explain each element of a SOAP note.

5.2 Identify elements of the history of present illness (HPI).

5.3 Identify elements of the Review of Systems (ROS).

5.4 Identify elements of the physical exam (PE).

5.5 Describe the process of traditional dictation and transcription.

5.6 Illustrate the advantages of speech recognition technology.

5.7 Outline the benefits of ePrescribing.

5.8 Evaluate the benefits of computerized physician order entry (CPOE).

5.9 Support the necessity to track physicians' orders.

5.10 Examine the benefits of a Problem List.

Key Terms

Assessment
Care provider
Chief complaint
Computerized Physician Order Entry (CPOE)
Discharge summary
ePrescribing
History of present illness (HPI)
History and Physical report (H&P)
Interface
Objective

Physical exam (PE)
Plan (of care)
Point of care (POC)
Problem list
Review of systems (ROS)
SOAP note
Subjective
Speech recognition technology
Voice recognition technology

What You Need to Know and Why You Need to Know It

In this chapter, the EHR is assessed from the care provider's perspective. In the PrimeSUITE demonstrations we will illustrate how a **care provider** captures clinical information, but in the exercises you will not be entering any information because only a physician, physician's assistant, nurse practitioner, or perhaps a midwife, all of whom are care providers, would be entering clinical data.

Knowing where in the record certain information resides is important because it is often necessary for the medical assistant, biller, or other healthcare professional to access a care provider's documentation to answer a question for another care provider or for an insurance company, or to complete forms.

5.1 | The SOAP Note

SOAP stands for **S**ubjective, **O**bjective, **A**ssessment, and **P**lan. It is a format for documentation that reflects a patient's visit (typically an office visit) in an orderly fashion—from the time the visit begins to the time it ends. The four areas are:

Subjective (S): This is the information the care provider learns from the patient. The **subjective** findings are the patient's description of his or her symptoms. For instance, Philip James is seen in Dr. Connors' office today; he tells the doctor that he has had a cold and terrible headache for three days.

Objective (O): **Objective** findings include information the care provider gathers from performing a physical exam. For example, upon conducting a physical exam on Philip James, he notes the patient has tenderness above the eyebrows and just beneath the cheek bones when touched and a green nasal discharge.

Assessment (A): At this **assessment** stage, the care provider *assesses* the patient's signs and symptoms and results of his physical exam in order to make a diagnosis or diagnoses. The documented diagnosis for Philip James is acute sinusitis.

Plan (P): The plan is also known as the **plan of care**. The care provider will order any tests he feels are medically necessary, prescribe medications or recommend over-the-counter medications, order consultations with other care providers if necessary, educate the patient about his condition, and advise the patient of follow-up instructions. So, in Mr. James' case, Dr. Connors wrote an order for a CT scan of the sinuses. His instructions to Mr. James included drinking plenty of fluids and taking the next two days off from work. A prescription for a Z-Pak was ordered and he was given printed educational material about sinusitis (from the EHR software). He was told to schedule a follow-up appointment for 10 days from now.

An example of an instruction screen for a patient is found in Figure 5.1.

In a paper record, the physician would handwrite the patient's record as seen in Figure 5.2.

In an electronic health record, these elements are documented, but rather than being handwritten, a combination of free-text writing and use of drop-down menus and standard text make documentation more thorough, consistent, easily retrievable, and legible. As you complete the following exercises, you will see that the SOAP elements described above are present in the EHR.

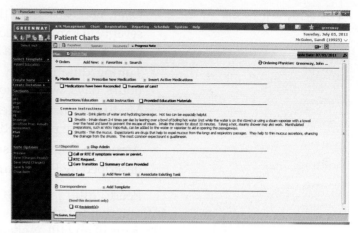

Figure 5.1 Example of patient instructions from PrimeSUITE

When a patient is admitted to a hospital, the care provider documents the subjective and objective findings, along with the results of a physical exam, in the **History and Physical** report, otherwise known as an **H&P**. The assessment and plan, as well as a recap of the patient's course in the hospital, would be documented in a **discharge summary** (or note).

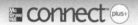 Go to http://connect.mcgraw-hill.com to complete this exercise.

 EXERCISE 5.1

Look up the Patient's Plan of Care

In this exercise, it is necessary to access the plan of care Dr. Ingram ordered for Juan Ortega. Dr. Ingram is on the phone and has asked you to look up the treatment plan for Juan Ortega, since he has to return a call to Mr. Ortega quickly and is not at a computer. Once the information is accessed, then you would read the documentation to Dr. Ingram.

Follow these steps to complete the exercise on your own once you have watched the demonstration and tried the steps with helpful prompts.

From the PrimeSUITE desktop, the patient's Facesheet is accessed and then the steps below are followed.

1. The **Documents** link is clicked on.
2. The entry for **06/07/2010** is clicked on.
3. Click the **scroll button.**
4. Note the information in the Plan section.

 You have completed Exercise 5.1

PrimeSUITE tip

The scroll bar itself does not move; instead, click on the arrow at the bottom of the scroll bar.

5.2 The History of Present Illness (HPI)

The **history of present illness**, or **HPI**, was introduced in Chapter 4; it is the patient's depiction of his or her current illness as told to the healthcare professional or care provider. The typical elements of an HPI are:

- Location of the condition (abdomen, arm, leg, head, etc.).
- Quality: pain is sharp, dull, or an ache, for example.
- Severity: rating of pain/itch/cough/nausea, etc. Often, patients are asked to rate their symptoms on a scale of one to 10 with one being

barely noticeable and 10 being intolerable. This may also mean the severity in terms of bleeding, vomiting, or diarrhea—for instance, profuse bleeding from a laceration versus a small amount of bleeding.

- Timing/duration: how long the condition has been present – hours, days, weeks, months, for example.
- Modifying factors: alternating ice and heat on a painful area;affect of pain medication, etc.
- Associated signs and symptoms: for instance, the cold symptoms described by Philip James in Figure 5.2.

Read Philip James' **SOAP note** in Figure 5.2 again. Match the information listed in the subjective portion of the note to the typical elements of an HPI. Not all elements are collected on all visits—only those that are necessary based on the patient's **chief complaint** would be documented.

Patient: Philip James	DOB: July 31, 1991	Date of Service: 05/11/2011
S		Mr. James presented today because he has had a headache for the past three days. He has not received any relief from OTC decongestants or antihistamines. He describes the pain as more of an ache, though when he pushes on his forehead, it is painful. He has had cold symptoms for about a week, but his symptoms are getting worse, and on a scale of 1 to 10, he says that his pain is an 8. He has also noted that he has had two minor nose bleeds in the past two days.
O		Vital signs noted in his chart. All within normal limits. Head and face: physical exam of nasal passages reveals a moderate amount of green discharge from both nares. The patient is tender to the touch above each eyebrow and cheek bone. Chest is clear to percussion and auscultation. Heart: Regular rate and rhythm. Abdomen: Non-tender. This is the third time Mr. James has been diagnosed with a sinus infection in the past 18 months.
A		Acute sinusitis.
P		CT scan of sinuses to be done today or tomorrow at Memorial Hospital (order given to patient). Instructed to drink plenty of fluids and bedrest for two days. To return to office in 10 days for follow-up. Z-Pak single-dose pack was sent to The Corner Pharmacy via ePrescribe. Patient was given sinusitis literature.
		Jared Connors, MD 5/11/2011

Figure 5.2   Handwritten SOAP note

EXERCISE   5.2   EHR

Go to http://connect.mcgraw-hill.com to complete this exercise.   connect plus+

Locate Juan Ortega's Blood Pressure

In this exercise, Juan Ortega stopped by the office and wants to know what his blood pressure was on his last visit. To look this up, you will access Juan Ortega's chart.

You will start by going to Juan X. Ortega's Facesheet. The Vital Signs are found there, and you do not need to leave the Facesheet to find his blood pressure readings.

Follow these steps to complete the exercise on your own once you have watched the demonstration and tried the steps with helpful prompts.

From the PrimeSUITE desktop, the patient's Facesheet is accessed and then the steps below are followed.

1. Click **Vital Signs.**

84 Copyright © 2012 The McGraw-Hill Companies

2. Note the BP readings.

Once you locate the vital signs, you will tell Mr. Ortega that on his visit of June 7, 2011, his blood pressure reading was 160/80.

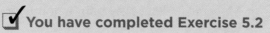 **You have completed Exercise 5.2**

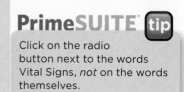

5.3 The Review of Systems (ROS)

The **review of systems (ROS)** is a body system by body system assessment of any signs or symptoms the patient is experiencing that may or may not be related to the reason for his visit. The ROS is not the same as a physical exam, because the ROS refers to the patient's own responses, not an objective assessment by the care provider. Often, the ROS is accomplished by the patient completing the medical history form that we discussed in Chapter 3. Or, the care provider may use that as a starting point and ask questions based on the patient's responses given on the form. The completion (or review) of the ROS is an integral component in assessing the patient's overall health as well as gaining a better picture of any additional signs or symptoms that may be related to the patient's chief complaint. In addition, the ROS plays a role in how much the patient will be charged for the visit, since it takes into account the care provider's time and medical expertise during an office visit. Regardless of whether the history form is already completed and the care provider reviews it or whether the care provider completes the form herself during an office visit, there must be some form of documentation to show that the ROS was done or reviewed in order to receive reimbursement for it. The particulars of procedure coding, charging, and reimbursement will be covered in another course.

Usually, a care provider will start at the head and work down through the body to the lower extremities. Listed below are the typical organs and/or body systems that may be reviewed as well as examples of questions that may be asked for each:

- General , also referred to as Constitutional (how the patient is feeling in general, any complaints or concerns, and a recap of vital signs)
- Skin (any rashes or wounds that will not heal, any unusual moles or markings that have appeared, etc.)
- Head, Eyes, Ears, Nose, and Mouth (headaches, double vision, blurring of vision, ringing of ears, earache, nosebleeds, dry mouth, dental issues)
- Throat (persistent sore throat, difficulty swallowing)
- Breasts (whether monthly self-exams are done, any changes, lumps, nipple discharge)
- Respiratory (difficulty breathing, shortness of breath)
- Cardiovascular (any chest pain, palpitations, or fluttering)
- Gastrointestinal (any problems with stomach pain, constipation, diarrhea; any changes in stool, signs of blood in stool)

- Genitourinary (any problems voiding, cloudiness of urine, changes in color or odor of urine, difficulty starting to urinate, nighttime urination, signs of blood in urine)
- Musculoskeletal (any pain in joints or extremities, difficulty walking)
- Neurologic (any dizziness, lightheadedness, difficulty with memory, cognition, coordination, or severe headaches)
- Endocrine (if female, any problems with menses, any swelling of the thyroid)
- Psychological (depression, changes in mood)
- Hematologic/Lymphatic (any unexplained or profuse bleeding, any swelling of lymph glands)
- Allergies (problems with environmental allergies; any known allergies or reactions to medications)

In PrimeSUITE and most EHR software, the ROS choices are determined by the patient's chief complaint or the body system it relates to. Not every ailment requires a thorough ROS. For instance, for a patient being seen with cold symptoms, the care provider may just review the head, eyes, ears, nose and throat (HEENT) and the chest (which essentially makes up the respiratory system) and would typically have no need to review the breasts, neurological, psychological, or reproductive systems. Figure 5.3 shows how the constitutional ROS looks in PrimeSUITE and Figure 5.4 shows the full ROS.

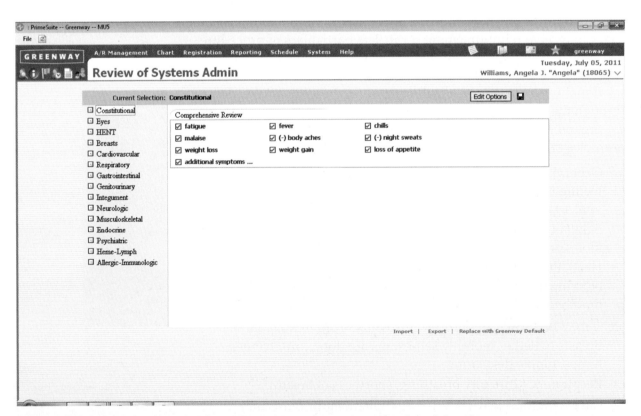

Figure 5.3   PrimeSUITE Review of Systems screen—Constitutional Section

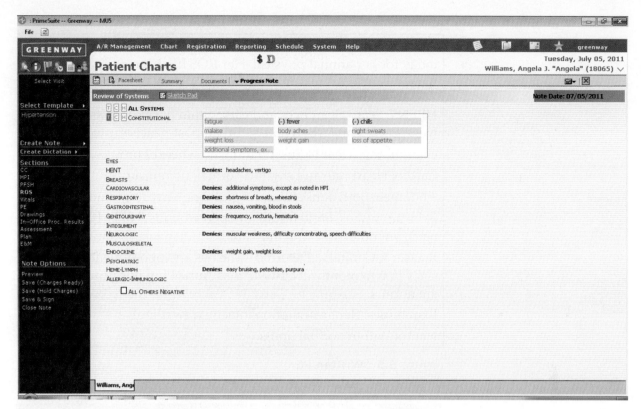

Figure 5.4   Completed ROS

<table>
<tr><td>5.4</td><td>**The Physical Exam**</td></tr>
</table>

The **physical exam (PE)** is performed by the care provider. As we discussed earlier, in a physician's office that would be the physician, physician's assistant, nurse practitioner, or nurse midwife. The extent of the physical exam is typically driven by the patient's chief complaint, or the reason the patient is being seen today. If a patient is being seen for an annual physical exam, then it will be more extensive than the PE performed for a patient who is being seen with a chief complaint of a splinter in the right ring finger.

The care provider will also determine the extent of the PE based on the patient's responses to the ROS questions. If the patient with the splinter in the right ring finger has also been falling more than usual, then the PE will be more extensive and may also include the musculoskeletal and neurologic systems.

Let's look at an example of a patient being seen for an annual physical exam (which will be in written form). (And, in Figure 5.6 you can see the PE of a patient, Ian Mikeals, in PrimeSUITE.)

The healthcare professional who needs to know the results of a patient's physical exam to answer questions, complete forms, or handle insurance issues will need to access the patient's physical exam, but will never have to actually enter information in this part of the patient's chart.

Alexis Shaw is a 25-year-old African American female being seen today for her annual physical. Her ROS has been reviewed; and is unremarkable.

HEENT: Scalp clear; eyes and ears within normal limits; Nose: Some congestion noted; throat: post-nasal drip noted.

Chest: Lungs clear to auscultation, no wheezes or rales.

Cardio: Heart rate and rhythm normal; no murmurs.

Abdomen: Soft, non-tender, no guarding or rebound noted.

Skin: No rashes, broken skin, or open wounds. Nails: bites her nails, but otherwise unremarkable.

Breasts & Genitalia: Deferred – she has an appointment with her GYN in two months. Her LMP was April 15 of this year. Periods are normal.

Extremities: Range of motion intact; no swelling.

Neuro: Within normal limits.

Figure 5.5   Written PE

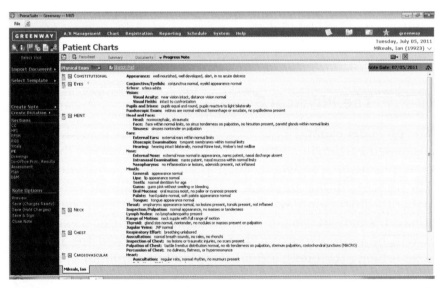

Figure 5.6   PE as seen in PrimeSUITE

5.5   Medical Dictation and Transcription

With a manual record system, most care providers choose to hand-write their charts. That's often been problematic since handwriting is often illegible. A chart that is not legible could cause safety concerns and negative patient outcomes, and wastes time for the healthcare professional who cannot read the writing and has to track down the care provider so that his or her writing can be deciphered. You have no doubt read or heard horror stories of wrong medications or wrong dosages being given to patients because of illegible handwriting. Health Insurance companies may also deny payment based on illegible handwriting.

One solution many physicians used in the past was to dictate their notes into a recorder (hand-held or into a larger system via telephone), and a transcriptionist would then transcribe the physician's words into a typed document. Dictation used as a business tool dates back to the early 20th century, when Thomas Edison, Inc. and Columbia Graphaphone Company distributed their first versions of voice recorders known as the Ediphone and Dictaphone respectively. Dictation has evolved considerably—from hand-held machines to less cumbersome systems that only require the use of a telephone.

The use of dictation and transcription software allowed for greater accuracy (because of better recording quality), faster turnaround time than the original dictation systems, and more advanced reporting capabilities, which allowed physicians' offices and hospitals to analyze the cost of dictation and transcription as a means of documentation.

The cost of dictation, and the required transcriptionists who translate the spoken word into the written word, are not inexpensive. As the technology progressed, so did the price of dictation systems. As the requirements of government agencies and insurance companies rose, as well as escalating malpractice and negligence cases, the need for better, faster documentation grew. But recording a physician's words on paper also needed to be done in a timely manner. The need for qualified transcriptionists grew, but were often in short supply.

5.6 | Voice (Speech) Recognition Technology

Over the past 15 years or so, voice (speech) recognition technology has replaced traditional dictation to a great degree. **Voice recognition technology** is software that "learns" as it is used. In other words, it learns the voice and tone inflections of the dictator, and accuracy improves with time. **Speech recognition technology**, on the other hand, does not recognize individual voices. Many of you may already be using speech recognition technology and do not even realize it. For instance, your cell phone has a feature that allows you to voice dial; or you call your local cable company and have to go through a series of questions that you can respond to by "saying or pushing 3." Both are forms of voice recognition. In these two examples, a command is carried out based on your speech response. With voice recognition used in the medical environment, as the care provider dictates, the words appear on the computer screen. In true voice recognition systems, the software "learns" the dictator's voice. The words that end up on screen are not perfect; for instance, "there" may be typed rather than "their" or Xanax may be heard as Zantac. But, since medicine requires accurate information, the transcriptionist's role has become more of editor than transcriber. The transcriptionist may listen to the entire piece of dictation and compare it against what appears on the screen, or, once the system learns that physician's voice and becomes more accurate, the transcriptionist may only read what is on the screen to look for obvious errors.

The quality of transcription is higher with voice recognition (if the software recognizes the words correctly). Once physicians are comfortable with the use of voice recognition software, it may be less time consuming than dictation, and long-term costs are lower since in most instances the transcription costs are lower (especially if a transcription service has been utilized in the past). The greatest advantage, though, is speed of documentation. With traditional transcription, days could pass between the time a chart note was dictated and transcribed (known as turnaround time). With voice recognition, the documentation is instant–as the words are spoken, they are documented in the chart simultaneously. Of course, the chart should be reviewed and edited before the care provider authenticates (signs) the note, but the fact that there is a draft copy in the record so quickly is a strong benefit.

Most EMR/EHR software solutions have a voice recognition component.

5.7 Electronic Prescribing (ePrescribing)

ePrescribing software is another component of the Meaningful Use requirements of HITECH. With ePrescribing, the care provider sends prescriptions to the patient's pharmacy electronically, at **point of care** (occurring at the time the patient is being seen). Electronically sending prescriptions speeds up the process for the patient as opposed to the traditional method where the care provider hands the patient a written prescription, the patient takes it to the pharmacy, and then waits for it to be filled (or returns at a later time). Even if the prescription is called in by the office, the process takes longer than using ePrescribing.

Most importantly, quality of care is greatly improved with electronic prescribing; not only does the prescription itself go directly to the pharmacy, but also the patient demographics, insurance information, allergies, and medication history are sent as well. Care providers and pharmacists are alerted to possible food and drug interactions between medications that are currently prescribed or that the patient is already taking, and drug allergies and sensitivities are flagged. Also, medication dosing errors are avoided—for instance, if the care provider orders 250 mg of a particular drug for a 15-year-old patient, but the recommended dosage for that drug is 25 mg for a 15-year-old, an alert message would automatically appear, so that the care provider can make the correction before the prescription is sent through to the pharmacy. Prescription renewal requests are handled more efficiently too since they are received electronically and there is no need to manually update the patient's chart. And of course, there are no more legibility issues—pharmacists do not have to make phone calls back to the office to ask what was written by the care provider; and the office staff does not have to take the time to track down the care provider or chart.

Using ePrescribe

Before we look at the steps involved in using ePrescribe, we will cover the parts of a prescription. They are:

Drug name: The name of the drug in brand or generic form. For instance, HydroDIURIL is the brand name for hydrochlorothiazide (the generic name).

Dosage: The measurement of the amount of drug that is being administered. HydroDIURIL is prescribed in 25 or 50 mg doses to treat adult hypertension.

Sig: The "label" or instructions that the pharmacist needs to list on the prescription label. A common Sig for HydroDIURIL would be "Take one tablet by mouth, once daily."

In our scenario for ePrescribe, Juan X. Ortega has called in for a refill of his prescription for Caduet (a medication for high blood pressure and angina).

Since this information would be found in the clinical part of the chart, Juan X. Ortega's Facesheet is first accessed and then the Medication List. The care provider would typically carry out these steps unless he or she has given the healthcare professional a verbal order to do so.

Follow these steps to complete the exercise on your own once you have watched the demonstration and tried the steps with helpful prompts. Use the information provided in the scenario above to complete the information.

1. Click **Medication List.**
2. Click **View Medication History.**
3. Click **(+) Caduet Oral Tablet 10-10 mg.**
4. Note the refill sent via ePrescribe.

Once we completed these steps, we found that Dr. Ingram ePrescribed a refill for Juan X. Ortega.

☑ **You have completed Exercise 5.3**

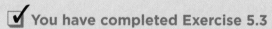

5.8 Computerized Physician Order Entry (CPOE)

No treatment, diagnostic test, or medication administration is performed on any patient without a care provider's order. Using paper records, orders were traditionally either written by the care provider or given verbally and written in the patient's record by a nurse. Orders may be in written form or may be electronically submitted. PrimeSUITE's functionality is called *Orders Requisition.* Through this function, orders can be printed or electronically submitted to an outside laboratory, medical equipment company, or hospital with **interface** capabilities with PrimeSUITE. The interface capability means that one computer system (or component) can accept and receive data from another system. The interface could refer to systems at different locations or within the same facility. Your office may have PrimeSUITE software for PM and EHR, but your laboratory system may be manufactured by a different vendor. If the computer programs for each are configured to exchange data without having to re-enter the data, then orders can flow directly to the laboratory system and the results can flow directly back to the EHR in PrimeSUITE.

A major advantage of CPOE functionality is built-in clinical decision support. Alerts appear when orders are entered for medications or treatment that may cause an adverse reaction to a drug or drugs that had previously been ordered for that patient. The same applies to dosing errors—if a care provider ordered 250 mg of a drug for a 10-year-old patient, but maximum dosage is 100 mg for that age group, then an alert would appear, and a potentially serious situation could be averted since the alert occurs prior to administration of the drug. Through use of CPOE, as long as the facility's data dictionary includes a comprehensive listing of medications and abbreviations used, the probability of medication errors is greatly reduced.

Regarding orders for diagnostic tests, once the order is carried out, for instance a Complete Blood Count (CBC), the results will be electronically sent to the care provider who ordered the lab test. Using CPOE is safer as well because there is no questionable handwriting or errors in transcribing the verbal orders of physicians to contend with—again, improving overall patient care.

5.9 Tracking Physicians' Orders

If a test is important enough to order, then learning the results of that test is equally important. Tests that are not carried out and reported in a timely manner can delay necessary care and also cause inefficiency in the business processes of an office. Having this functionality in an EHR system prevents communication breakdowns and unnecessary rework.

When an order has been completed and the results are ready for the care provider's review, she will receive notification on her Desktop. In Figure 5.7, note on the left side of the screen that the Lab Flowsheet tab shows one resulted order and has a red star next to it,

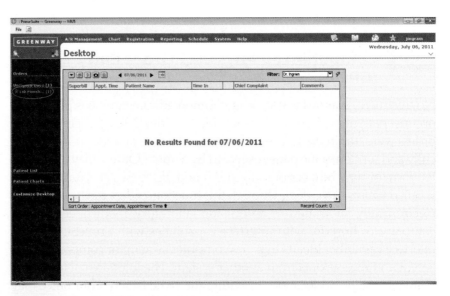

Figure 5.7 Results ready for review

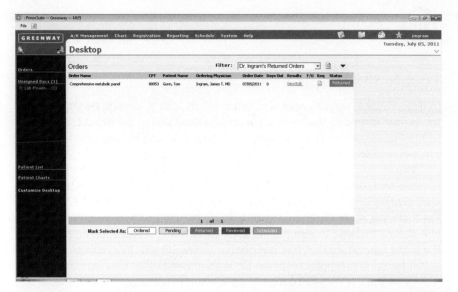

Figure 5.8 Resulted order

meaning it is high priority. The care provider would click on the Orders tab to review the returned results.

Once the care provider clicks the Orders tab, all resulted orders will appear on the screen. In Figure 5.8 you can see that there is one order that has been resulted, and it is for a metabolic panel on Dr. Ingram's patient, Tom Gunn.

Dr. Ingram will want to see the detailed results, and to do so he clicks on View/Edit and will see the complete report; at that time he will also click Sign Note on the report to document that he has reviewed the results. Figure 5.9 illustrates a detailed report.

If, based on the results of the lab test, Dr. Ingram wants to order additional tests, prescribe a particular medication, or follow up with the patient soon, he will give additional orders to the healthcare professional to handle the situation accordingly.

Figure 5.10 represents the final screen the care provider sees. From it he can note whether the results were normal, abnormal, or a specific assessment, and can also send a follow-up task to one of the healthcare professionals in the office or to another care provider in the practice for review. These tasks can be done directly from the Order screen without having to exit that function and find another.

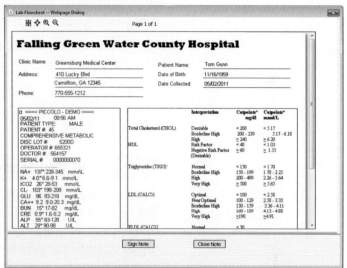

Figure 5.9 Detailed report and option to sign note

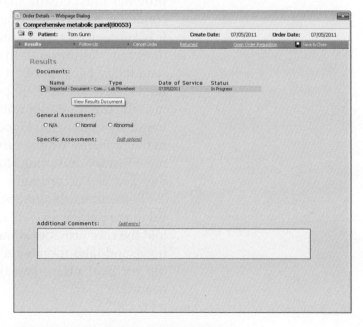

Figure 5.10 Order details screen

Go to http://connect.mcgraw-hill.com
to complete this exercise.
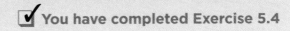

Locate the Status of an Order

In this exercise, a lipid panel was ordered for Juan X. Ortega by Dr. Ingram. Dr. Ingram is asking the healthcare professional about the results. By going to the Facesheet and then looking at Orders Tracking History, the healthcare professional found that those results are still pending.

The results could be pending because Mr. Ortega did not go to the lab to have his blood drawn, or the results may not be ready yet. It is the healthcare professional's responsibility to follow up with the lab and/or Mr. Ortega. For instance, if Mr. Ortega has not gone to the lab to have his blood drawn, she should express to him the importance of doing so as soon as possible. If it is the laboratory that has not posted the result yet, then she should ask that it be done promptly because Dr. Ingram needs the results.

Once the Facesheet of the patient's chart is accessed, follow these steps to complete the exercise on your own once you have watched the demonstration and tried the steps with helpful prompts.

1. Click **Orders Tracking History.**
2. Note the Status.

✔ **You have completed Exercise 5.4**

5.10 The Problem List

Another requirement of Meaningful Use is an up-to-date **problem list** of current and active diagnoses. Providing quality care means that current diagnoses or conditions should be followed on an ongoing basis until the problem is resolved, or at least until it is stable. Of course, there are some medical conditions, such as asthma or coronary artery disease, that may never resolve completely, but the care provider must ensure that the patient is stable and that his or her condition is not worsening. With the use of a problem list, as long as it is kept current, necessary testing or assessment of the condition does not "fall through the cracks." For instance, a patient may be seen today because of an upper respiratory infection, but has also been treated by the care provider for hypertension, and on today's visit the care provider notes that the patient's blood pressure is elevated. By clicking on Hypertension in the list of diagnoses included in the problem list, the care provider is able to quickly see the treatment history and prior blood pressure readings on that patient and then proceed accordingly.

Sometimes, the information included in the problem list is helpful to the patient as well as the care provider. The patient may have told the care provider something about his treatment or hospitalizations, and later forgets the details. By having this complete history, the medical office has the information readily available when needed.

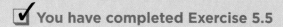
Utilizing the Problem List

In the scenario we are about to view, Juan X. Ortega has been treated for angina over the past few years. He was first diagnosed in 2005 and has been hospitalized at Memorial Hospital twice for it—once on August 31, 2010, and once on June 17, 2009. Mr. Ortega has asked the office staff to complete a form that he needs for his employer. His employer needs to know if he has ever been hospitalized for angina and when. He does not recall the dates but does remember giving that information to Dr. Ingram on his last visit, so he hopes the information can be found in his record.

From the Facesheet of Juan X. Ortega, the healthcare professional will click on angina from the Problem List area in order to get Mr. Ortega the information he needs.

Once the Facesheet of the patient's chart is accessed, follow these steps to complete the exercise on your own once you've watched the demonstration and tried the steps with helpful prompts.

1. Under Problem List, click on **Angina.**
2. Click **OK.**
3. Note the hospitalization dates.

☑ **You have completed Exercise 5.5**

chapter 5 **summary**

LEARNING OUTCOME	CONCEPTS FOR REVIEW
5.1 Explain each element of a SOAP note. pp. 82–83	– Subjective—the patient's description of the problem – Objective—the care provider's results of physical examination – Assessment—the diagnosis or diagnoses – Plan—the diagnostic tests or treatment plan for the patient
5.2 Identify the elements of the history of present illness (HPI). pp. 83–85	– Location of the condition (abdomen, arm, leg, head, etc.) – Quality of the symptoms – Severity of the symptoms – Duration/timing of the symptoms – Context under which symptoms occur – Modifying factors – Associated signs and symptoms
5.3 Identify elements of the review of systems (ROS). pp. 85–87	– Body system by body system assessment of any signs or symptoms the patient is experiencing that may or may not be related to the reason for his or her visit – Not the same as the physical exam
5.4 Identify the elements of the physical exam (PE). pp. 87–88	– The extent of the exam is dependent on the patient's presenting symptoms (the chief complaint) – The physical exam relates to the findings of the care provider, not the patient, as in the ROS; for example, the patient complains of pain in the right lower abdomen, yet when the care provider presses on the right lower abdomen, the patient does not express feelings of pain
5.5 Describe the process of traditional dictation and transcription. pp. 88–89	– Physician dictates medical notes into a recording device – Transcriptionist types the words using word processing software – Often takes days for the transcribed report to be filed in the patient's record
5.6 Illustrate the advantages of speech recognition technology. pp. 89–90	– The provider's documentation immediately appears in the patient's record; no lag time between dictation and transcription – In the long term, may be less expensive than traditional dictation and transcription – Quality is higher than with traditional transcription (in most cases)

LEARNING OUTCOME	CONCEPTS FOR REVIEW
5.7 Outline the benefits of ePrescribing. pp. 90–91	– Less chance for medication errors – Potential food/drug interactions are identified – Fewer man-hours to complete the process – More convenient and less wait time for patients – Overall, better-quality care
5.8 Evaluate the benefits of computerized physician order entry (CPOE). pp. 91–92	– Fewer errors in carrying out orders because they are no longer handwritten – Orders can be sent directly from the office to the laboratory or hospital – Safer for the patient—the order is sent by the care provider rather than verbally given to another healthcare professional to send on to the laboratory or hospital – If an interface exists, the results automatically come back to the ordering physician.
5.9 Support the necessity to track physicians' orders. pp. 92–94	– Patient care—knowing the results of the test in a timely manner, proper treatment can be started quickly
5.10 Examine the benefits of a problem list. pp. 94–95	– Timely follow-up of conditions – Serves as a reminder to the care provider to address problems on the patient's problem list – Information about each problem is located in one place

chapter review

MATCHING QUESTIONS

Match the terms on the left with the definitions on the right.

_____ 1. **[LO 5.1]** objective

_____ 2. **[LO 5.8]** interface

_____ 3. **[LO 5.4]** physical exam

_____ 4. **[LO 5.6]** voice recognition

_____ 5. **[LO 5.9]** order tracking

_____ 6. **[LO 5.2]** history of present illnes

_____ 7. **[LO 5.5]** transcriptionist

_____ 8. **[LO 5.10]** problem list

_____ 9. **[LO 5.7]** ePrescribing

_____ 10 **[LO 5.3]** review of systems

a. patient's description of her current illness

b. EMR feature that is part of HITECH's Meaningful Use requirements

c. comprehensive inventory of patient symptoms such as headaches, vision, heart palpitations, swelling of joints, etc.

d. staff member responsible for creating typed documentation of a doctor's spoken notes

e. comprehensive record of a patient's complaints and conditions

f. section of a SOAP note that contains information gathered during a physician's exam

g. the ability to access and use another provider's practice management software

h. set of steps performed by a medical provider to assess a patient

i. software that automatically turns spoken words into text

j. periodically checking the status of procedures requested by a provider

MULTIPLE-CHOICE QUESTIONS

Select the letter that best completes the statement or answers the question:

1. **[LO 5.2]** Which of the following is an element of the history of present illness?
   a. Duration
   b. Prevention
   c. Medication
   d. Treatment

2. **[LO 5.3]** Which of the following would most likely require a complete review of systems?
   a. Annual exam
   b. Headache
   c. Mole on back
   d. Sore throat

3. **[LO 5.1]** Notes about a prescription ordered for a patient would appear in the _____ section of a SOAP note.
   a. subjective
   b. objective
   c. assessment
   d. plan

4. **[LO 5.3]** An ROS covers information likely documented in the:
   a. history of present illness.
   b. medical history form.
   c. physical exam.
   d. SOAP note.

5. **[LO 5.9]** PrimeSUITE has the capability to _____ the status of an order.
   a. assign
   b. generate
   c. query
   d. track

6. **[LO 5.6]** The biggest advantage of voice recognition software over manual transcription is:
   a. clarity.
   b. cost.
   c. ease.
   d. speed of turn-around-time.

7. **[LO 5.1]** Creating an electronic SOAP note in an EHR makes use of:
   a. drop-down menus.
   b. free-text fields.
   c. standard text.
   d. all of the above.

8. **[LO 5.1]** Information gathered during a provider's physical exam would appear in the _____ section of a SOAP note.
   a. subjective
   b. objective
   c. assessment
   d. plan

9. **[LO 5.6]** The more voice recognition software is used, the:
   a. faster it corrects mistakes.
   b. quicker it gets.
   c. more it learns voice inflections.
   d. slower it gets.

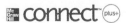 Enhance your learning by completing these exercises and more at http://connect.mcgraw-hill.com!

10. **[LO 5.8]** There must be a _____ to perform any tests or treatments.
    a. diagnosis
    b. referral
    c. order by the care provider
    d. SOAP note

11. **[LO 5.5]** A person hired to manually record a physician's spoken words is known as a:
    a. dictator.
    b. recorder.
    c. stenographer.
    d. transcriptionist.

12. **[LO 5.2]** Which of the following elements of an HPI are collected at a visit?
    a. All of them
    b. Duration, quality, and severity
    c. Location and severity
    d. Only those that apply to the patient's chief complaint

13. **[LO 5.4]** The extent of a physical exam largely depends upon which of the following?
    a. Age of patient
    b. Amount of time available
    c. Patient's chief complaint
    d. Patient's medical history

14. **[LO 5.10]** Meaningful Use regulations require the keeping of an up-to-date:
    a. exam registry.
    b. order queue.
    c. problem list.
    d. provider note.

15. **[LO 5.7]** The use of ePrescribing is part of the requirements for:
    a. HIPAA
    b. HITECH
    c. HIM
    d. HPI

SHORT ANSWER QUESTIONS

1. **[LO 5.2]** List the typical elements of a History of Present Illness.

2. **[LO 5.5]** List at least three drawbacks of handwritten patient charts.

3. **[LO 5.7]** List five benefits of using ePrescribing.

4. **[LO 5.3]** In order for a practice to receive reimbursement for an ROS, what must happen?

5. **[LO 5.4]** Explain the factors that might influence the extent of a physical exam.

6. **[LO 5.1]** List the four sections of a SOAP note and give an example of each.

7. **[LOs 5.5, 5.6]** Why is there still a need for medical transcriptionists in an age of voice-recognition software?

8. **[LO 5.3]** List the typical organs and body systems that would be covered in a complete review of systems.

9. **[LO 5.10]** List one reason a provider might use a patient's problem list.

10. **[LOs 5.3, 5.4]** Contrast an ROS with a PE.

11. **[LO 5.4]** List four types of medical providers who might perform a physical exam.

12. **[LO 5.8]** Explain what it means to have interface capabilities with PrimeSUITE. What benefits does interfacing have?

13. **[LO 5.9]** List three benefits of PrimeSUITE's order tracking capabilities.

14. **[LO 5.4]** Based on Alexis Shaw's physical exam as documented in the text, what is her chief complaint?

15. **[LO 5.6]** Contrast voice recognition with speech recognition.

APPLYING YOUR KNOWLEDGE

1. **[LOs 5.1, 5.2, 5.3, 5.4]** Patient James Frank presents for his appointment. He is complaining of fatigue and headaches. When Dr. Ingram examines him, he finds that James has an enlarged lymph node on the right side of his throat; his lungs are clear; his blood pressure is a little low at 100/68. Dr. Ingram suspects anemia or an underactive thyroid as the causes of James's fatigue, so he orders a comprehensive blood panel be done. Create a SOAP note that properly documents each piece of James Frank's visit with Dr. Ingram.

2. **[LO 5.6]** Your office is preparing to implement new voice recognition technology, and you have been tasked with creating some talking points and benefits to share with your peers. How could you go about explaining the benefits of voice recognition software?

3. **[LOs 5.7, 5.10]** Why would ePrescribing and an up-to-date problem list be addressed under Meaningful Use requirements?

4. **[LOs 5.7, 5.8, 5.9, 5.10]** Of the following PrimeSUITE capabilities—ePrescribing, CPOE, order tracking, and the problem list—which do you think is the most beneficial? Explain your answer.

5. **[LO 5.7]** Create two flowcharts: one that shows the progression of a manually written prescription, and one that shows the progression of a prescription entered using ePrescribing.

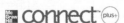 Enhance your learning by completing these exercises and more at http://connect.mcgraw-hill.com!

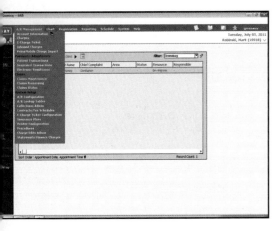

chapter **six**

Financial Management: Insurance and Billing Functions

Learning Outcomes

At the end of this chapter, the student should be able to:

6.1 Illustrate the need for a claims management process.

6.2 List the information contained in a Superbill.

6.3 Apply procedures to update a patient's account in PrimeSUITE.

6.4 Demonstrate coding using ICD-9-CM and CPT codes in PrimeSUITE.

6.5 Examine the correlation between documentation and code assignment.

6.6 Support the need for the conversion to ICD-10-CM/PCS.

6.7 Describe the information contained in a Remittance Advice or Explanation of Benefits.

6.8 Apply procedures to manage accounts receivable in PrimeSUITE.

6.9 Demonstrate the need for a compliance plan.

Key Terms

Abuse

Accounts payable

Accounts receivable

CMS-1500 claim form

Co-payment (co-pay)

Compliance plan

Current Procedural Terminology (CPT)

Deductible

Encounter

Encounter form

Evaluation and Management (E&M)

Explanation of benefits (EOB)

Fee schedule

Fraud

Healthcare Common Procedure Coding System (HCPCS)

International Classification of Diseases-9th revision, Clinical Modification (ICD-9-CM)

International Classification of Diseases, 10th revision, Clinical Modification/Procedure Coding System (ICD-10-CM/PCS)

Insurance plan

Insurance verification

Library

Managed care plan

Medical necessity

National Provider Identifier (NPI)

Plan

Remittance advice (RA)

Subscriber

Superbill

Transactions

What You Need to Know and Why You Need to Know It

Physicians, hospitals, and any other healthcare facility are in business to take care of patients, first and foremost. However, they are also businesses. They have bills to pay just like any other business—payroll, rent or mortgage, utilities, supplies, insurance, and, yes, the providers themselves also need to be paid as well. The efficiency we have discussed in terms of providing patient care also applies to collecting monies owed to the office. The billing and collections process will be discussed in this chapter. Remember, though, that this is not a course on billing procedures. From this chapter you will gain an awareness of how billing and EHR applications are intermeshed using PrimeSUITE. The specifics of *how* to complete and file insurance claims, manage accounts, collect unpaid bills, and handle financial management in general will be covered in another course. The coding of diagnoses and procedures will also be covered in other classes, but when you finish this chapter you will understand how documentation, coding, and reimbursement are related.

6.1 Claims Management—Why and How

Every patient seen in a healthcare facility is charged for the care he or she receives. Yes, some accounts are "written off"; in other words, the patient does not pay, but there still needs to be an accounting of the visit and the charges that were incurred for the visit. If this is not done, the business profile of the office would show an inaccurate picture of the number of patients seen, the procedures carried out, the charges incurred, and the amount of money collected. In other words, the statistics collected for that medical practice would not be valid because not all of the patients were included in the entire picture.

The financial well-being of a medical office is of great importance if the practice is to stay in business. Therefore, a process, or to be specific, a written claims management process, is necessary. Each step of the process must be carried out efficiently and effectively. This process includes written policies—how much is charged per service (**fee schedule**), the timing of filing claims, follow-up on unpaid claims, and collections procedures when claims are not paid must all be in writing. The importance of written policies will be addressed in the compliance section of this chapter.

The use of practice management (PM) software greatly improves the efficiency of a claims process because it allows for more accurate capturing of charges, submits automatic reminders, offers a variety of reporting options, and provides automatic follow-up of each account. There is far less chance of missed charges, missed payments, and payments being posted to the wrong account with a computerized system than a manual one. Just the ability to run reports on daily charges, daily payments, and accounts in collections increases the efficiency of the business processes.

Remember that each patient is entered only once in the practice's database of patients, but each patient may have more than one encounter (visit) attached to that master entry. Each visit has an account attached to it, and therefore, the claims process must be fulfilled for each of those accounts. Without PM software, just tracking insurance payments on one patient who is seen a couple of times a month would be a daunting task!

See Figure 6.1, which shows one patient who has been seen several times; each visit is listed separately.

The patient's account for each visit begins when the patient makes the appointment. The healthcare professional asks for the expected source of payment at that time. If the patient is going to be paying out of pocket (no insurance), the payment policies of the office are discussed with the patient. If the office does provide for payment options, that will be discussed as well. Many patients have some type of insurance coverage, whether it be Medicare, Medicaid, TRICARE, private insurance, or group insurance, including managed care plans. **Managed care plans** promote quality, cost-effective health-care through monitoring of patients, preventive care, and performance measures of providers. Physicians contract with managed care plans to provide care at a pre-determined rate. If the patient is covered by insurance, **insurance verification** is completed by the office staff, usually before the patient arrives for his appointment, so that the office is reasonably sure that the patient is covered and that payment will come from some source. Verifying insurance is the process of contacting the insurance carrier and receiving validation of coverage for that patient, whether he owes a co-pay amount (due from the patient at the time of the visit), whether the visit and services ordered are covered by the insurance, and whether he has met his **deductible** (the out-of-pocket payment amount that a policyholder or patient must meet before insurance covers the services).

Once the patient arrives for his appointment he checks in at the front desk. The patient is then seen by the care provider and charges are applied to his bill. When the visit is complete, he checks out (in a hospital this is called *discharged*). The patient now has an account for that visit to which charges have been applied.

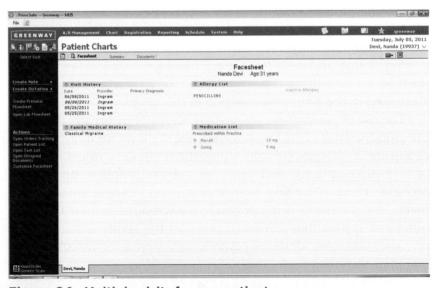

Figure 6.1 Multiple visits for one patient

In a hospital setting, all of the above tasks are performed; however, there are specific rules that apply to insurance verification, especially if the patient presents through the emergency department and/or is in labor. Hospital billing is beyond the scope of this worktext, but a claim is filed with insurance, when applicable..

6.2 | Use of a Superbill

The Paper Superbill

A document that is often used in medical offices to capture the diagnoses and services or procedures performed, either as a hard copy piece of paper or is computer generated by the PM system is known as a **Superbill** or an **encounter form** (this concept was introduced in Chapter 1). The information on the Superbill will be transferred to a form known as the **CMS-1500 claim form** and used to bill an outpatient **encounter**. An encounter is synonymous with a visit and was also discussed in Chapter 1.

Typically, a hard-copy Superbill (Figure 6.2) includes the following information, though it may contain more elements than those listed below:

- Name and address of the medical practice
- National Provider Identification number (NPI) number
- Patient's name
- Patient's chart number
- Date and time of visit
- CPT codes for common procedures performed in that office
- Diagnosis narrative (as written by the care provider)
- ICD-9-CM codes corresponding to each written diagnosis (not on all Superbills)

On this form, the provider documents the services that were rendered during the encounter. Even if a PM system is computerized, the paper form may still be printed. The patient's identifying information is already completed for the provider, and he or she checks off the CPT codes for the procedures that were performed and writes in the diagnosis or diagnoses the patient was treated for during that particular visit.

The Electronic Superbill

Figure 6.3 shows a Superbill Summary in PrimeSUITE for a patient, Tom E. Gunn, who is being seen for cholelithiasis (gall stones).

Notice that the charges are listed just under the visit information. There are five (5) CPT codes listed; these were introduced in Chapter 1 and will be discussed in more detail later in this chapter. Each CPT code must "map" to a diagnosis code because the diagnosis code shows **medical necessity** (the fact that there is a medical reason to perform that procedure). To the left of the CPT code column, notice that there are symbols. There are many coding rules set down by Medicare and Medicaid, and most insurance companies have additional rules as well. The symbols you see are an advantage of using

Lakeridge Medical Group
262 East Pine Street, Suite 100
Santa Cruz, CA 95062

☐ **PRIVATE**   ☐ **BLUECROSS**   ☐ **IND.**   ☐ **MEDICARE**   ☐ **MEDI-CAL**   ☐ **HMO**   ☐ **PPO**

PATIENT'S LAST NAME		FIRST		ACCOUNT #	BIRTHDATE / /	SEX ☐ MALE ☐ FEMALE	TODAY'S DATE / /
INSURANCE COMPANY		SUBSCRIBER			PLAN #	SUB. #	GROUP

ASSIGNMENT: I hereby assign my insurance benefits to be paid directly to the undersigned physician. I am financially responsible for non-covered services. SIGNED: (Patient, or Parent, if Minor) DATE: / /	RELEASE: I hereby authorize the physician to release to my insurance carrers any information required to process this claim. SIGNED: (Patient, or Parent, if Minor) DATE: / /

✔	DESCRIPTION	M/Care	CPT/Mod	DxRe	FEE	✔	DESCRIPTION	M/Care	CPT/Mod	DxRe	FEE	✔	DESCRIPTION	M/Care	CPT/Mod	DxRe	FEE
	OFFICE CARE						PROCEDURES						INJECTIONS/IMMUNIZATIONS				
	NEW PATIENT						Tread Mill (In Office)		93015				Tetanus		90718		
	Brief		99201				24 Hour Holter		93224				Hypertet	J1670	90782		
	Limited		99202				If Medicare (Set up Fec)		93225				Pneumococcal		90732		
	Intermediate		99203				Physician Interpret		93227				Influenza		90724		
	Extended		99204				EKG w/Interpretation		93000				TB Skin Test (PPD)		86585		
	Comprehensive		99205				EKG (Medicare)		93005				Antigen Injection-Single		95115		
							Sigmoidoscopy		45300				Multiple		95117		
	ESTABLISHED PATIENT						Sigmoidoscopy, Flexible		45330				B12 Injection	J3420	90782		
	Minimal		99211				Sigmoidos. , Flex. w/Bx.		45331				Injection, IM		90782		
	Brief		99212				Spirometry, FEV/FVC		94010				Compazine	J0780	90782		
	Limited		99213				Spirometry, Post-Dilator		94060				Demerol	J2175	90782		
	Intermediate		99214										Vistaril	J3410	90782		
	Extended		99215										Susphrine	J0170	90782		
	Comprehensive		99215				LABORATORY						Decadron	J0890	90782		
							Blood Draw Fee		36415				Estradiol	J1000	90782		
	CONSULTATION-OFFICE						Urinalysis, Chemical		81005				Testosterone	J1080	90782		
	Focused		99241				Throat Culture		87081				Lidocaine	J2000	90782		
	Expanded		99242				Occult Blood		82270				Solumedrol	J2920	90782		
	Detailed		99243				Pap Handling Charge		99000				Solucortef	J1720	90782		
	Comprehensive 1		99244				Pap Life Guard		88150-90				Hydeltra	J1690	90782		
	Comprehensive 2		99245				Gram Stain		87205				Pen Procaine	J2510	90788		
	Dr.						Hanging Drop		87210								
	Case Management		98900				Urine Drug Screen		99000				INJECTIONS - JOINT/BURSA				
													Small Joints		20600		
	Post-op Exam		99024										Intermediate		20605		
							SUPPLIES						Large Joints		20610		
													Trigger Point		20550		
													MISCELLANEOUS				

DIAGNOSIS:	ICD-9											
Abdominal Pain	789.0	Gout	274.0	C.V.A. - Acute	436.	Electrolyte Dis.	276.9	Herpes Simplex	054.9
Abscess (Site)	682.9	Asthma	493.90	Cere. Vas. Accid. (Old)	438	Fatigue	780.7	Herpes Zoster	053.9
Adverse Drug Rx	995.2	Asthmatic Bronchitis	493.90	Cerumen	380.4	Fibrocys. Br. Dis	610.1	Hydrocele	603.9
Alcohol Detox	291.8	Atrial Fib.	427.31	Chestwall Pain	786.59	Fracture (Site)	829.0	Hyperlipidemia	272.4
Alcoholism	303.90	Atrial Tachi.	427.0	Cholecystitis	575.0	Open/Close		Hypertension	401.9
Allergic Rhinitis	477	Bowel Obstruct.	560.9	Cholelithiasis	574.00	Fungal Infect. (Site)	110.8	Hyperthyroidism	242.9
Allergy	995.3	Breast Mass	611.72	COPD	492.8	Gastric Ulcer	531.90	Hypothyroidism	244.9
Alzheimer's Dis.	290.1	Bronchitis	490	Cirrhosis	571.5	Gastritis	535.0	Labyrinthitis	386.30
Anemia	285.9	Bursitis	727.3	Cong. Heart Fail.	428.9	Gastroenteritis	558.9	Lipoma (Site)	214.9
Anemia - Pernicious	281.0	Cancer, Breast (Site)	174.9	Conjunctivitis	372.30	G.I. Bleeding	578.9	Lymphoma	202.8
Angina	413.9	Metastatic (Site)	199.1	Contusion (Site)	924.9	Glomerulonephritis	583.9	Mit. Valve Prolapse	424.0
Anxiety Synd.	300.00	Colon	153.9	Costochondritis	733.99	Headache	784.0	Myocard. Infarction (Area)	410.9
Appendicitis	541	Cancer, Rectal	154.1	Depression	311.	Headache, Tension	307.81	M.I., Old	412
Arterioscl. H.D.	414.0	Lung (Site)	162.9	Dermatitis	692.9	Migraine (Type)	346.9	Myositis	729.1
Arthritis, Osteo.	715.90	Skin (Site)	173.9	Diabetes Mellitus	250.00	Hemorrhoids	455.6	Nausea/Vomiting	787.0
Rheumatoid	714.0	Card. Arrhythmia (Type)	427.9	Diabetic Ketosis	250.1	Hernia, Hiatal	553.3	Neuralgia	729.2
Lupus	710.0	Cardiomyopathy	425.4	Diverticulitis	562.11	Inguinal	550.9	Nevus (Site)	216.9
		Cellulitis (Site)	682.9	Diverticulosis	562.10	Hepatitis	573.3	Obesity	278.0

DIAGNOSIS: (IF NOT CHECKED ABOVE)

SERVICES PERFORMED AT: ☐ Office ☐ E.R. ☐ ☐	☐ CLAIM CONTAINS NO ORDERED REFERRING SERVICE	REFERRING PHYSICIAN & I.D. NUMBER

RETURN APPOINTMENT INFORMATION: 5 - 10 - 15 - 20 - 30 - 40 - 60 [DAYS] [WKS.] [MOS.] [PRN]	NEXT APPOINTMENT M - T - W - TH - F - S DATE / / TIME:	AM PM	ACCEPT ASSIGNMENT? ☐ YES ☐ NO	DOCTOR'S SIGNATURE

INSTRUCTIONS TO PATIENT FOR FILING INSURANCE CLAIMS: 1. Complete upper portion of this form, sign and date. 2. Attach this form to your own insurance company's form for direct reimbursement. **MEDICARE PATIENTS - DO NOT SEND THIS TO MEDICARE. WE WILL SUBMIT THE CLAIM FOR YOU.**	☐ CASH ☐ CHECK # ___ ☐ VISA ☐ MC ☐ CO-PAY	TOTAL TODAY'S FEE	
		OLD BALANCE	
		TOTAL DUE	
		AMOUNT REC'D. TODAY	

INSUR-A-BILL ® BIBBERO SYSTEMS, INC. • PETALUMA, CA • UP. SUPER. © 6/94 (BIBB/STOCK)

Figure 6.2   Paper Superbill

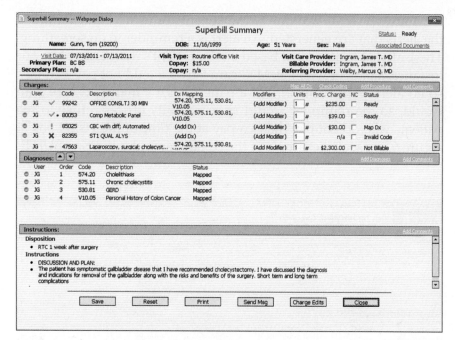

Figure 6.3   PrimeSUITE Superbill

PM software; cash flow is not adversely affected when potential coding problems leading to denied claims are taken care of before the claim is filed. In Figure 6.4 you will find the legend for these symbols. For instance, a green checkmark denotes that there are no problems with that code and charges can be posted. A yellow exclamation point, on the other hand means that no diagnosis code is mapped to that procedure code that would justify payment of the claim; until that is resolved, cash flow would be affected because the claim would be denied or returned for more

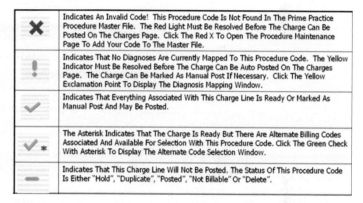

✖	Indicates An Invalid Code! This Procedure Code Is Not Found In The Prime Practice Procedure Master File. The Red Light Must Be Resolved Before The Charge Can Be Posted On The Charges Page. Click The Red X To Open The Procedure Maintenance Page To Add Your Code To The Master File.
!	Indicates That No Diagnoses Are Currently Mapped To This Procedure Code. The Yellow Indicator Must Be Resolved Before The Charge Can Be Auto Posted On The Charges Page. The Charge Can Be Marked As Manual Post If Necessary. Click The Yellow Exclamation Point To Display The Diagnosis Mapping Window.
✔	Indicates That Everything Associated With This Charge Line Is Ready Or Marked As Manual Post And May Be Posted.
✔*	The Asterisk Indicates That The Charge Is Ready But There Are Alternate Billing Codes Associated And Available For Selection With This Procedure Code. Click The Green Check With Asterisk To Display The Alternate Code Selection Window.
—	Indicates That This Charge Line Will Not Be Posted. The Status Of This Procedure Code Is Either "Hold", "Duplicate", "Posted", "Not Billable" Or "Delete".

Figure 6.4   Symbols used on PrimeSUITE Superbill summary

information by the insurance company. A red "X" indicates that an invalid code appears on the Superbill and that payment would be denied or returned for more information.

6.3   The Claims Process Using PrimeSUITE

As noted above, the process begins when the patient makes an appointment. But the charges do not start accruing until the patient presents for the appointment and services are rendered.

The first step, if the patient has insurance, is to collect the **co-payment**, otherwise known as the **co-pay**. In managed care plans particularly, this is the portion of the bill that is the responsibility of the patient. It is due at the time of the office visit. Many offices collect the co-pay at the time of arrival; others collect it when the patient checks out at the conclusion of the visit. For inpatient hospital visits, co-pays do not exist.

You will recall that one of the benefits of using PM software is the alerts that are generated. An alert is a reminder to do something. These alerts are generated based on the patient's **insurance plan**. For instance, a patient who has Medicare Part B would not pay a co-pay, so no alert would appear, but a patient with a managed care plan would, so the reminder would appear. Many offices refuse to see patients who do not pay their co-pay at the time of the visit. Look at Figure 6.5 to see an example of the co-pay reminder in PrimeSUITE.

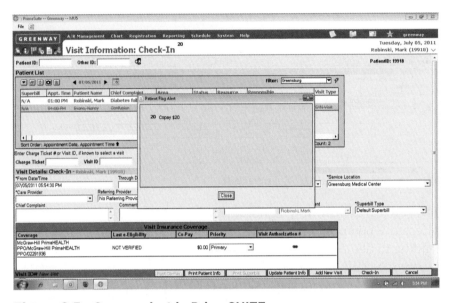

Figure 6.5   Co-pay alert in PrimeSUITE

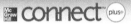

EXERCISE   6.1   PM

Go to http://connect.mcgraw-hill.com to complete this exercise.

Post a Co-payment to an Account

In this scenario, a patient, Mark Robinski, has just come in for his 1:00 p.m. appointment and has checked in at the front desk. The healthcare professional noted his arrival in PrimeSUITE by using the Visit Information Check-in screen. Mr. Robinski has a $20 co-pay, which he is paying for with his VISA® credit card, account number 7708363100. The credit payment itself is run through a different system; only the fact that it was paid with a credit card is noted in PrimeSUITE.

Follow these steps to complete the exercise on your own once you have watched the demonstration and tried the steps with helpful prompts in practice mode. Use the information provided in the scenario above to complete the information.

1. Click **01:00 PM.**
2. Click **Close.**
3. Click **Post Co-Pay.**
4. Click **Method** drop-down menu.
5. Clicking the entry **Credit Card** selects it.
6. Click **Supplier** drop-down menu.
7. Clicking the entry **Visa** selects it.
8. The **Additional Info** field is filled out, which is the Visa® account number. Press the tab key to confirm your entry.

9. The **Amount** field is filled out with the amount paid by the patient. Press the tab key to confirm your entry.

10. Click **Save.**

11. Click **Yes.**

12. Click **OK.**

13. Click **Close** (the red "X").

14. Click **Save.**

 You have completed Exercise 6.1

In the next exercise, we will be checking on the status of a claim for Mark Robinski for an earlier appointment he had at Greensburg Medical Center. This might be done for any number of reasons—the patient may be inquiring, the billing staff may be investigating because his name and visit date appeared on an unpaid accounts report, or an office manager may be doing a quality check of the work performed by a member of the staff.

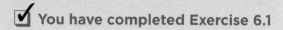

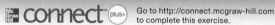 Go to http://connect.mcgraw-hill.com to complete this exercise.

EXERCISE 6.2

Given a Scenario, Look Up the Status of an Insurance Claim

The scenario is that Mark Robinski, while being seen on May 9, 2011, asks if the claim from his May 2 visit has been paid.

The healthcare professional will investigate by accessing the **Accounts Receivable (A/R)** Management menu, and then the claims management function. Accounts receivable includes money that is received by the medical practice including insurance payments or payments made by the patient. The patient's identification number (chart number) is needed for this step, and it is found in the upper right corner of every screen. Mr. Robinski's chart (ID) number is 19918.

Follow these steps to complete the exercise on your own once you have watched the demonstration and tried the steps with helpful prompts. Use the information provided in the scenario above to complete the information.

1. Click **Search for Patient.**

2. The *Last Name** field is filled out. Press the tab key to confirm your entry.

3. Click **Search.**

4. Click **Select.**

5. Click **Claims Maintenance.**

6. Click **Patient ID.**

7. The **Patient ID** field is filled out. Press the tab key to confirm your entry.

8. Click **Search.**

9. Click the **horizontal scroll button** on the right.

10. Click **U - New/No EOB.**

11. Look at the final screen and note the claim status.

In the exercises above, we have seen how to perform the co-pay posting function as well as how to find the status of a patient's claim using PrimeSUITE.

 You have completed Exercise 6.2

In the medical field, care providers diagnose patients using medical terms, for instance, a myocardial infarction (heart attack), an upper respiratory infection (a common cold), or cholelithiasis (gall stones). They also perform tests to make a diagnosis, such as an EKG, a strep screen (for strep throat), or a lower GI series (x-rays to detect abdominal conditions). Therapeutic procedures (those that are done to alleviate symptoms or correct a condition) are done as well, for example, suturing a laceration, packing the nose to stop a severe nosebleed, or removing cyst. Supplies are necessary to complete procedures or for treatment purposes. For instance, a suture kit is used to suture a laceration, serum is used to administer an injection, and a sling may be ordered for a patient with a sprain.

Though the care provider documents the diagnoses, procedures, or services in words, those words have to be converted to a numeric form in order to file claims to insurance companies and to keep statistics of the conditions treated and procedures performed at the office or facility.

We will discuss three types of codes that are used, and one new one that will be used beginning in October 2013.

First, let's look at diagnosis coding. The current coding system used to convert written diagnoses into numeric form is the ***International Classification of Diseases, 9th revision, Clinical Modification***, better known as **ICD-9-CM**. It has been in use since 1979. A yearly update each October (and sometimes April) occurs when new codes are added (for instance, to account for West Nile Virus, or H1N1 influenza), codes are changed in some way, and obsolete codes are omitted. ICD-9-CM is used in physicians' offices to code diagnoses only. In a hospital setting, it is used to code diagnoses and procedures.

Some examples of ICD-9 codes frequently used in the physician's office setting are:

Code	Description
034.0	Streptococcal sore throat (strep throat)
784.7	Epistaxis (nosebleed)
708.0	Urticaria (hives)
786.50	Chest pain
250.00	Diabetes mellitus
V70.0	Routine general medical exam

Examples of ICD-9-codes frequently used in a hospital setting are:

Code	Description
410.11	Acute anterior wall myocardial infarction (heart attack)
574.20	Cholelithiasis (gall stones)
820.03	Fracture, neck of femur (hip fracture)
430	Subarachnoid hemorrhage (stroke)

Patients may have one diagnosis code or many for each encounter. Any conditions that were diagnosed, were treated, or required more nursing or care provider attention should be coded. The first listed diagnosis is most closely related to the reason the patient was seen for that encounter (the chief complaint).

The second code set we will discuss is **Current Procedural Terminology**, or **CPT**. It is Level 1 of the **Healthcare Common Procedure Coding System**, known as **HCPCS**.

In the physician's office setting, CPT codes are used to code procedures or services given to a patient. In a hospital setting, they are used for outpatient coding (emergency room, outpatient diagnostic testing, or ambulatory surgery, for example).

Examples of CPT codes in a physician's office include:

Code	Description
87430	Strep test
90703	Tetanus injection
71010	Chest x-ray
11100	Skin biopsy
99213	Detailed office visit of an established patient
99202	Low complexity office visit of a new patient

HCPCS Level 2 codes are codes used to show tangible items provided such as suture kits, ambulance services, and orthotic devices (cane, splint, etc.). They are used in any healthcare setting.

Examples of HCPCS level 2 codes include:

Code	Description
A0998	Ambulance response and treatment without transport
E0105	Cane, triple or quad
A6453	Self-adherent elastic bandage

Services rendered to a patient—whether they involve the face-to-face time with the physician, treatment, or diagnostic tests and procedures—cannot be billed to insurance unless they are medically necessary. That is to say, there need to be sufficient signs, symptoms, or history to warrant the services given. Therefore, the documentation in the record must support the need for any and all services and procedures. The EHR has been instrumental in making it possible for care providers to spend beneficial face-to-face time with their patients rather than spend time completing their records. Of course, documenting the patient's record while the patient is in the room also takes some finesse. The provider does not want to appear to be paying more attention to the computer screen than to the patient, but the longer the provider uses the computer to document, the more easily she is able to document, listen attentively, and converse with her patients all at the same time.

Performing services that are not necessary or coding services that were not actually performed both constitute insurance (including Medicare and Medicaid) **fraud**. Fraud is intentional or unintentional deception, which in healthcare takes advantage of a patient, an insurance company, or Medicare or Medicaid.

Whether you are studying to become a health information professional, a medical assistant, or a medical coder and biller, you will take courses that are specific to coding, and you will spend a significant amount of time discussing accurate, appropriate coding as well as the guidelines that apply to the coding and billing functions.

In the next exercise, you will see how ICD-9 and CPT coding are assigned using the PrimeSUITE software.

EXERCISE 6.3   Go to http://connect.mcgraw-hill.com to complete this exercise.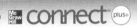

Enter Diagnoses and Procedures to Locate ICD-9 and CPT Codes

Once a patient has been seen and examined by the care provider, a diagnosis is made. The written diagnosis is then transformed into a numeric code. In our example, it is done using a function of PrimeSUITE, but it can also be done manually, using code books. As we mentioned earlier, the diagnosis coding is done using ICD-9-CM and the procedures or services are coded using CPT and/or HCPCS Level 2.

In the example that follows, Dr. Rodriguez has just seen a patient, Mark Robinski. Remember, only the care provider can make a diagnosis. So, from the Patient Notes Progress Note screen, Dr. Rodriguez will be using the Assessments tab (found on the left side of the screen) to add a diagnosis for Mark Robinski.

Mark Robinski's diagnosis is diabetes mellitus, type 2, and Dr. Rodriguez ordered a fasting blood sugar. A diagnosis code (ICD-9-CM) and a procedure code (CPT) will be assigned in the following exercise. The software will automatically assign the codes, but it is important to read the description of the codes and compare it to the narrative diagnosis the care provider has made. You should never code more than what the care provider has documented.

Follow these steps to complete the exercise on your own once you have watched the demonstration and tried the steps with helpful prompts in practice mode. Use the information provided in the scenario above to complete the information.

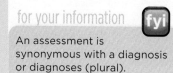

1. Click **Assessment.**
2. Click **Add Diagnosis.**
3. Click **Search.**
4. The **Diagnosis Search** field is filled out with **diabetes.** Press the tab key to confirm your entry.
5. Click **Search.**
6. Click **Type Two Diabetes Mellitus Without Mention of Complication.**
7. Click **OK.**
8. Click **Plan.**
9. Click **Search.**
10. Click **Search For Code.**
11. The **Procedure Code Search** field is filled out with **fasting blood.** Press the tab key to confirm your entry.
12. Click **Search.**
13. Click **Fasting Blood Sugar.**
14. Click the ***Category** drop-down menu.
15. Click **Labs.**
16. Click **OK.**
17. Look at the information in the **Orders** section.

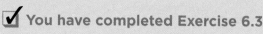 You have completed Exercise 6.3

6.6 The Conversion to ICD-10-CM/PCS

The current classification system, ICD-9-CM has been in use since 1979. Though it is updated yearly to reflect new diagnoses, remove obsolete ones, and capture the advances in technology, it is far overdue for a complete revision because it is simply not up to date with current medical diagnoses or available treatment options. The World Health Organization, in 1990, endorsed the newest version, ICD-10, and since 1994 it has been used in many nations, although the United States has yet to require its use, other than in the reporting of morbidity (death).

The *International Classification of Diseases* (ICD) is used to classify diseases and conditions that are diagnosed in any healthcare setting. It is also used to record cause of death on death certificates. The United States continues to use ICD-9, though the implementation date for *International Classification of Diseases, 10th revision, Clinical Modification/Procedure Coding System* (ICD-10-CM/PCS) has been set for October 1, 2013.

There are many reasons that the United States has not adopted ICD-10 for use in healthcare settings, but main factors include cost of converting current computer systems to accept ICD-10 rather than ICD-9 codes, time and cost involved in training staff in the use of ICD-10, and general questions of whether or not ICD-10 will meet the needs of the U.S. healthcare system. In the United States, coding enables the storage and retrieval of diagnostic information for clinical, epidemiological, and quality purposes as well as the compilation of morbidity and mortality statistics. This is its use in other nations as well, but in this country ICD-9 is also used for reimbursement purposes. The amount a hospital is reimbursed per patient stay is tied in part to each patient's diagnosis codes, or a combination thereof. In hospital and outpatient settings, the ICD code correlates to the medical necessity of the procedures and services being done to or for patients. ICD-9 does not address the severity of a patient's condition, whereas ICD-10, though not perfect, does a better job of capturing a truer picture of the resources needed to care for a patient during a particular stay or encounter.

Another issue that has held up implementation in this country is the coding of procedures, which is done now using ICD-9-CM. The "CM" stands for clinical modification and includes procedure codes. In other countries, the CM portion is not used. With ICD-10-PCS, the PCS stands for Procedural Coding System, and contains the procedure codes that will be used by hospitals. Outpatient facilities, including physicians' offices, will continue to code procedures with CPT.

Let's look at the diagnoses we coded earlier using ICD-9 and see how they look with ICD-10 codes.

ICD-9 Code	ICD-10 Code	Narrative Diagnosis
784.7	R04.0	Epistaxis (nosebleed)
708.0	L50.0	Urticaria (hives)
786.50	R07.9	Chest pain
250.00	E11.9	Diabetes mellitus
V70.0	Z00.00	Routine general medical exam

In the time leading up to October 1, 2013, experienced coders will be re-learning how to code with this new classification system. Health Information Management students, medical assisting students, and medical billing and coding students who are currently in educational programs will gradually learn ICD-10 as the main code set; ICD-9 will be covered, but not to the extent that ICD-10 will be.

6.7 Accounts Receivable—Getting Paid

You may have heard the terms **accounts payable** and **accounts receivable** at some point in time. Accounts payable is money going out—paying the bills. Accounts receivable, on the other hand, is money coming in—in this context, it is the insurance companies' payment of claims that have been filed by Greensburg Medical Center. Of course, it is imperative that what is billed is paid, and that there is an accurate accounting of all **transactions**. Transactions are the posting of charges and the payment of claims.

Insurance companies submit payments to care providers and hospitals electronically (electronic claims transactions or submissions), by check, or by automatic deposit into the bank account of the office. But the amount of the payment may be for more than one patient's care. The insurance company submits the payment with a detailed accounting of the claims for which payment is being made. The document that accompanies the payment is called a **remittance advice (RA)** (see Figure 6.6). It may also be called an **explanation of benefits (EOB)**. Many insurance companies use the term remittance advice to describe the document that accompanies payment to the provider, and the explanation of benefits is generally the form the **subscriber** (the primary person covered by the insurance) receives to notify him of what was billed, what was paid, and what is owed by him.

Regardless of what it is called, the information typically included on an RA or EOB is listed below. Again, this is not a billing class; there will be more than one patient included, typically, and many insurance companies include more information than is listed below:

- Provider's name and **National Provider Identification (NPI)** number
- Patient's name
- Claim number
- Medical record number
- Date(s) of service
- Claim status (open, denied, more information needed, paid, etc.)
- Electronic Transaction Number (if RA and payment have been sent via electronic means)
- Service detail
  - Each CPT code billed (as submitted on the claim form)
  - Amount charged for each code
  - Allowed amount (amount the insurance carrier has agreed to pay) for each code
  - Co-pay paid by patient
  - Adjusted amount (difference between what was charged and the allowed amount)
- Recap of charges and payments include
  - Total reported charges amount
  - Charges not covered amount
  - Charges denied amount
  - Covered charge amount

6.8 Managing Accounts Receivable in PrimeSUITE

The management of patient accounts, from charging patients for services to tracking accounts receivable and collections, begins by setting up the parameters of each insurance carrier and each plan within the insurance. The **plan** refers to the extent of coverage offered. For instance, 400 patients in your office may have Blue Cross/Blue Shield

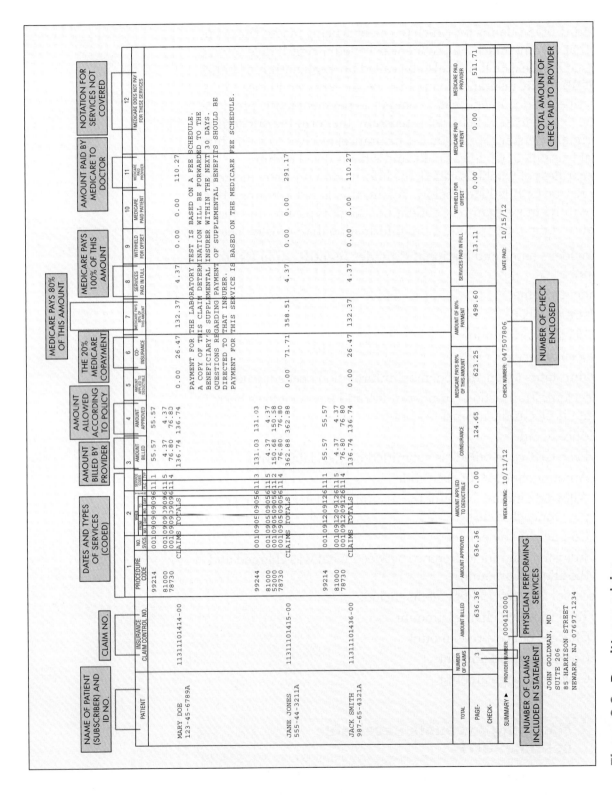

Figure 6.6 Remittance advice

insurance, but for those 400 patients, there may be more than 20 plans. Plans differ regarding:

- Co-pay requirement—Some plans require a co-pay, others do not, and the dollar amounts vary by plan. Let's look at an example: Neil Holt is an engineer for Johnsontown Analytics, and his insurance is McGraw-Hill Prime. He is responsible for a $20 co-pay, and he is responsible for 20 percent of all outpatient service charges. Lisa Haver also works for Johnsontown Analytics, and she too has McGraw-Hill insurance, but she works at a different location in a different state, and her plan requires a $25 co-pay, plus 20 percent of all outpatient services.

- Extent of coverage and whether or not services are covered at all—for example, Neil Holt's plan may cover outpatient mental health services, while Lisa Haver's does not.

- Rules regarding filing of claims—may differ from plan to plan, and they certainly differ from insurance company to insurance company

Because of these differences, it is imperative that the medical office or hospital use a system that efficiently applies the various policies to the correct patients.

When a medical office purchases any type of software, in this case PM software, an administrative staff member (the office manager, office administrator, or business manager) works with an installation specialist from the software company to build **libraries** that are used to perform functions within the different applications (accounts receivable, patient chart, etc.).

Common libraries include:

- Insurance company library—includes all of the insurance companies and the individual plans that are represented by the patients in the practice. These can be created, edited, or deleted within PrimeSUITE.

- ICD-9-CM, CPT, and HCPCS Level 2 code tables—must be maintained every year to account for additions, deletions, and amendments to codes. In order to get paid in a timely manner, only active, valid codes can be submitted; otherwise the claim will be rejected.

- Fee schedule—listed by CPT code and done for Medicare, group insurance, and by individual contracts for managed care plans. The charge for each service is documented in a fee schedule.

- Reports—in particular, aging reports (length of time a claim has remained unpaid) are set up to allow for timely tracking and follow-up of claims.

- Alerts—reminders to the office staff related to the billing functions. Some examples are co-pay alert, write-off, and overdue balance, just to name a few. Alerts assist the staff in collections processes in particular.

Using PM software to accomplish the filing of, follow-up, and collection of claims also allows electronic remittance of claims as well as electronic receipt of payment from insurance carriers. The healthcare professional can see at a glance exactly what is happening with a claim or claims at any given time in the process. Collections procedures are also streamlined using PM software. Many offices use an outside collections agency to collect overdue balances. With the use of PM software, a report of accounts ready for collections is sent electronically, the office is able to see the status of the account, and paid claims are sent to the office, often electronically.

Greater billing accuracy is an advantage of using PM software, and there is less chance of lost charges. Each time a patient is seen, and the care provider documents the progress note in PrimeSUITE and orders tests that are done on-site, she is prompted to select the ICD-9 code and the CPT codes that correspond to the diagnosis and procedures.

The face-to-face time between a patient and the care provider is charged with a CPT code known as an **Evaluation and Management (E&M)** code. It is generated based on documentation made by the care provider. The E&M code is dependent on whether the patient is new to the practice (not seen within the past three years) or an established patient (seen within the last three years); the level of history (including chief complaint and review of systems); the level of physical exam performed; and the depth of medical decision-making necessary.

Two examples of E&M codes are:

99213 An office visit for an established patient, 20 years old, who was seen for exercise-induced asthma.

99203 Initial office visit for a 30-year-old patient who has recently been complaining of rectal bleeding.

In your CPT coding class, you will learn the intricacies of assigning E&M codes, but at this point it is important to know that E&M codes are CPT codes that reflect the professional services rendered to a patient.

Once the claim has been filed and payment has been sent to the office (either by mail, direct deposit into the practice's account, or sent electronically), the payment is posted to the patient's record for that particular date of service.

We will now follow the steps to post a payment using PrimeSUITE.

EXERCISE 6.4

Go to http://connect.mcgraw-hill.com to complete this exercise. Mc Graw Hill connect plus+

Post an Insurance Payment to an Account

In our scenario, Dr. Rodriguez's office has received an RA, which includes payment to cover the claim for Mark Robinski for date of service May 2, 2011. There are two charges for the May 2nd account. They are CPT code 99214, which is an Evaluation and Management code for the face-to-face time he spent with the doctor, and code 82951, which is for a glucose tolerance test. The total amount of the remittance for Mark Robinski is $75. Fifty dollars of the $75 is for the services under the 99214 code. Twenty-five dollars of it is for the services billed under code 82951. We will be working in the A/R Management module under the insurance transactions function. The objective is to mark the services as paid, based on the amount of money received.

Follow these steps to complete the exercise on your own once you have watched the demonstration and tried the steps with helpful prompts in practice mode. Use the information provided in the scenario above to complete the information.

1. Click **Search for Patient.**
2. The ***Last Name** field is filled out. Press the tab key to confirm your entry.
3. Click **Search.**
4. Click **Select.**
5. Click **Insurance Transactions.**
6. The **Amount** field is filled out with **$50.** Press the tab key to confirm your entry.
7. The **Amount** field is filled out with **$25.** Press the tab key to confirm your entry.
8. Click **Save.**

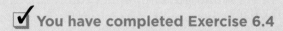 **You have completed Exercise 6.4**

The Medical Billing Process is shown in Figure 6.7. Some steps may be repeated two or three times, but the goal is payment of the claim.

Medical Billing Cycle

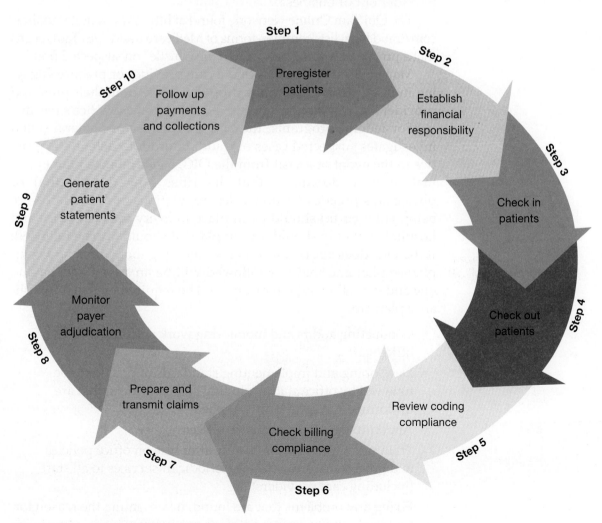

Figure 6.7   Billing and reimbursement cycle

Medicare, Medicaid, TRICARE, Worker's Compensation, group health insurance, and managed care plans are all examples of types of insurance coverage. Each has rules and regulations related to the coding, billing, and collection of healthcare claims. Intentionally or unintentionally not following those rules and regulations can result in allegations of fraud, or at the very least, **abuse**. Fraudulent coding or billing is done to intentionally or unintentionally deceive or misrepresent services that were actually performed. Abusive coding and billing practices are inconsistent with typical coding and billing practice. Either can be done intentionally or unintentionally, though they are still considered fraud or abuse. Being found guilty of either can result in monetary fines or in the worst-case scenario a sanction from any one or more of the above insurance plans. If a care provider is sanctioned from Medicare, that means he is forbidden to accept Medicare patients into his or her practice. If the practice is an internal medicine practice, Medicare enrollees most likely make up a good percentage of the patient population in the practice. Needless to say, being sanctioned from Medicare will impact his practice to the point where it may put the provider out of business.

The Qui Tam Online Network, found at http://www.quitamonline.com/fraud.html lists common forms of Medicare fraud. Qui Tam means that a private individual has "blown the whistle" on suspected fraud.

Managed care plans that find a care provider or practice engaging in fraudulent activity may drop that office from their preferred provider list, resulting in a negative impact to the practice's income.

For federal programs, the Office of Inspector General (OIG) investigates suspected cases of fraud. In order to defend the practice in the event of a visit from the OIG, a **compliance plan** (a formal, written document that describes how the hospital or physician's practice ensures rules, regulations and standards are being adhered to) should be in place in every medical office and hospital. Not only should it be in place, it should also be followed. If the OIG does audit your practice, showing that you have a compliance plan and that it is followed will be an advantage; having one and *not* following it may not be. The requirements of a compliance plan are:

- Conducting audits and monitoring work performed by the office staff
- Developing and implementing standards of practice to be followed by office staff (including care providers) that are uniformly and consistently applied
- Appointment of a compliance officer
- Training new staff immediately after hire on office policies and procedures and offering periodic in-services to all staff (including care providers)
- Fixing any problems that are found, investigating the reason for problems, and re-training staff as necessary

- Encouraging staff to bring any compliance issues to the office administration
- Enforcing the office's policies and procedures and not making exceptions

Having, following, and referencing a practice's written policies, procedures, and compliance plan will assure sound fiscal practices within a practice or facility, and may be a sound defense should the practice ever be involved in fraud or abuse allegations.

chapter 6 **summary**

LEARNING OUTCOME	CONCEPTS FOR REVIEW
6.1 Illustrate the need for a claims management process. pp. 103 – 105	– Though in business to provide patient care, a medical office is still a business. – Written policies are necessary to run the office effectively and efficiently. – Use of PM software improves efficiency. – A patient account for a visit begins when the appointment is made. – Insurance verification should be completed—either before the day of the visit or when the patient arrives (prior to is preferred). – Patient check-out occurs once the visit is complete.

6.2 List the information contained in a Superbill. pp. 105–107	– A Superbill is otherwise known as an encounter form and includes at least:
	  • name and address of medical practice
	  • NPI number
	  • Patient's name
	  • Patients charge number
	  • Date and time of visit
	  • CPT codes
	  • Diagnosis narrative by care provider
	  • ICD-9-CM diagnosis codes
	– It can be hard-copy or electronic.
	– The information on the Superbill transfers to the CMS-1500 claim form.
	– It includes some identifying information about the encounter as well as the diagnosis and procedure codes using ICD-9 and CPT code sets.

6.3 Apply procedures to update a patient's account in PrimeSUITE. pp. 107–109	– Co-payment may be collected at the time of check-in or check-out, depending on office policy. – Financial alerts appear when the patient is checked into Prime-SUITE at the time of arrival. The insurance plan entered in the system determines which, if any, alerts appear. – Once paid, the co-pay is immediately posted in PrimeSUITE. – Charges start to accrue once the patient is taken to the examining room and is seen by a healthcare professional. – Insurance status may be looked up at any time.
6.4 Demonstrate ICD-9-CM and CPT codes in PrimeSUITE. pp. 110–111	– The provider's assessment is otherwise known as the diagnosis (or diagnoses, plural). – Services rendered may be diagnostic (x-rays, lab tests) or therapeutic (sutures, cleansing of a wound, injections). – Diagnoses are coded using the ICD-9-CM code set and are used in both hospital and outpatient (physicians' offices) settings. – The first listed diagnosis is the one most closely related to the reason the patient was seen. – Any conditions that were diagnosed, treated, or required more nursing or provider attention should be documented. – Procedures are coded using CPT in the physician's office. – Procedures are coded using ICD-9-CM in the hospital setting. – HCPCS level 2 codes are used to code equipment or supplies. – Coding is done for statistical and reimbursement purposes.

LEARNING OUTCOME	CONCEPTS FOR REVIEW
6.5 Examine the correlation between documentation and code assignment. pp. 112–113	– All services and procedures performed must be medically necessary. – The diagnoses support the medical necessity for the procedure(s) and service(s). – Performing services that aren't medically necessary and billing for them is considered fraud.
6.6 Support the need for the conversion to ICD-10-CM/PCS. pp. 113–114	– ICD-9-CM is outdated and has not kept up with the needs of healthcare. – ICD-10-CM/PCS will become effective October 1, 2013. – Experienced coders will need new training on the use of ICD-10-CM/PCS. – Current students will see a change from an ICD-9-CM focus to an ICD-10-CM/PCS focus over the next several months.
6.7 Describe the information contained in a Remittance Advice or Explanation of Benefits. pp. 114–115	– Accounts receivable—money paid to the office by insurance carriers. – Transactions—documentation of all money paid and applying it to the correct patient's balances. – Remittance Advice (RA), also referred to as an Explanation of Benefits (EOB), accompanies the payment and explains the claims to which the payments apply. – The subscriber is the person who is covered under the group insurance plan.
6.8 Apply policies and procedures to manage accounts receivable in PrimeSUITE. pp. 115–119	– Efficiency and effectiveness of a managing the financial aspects start with accurately setting up the parameters of each insurance carrier and the plans within each in the PM software. – The type of plan a patient has determines the extent of coverage and the co-pay requirements. – Each insurance carrier (and the plans within) has rules and regulations regarding filing of claims. – Libraries are built within the PM software for each insurance carrier.
6.9 Demonstrate the need for a compliance plan. pp. 120–121	– All offices should have written policies and procedures for all processes in the office, but in particular for the financial aspects. – All policies should be complied with uniformly and consistently. – Each insurance carrier also has rules and regulations that must be followed. – Not following the rules and regulations may constitute fraud or abuse. – The Office of Inspector General enforces the rules and regulations set forth by any federal insurance plans. – The office should have a compliance plan to assure all rules and regulations are being followed. The plan should include: • conducting internal audits of work performed • developing standards of practice • appointment of a compliance officer • training of new personnel; updates for experienced personnel • Correcting any known problems; re-training staff as necessary • encouraging open communication from staff regarding compliance issues • enforce all policies and procedures

chapter **review**

chapter 6 review

MATCHING QUESTIONS

Match the terms on the left with the definitions on the right.

_____ 1. **[LO6.5]** fraud

_____ 2. **[LO6.2]** encounter

_____ 3. **[LO6.6]** ICD-10-CM/PCS

_____ 4. **[LO6.7]** accounts receivable

_____ 5. **[LO6.8]** Evaluation and Management codes

_____ 6. **[LO 6.1]** fee schedule

_____ 7. **[LO6.4]** Current Procedural Terminology [CPT]

_____ 8. **[LO6.9]** compliance

_____ 9. **[LO6.3]** co-payment

_____ 10. **[LO6.7]** explanation of benefits

a. list of how much is charged per service by CPT code

b. document sent from an insurance company to a subscriber outlining payment decisions

c. portion of a bill that is usually the responsibility of the patient; typically collected upon check-in

d. code set that is used to code procedures or services given to a patient

e. conscious decision to follow established rules and guidelines

f. a unit of service in the healthcare setting such as an office visit or trip to the emergency room

g. codes representing the face-to-face time spent with a provider

h. process of receiving and posting payments for medical claims

i. an act of deception, intentional or unintentional, which takes advantage of another person or entity

j. revised coding system scheduled for release in 2013

MULTIPLE-CHOICE QUESTIONS

Select the letter that best completes the statement or answers the question:

1. **[LO 6.2]** The information contained in the Superbill is eventually transferred to the _____ form for submission.
   a. claim
   b. encounter
   c. insurance
   d. registration

2. **[LO 6.5]** Only services deemed medically _____ can be billed to insurance.
   a. necessary
   b. progressive
   c. restorative
   d. useful

3. **[LO 6.4]** The ICD-10-CM code sets go into effect in:
   a. 2011
   b. 2012
   c. 2013
   d. 2014

4. **[LO 6.6]** What does the "CM" stand for in the abbreviation ICD-9-CM?
   a. Care management
   b. Clinical modification
   c. Code management
   d. Coding methodology

5. **[LO 6.8]** The amount of a patient's co-pay may vary by:
   a. care provider.
   b. insurance plan.
   c. office location.
   d. visit type.

6. **[LO 6.3]** Charges begin to accrue once the _____.
   a. appointment is made
   b. patient checks in at the reception area
   c. MA or care provider interacts with patient
   d. claim has been filed

7. **[LO 6.7]** A remittance advice is typically given to a _____, whereas an explanation of benefits is typically given to a _____.
   a. patient; provider
   b. provider; patient
   c. insurance company; patient
   d. provider; insurance company

8. **[LO 6.2]** In PrimeSUITE, a red "X" on a Superbill summary indicates:
   a. an absent diagnosis.
   b. an invalid code assignment.
   c. a charge line will not be posted.
   d. a charge is ready.

9. **[LO 6.9]** To avoid negative consequences, a compliance plan should be _____ in every hospital and medical office.
   a. discussed
   b. followed
   c. used as a guide
   d. written

10. **[LO 6.8]** The _____ is usually the person to set up information libraries within Practice Management software programs.
    a. care provider
    b. healthcare professional
    c. medical assistant
    d. office manager

McGraw Hill connect (plus+) Enhance your learning by completing these exercises and more at http://connect.mcgraw-hill.com!

11. **[LO 6.5]** Who is the only person authorized to make a diagnosis?
    a. Care provider
    b. Healthcare professional
    c. Medical assistant
    d. Office manager

12. **[LO 6.3]** To check if a claim has been paid, which menu will the healthcare professional look at?
    a. Accounts payable
    b. Accounts receivable
    c. Claims processing
    d. Claim updates

13. **[LO 6.6]** An advantage of the ICD-10 over the ICD-9 is that the ICD-10 helps to address the:
    a. length of illness.
    b. patient's chief complaint.
    c. severity of a patient's condition.
    d. time spent in a physician's care.

14. **[LO 6.1]** Depending on the terms of a patient's insurance coverage, the balance remaining after insurance has paid may be:
    a. written off as paid in full.
    b. removed from the master index.
    c. sent to collections.
    d. both A & C are correct.

15. **[LO 6.1]** Expected methods of payment are discussed when a patient:
    a. checks in.
    b. is seen by the provider.
    c. is discharged.
    d. makes an appointment.

SHORT ANSWER QUESTIONS

1. **[LO 6.1]** List four ways Practice Management software improves claim management.

2. **[LO 6.7]** Contrast accounts receivable with accounts payable.

3. **[LO 6.8]** What is the difference between an insurance provider [carrier] and an insurance plan?

4. **[LO 6.2]** List at least five items that are typically included on a hard-copy Superbill.

5. **[LO 6.3]** What is an alert?

6. **[LO 6.5]** How have EHRs improved the face-to-face time between patients and care providers?

7. **[LO 6.2]** Explain how the icons available in practice management software make claim management easier and more accurate.

8. **[LO 6.6]** Briefly summarize why the United States has not begun to use ICD-10, even though it is in use in many other nations.

9. **[LO 6.5]** Explain fraud in terms of the healthcare profession.

10. **[LO 6.3]** List three reasons why you might need to check the status of an insurance claim.

11. **[LO 6.8]** What is an aging report?

12. **[LO 6.7]** What four items are included in the recap of charges and payments found on an EOB?

13. **[LO 6.4]** List the three types of codes that are used, and give an example of how each is used.

14. **[LO 6.6]** Discuss how the ICD-9 influences reimbursement in both a hospital and an outpatient setting.

15. **[LO 6.9]** What is the difference between fraud and abuse?

APPLYING YOUR KNOWLEDGE

1. **[LO 6.3]** Discuss why many healthcare practices refuse to see patients who do not pay their co-pays at the time of their visit.

2. **[LO 6.5]** Research two recent cases of medical/insurance fraud and discuss the outcome of each case. Provide specifics about your sources [Internet, medical journals, textbooks, etc.].

3. **[LOs 6.2, 6.4, 6.5, 6.6]** Based on the information about coding discussed in the text, is moving to the ICD-10 code sets a good idea for the United States? Why or why not?

4. **[LOs 6.1, 6.8]** Why might an office need to use a collections agency to pursue overdue accounts?

5. **[LO 6.7]** Why is there so much information contained on an RA or EOB form?

6. **[LOs 6.4, 6.5, 6.9]** Anna Devlan is a healthcare professional. Recently she posted some patient claims; when performing the coding process, Anna could not find a code that exactly matched the diagnosis made by the care provider. So she found the closest match and coded that. Did Anna commit fraud and/or abuse? Explain your answer.

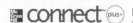 Enhance your learning by completing these exercises and more at http://connect.mcgraw-hill.com!

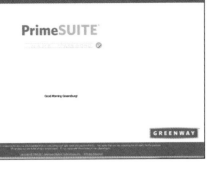

Privacy, Security, Confidentiality, and Legal Issues

Learning Outcomes

At the end of this chapter, the student should be able to:

7.1 Identify the HIPAA privacy and security standards.

7.2 Evaluate an EHR system for HIPAA compliance.

7.3 Describe the role of certification in EHR implementation.

7.4 Apply procedures to set up security measures in PrimeSUITE.

7.5 Apply procedures to ensure data integrity.

7.6 Apply procedures to release health information using PrimeSUITE.

7.7 Account for data disclosures using PrimeSUITE.

7.8 Exchange information with outside healthcare providers for continuity of care using PrimeSUITE.

7.9 Outline the content of compliance plans.

7.10 Appraise the importance of contingency planning.

Key Terms

Access report
Accounting of disclosures
Audit trail
Blog
Breach of confidentiality
Compliance plan
Confidentiality
Contingency plan
Covered entity
Data Integrity
Disaster recovery plan
Directory information
Encryption
Firewall

Hardware
Health Information Exchange (HIE)
HIPAA
HITECH
Malware
Minimum necessary information
Notice of Privacy Practices
Password
Protected health information (PHI)
Privacy
Social media
User rights
Virus

What You Need to Know and Why You Need to Know It

No matter what type of healthcare professional you become—a nurse, medical assistant, health information manager, coder, biller, registration clerk, receptionist, or care provider—you will come in contact with patients' health information. In healthcare, and particularly with electronic healthcare, privacy and security are on everyone's minds—the patients', the providers', the media's, and the government's. There is concern that computer hackers and personnel who work in healthcare facilities will gain access to records that they have no legitimate need to access. The concern is justified, but even in a paper system, frequent privacy breaches have occurred. It is just as easy for a healthcare professional to look in a patient's chart at the nurses' station as it is to sit down at a computer that is left open to a patient's record and read it. In this chapter we will discuss laws that protect privacy and security as well as methods to lessen the chances of privacy breaches occurring. It is the responsibility of all healthcare professionals and care providers to maintain patient privacy and confidentiality and to access the health information only on a need-to-know basis.

7.1 The HIPAA Privacy and Security Standards

You were introduced to **HIPAA** in Chapter 2, but to recap, HIPAA was passed in 1996. It contains several rules, though for our purposes, we will be concentrating on the privacy and security rules. In addition, in 2009, the Health Information Technology for Economic and Clinical Health Act (**HITECH**) went a step further, making the original privacy and security rules under HIPAA more stringent. HITECH also gives more power to federal and state government authorities to enforce the privacy and security rules.

The intent of both is to ensure that **protected health information (PHI)** is kept private and secure. They give patients the right to determine who sees their health information, but still gives **covered entities** (a healthcare provider, a clearinghouse, or a health insurance plan) the leeway to access PHI needed to care for patients, collect payment for services rendered, and operate a business. Protected health information is any piece of information that identifies a patient—it includes a patient's name, DOB, address, e-mail address, and telephone number; his employer; any relatives' names; social security number; medical record number; account numbers tied to the patient's account; fingerprints; any photographs of the patient; and any characteristics about the patient that would automatically disclose his or her identity (for instance, "the governor of the largest state in the United States."

In addition, PHI includes the medical information that is tied to the person, including diagnosis, test results, treatments, and prognosis; documentation by the care provider and other healthcare professionals; and billing information.

Covered entities include any healthcare entity that captures or utilizes health information. These include healthcare plans (insurance companies), clearinghouses that process healthcare claims, individual physicians and physicians' practices, any type of therapist (mental health, physical, speech, occupational) and dentists; the staffs of hospitals, ambulatory facilities, nursing homes, home health agencies, and pharmacies; and employers.

HIPAA states (and HITECH enhances) that only persons who have a need to know may have access to a patient's PHI. And, to take it a step further, they are only entitled to access to the **minimum necessary information** required to do their jobs. An example would be a covered entity such as a health insurance company that is working on a claim for a patient who underwent coronary artery bypass three months ago. Unless they can prove otherwise, the minimum necessary information they need is the supporting documentation related to the bypass surgery. The fact that the patient delivered a child in 1980 has nothing to do with the bypass surgery, and therefore they do not need access to those records.

There are many ways that facilities protect the **privacy** and **confidentiality** of their patients. Privacy is the right to be left alone; in other words, no one should infringe upon a patient's time or personal space while being treated. Confidentiality is keeping a secret; in healthcare, it means keeping information about a patient to oneself. Patients have the right to expect that their medical information is going to be kept confidential. Written policies and ongoing education of staff are two very important aspects of complying with the HIPAA and HITECH rules.

Privacy and confidentiality policies should address, at a minimum:

- Release (disclosure) of information to outside sources only upon written authorization of the patient/legal representative. Release to inside sources (access) is only on a need-to-know basis. The policy should also address any exceptions, for instance to an insurance company, to public health officials in cases of mandatory reporting (infectious diseases, for example), and to licensing and accrediting agencies.
- Release of **directory information** without a written authorization. Directory information includes the fact that the patient is in the hospital (or is being treated at an ambulatory facility) and his or her room number.
- Written guidelines and examples of what is considered minimum necessary information.
- Faxing of documentation—information that can and cannot be faxed and also the protocol to be followed should information be faxed to the wrong location!
- Computer access and lockdown—policy requires staff to lock their computers down (sign out) if they are going to be away from their desk for any length of time.

- Password sharing—makes it a disciplinary offense to share one's password with another.
- Computer screens—should be kept out of view of the public or anyone else who might have access to areas with computers.
- Shredding any hard-copy documents (where applicable) rather than just discarding them.
- Signing by patients of a **Notice of Privacy Practices** so that they are aware of how their personal health information will be used. The Notice of Privacy Practices must be in writing, signed by the patient, and informs the patient how his or her health information will be used, reasons it may be released, notice that he or she may view or have copies of the health record and may request amendments to it, and the procedure for filing a complaint with the Department of Health and Human Services.
- Requirement that all staff (including care providers) sign a document committing themselves to keeping private and confidential the information that is written, spoken, or overheard about any and all patients.

An example of a shredding policy statement in an office that no longer keeps hard-copy records (a "paperless environment") is:

The electronic health record is the legal health record at Greensburg Medical Center. Printed copies should only be made when there is a need to refer to the printed document rather than the computerized image. Once the printed document is no longer needed, it is to be placed in the marked shred bins immediately. Shred bins are located in the business office and in the secure area of the front office. The only exception to this policy is the printed copies made for patients' requests, or that are to be mailed by the Release of Information Specialist.

In addition to the policies noted above, security-specific policies should address:

- Password Protection—Every computer user must have a unique code or **password** that is known (and used) only by the user. Passwords should not be something that can be easily discerned; for instance, the user's birthdate, spouse's name, child's name, phone number, etc., would not be secure passwords. Instead, the password should be a combination of numbers and letters, at least six digits in length, and the system should be set up to prompt users to change their password at least every 90 days. Individual offices and facilities will set policies regarding their password configuration requirements.
- Appointment of a security and/or privacy officer—someone in the facility must be named as privacy and security officer, though these may be two different individuals. The privacy/security officer is ultimately responsible for setting, monitoring, updating, investigating, and enforcing all privacy and security policies.

- Log-in attempts—the system set-up should include automatic lock-out when a user attempts to log in a certain number of times (usually three) with the wrong password. The policy and procedure should also address how to regain access.
- Protection from computer **viruses** and **malware**. This should include the facility's policy on downloading music or other attachments that may carry viruses and malware. A virus is a "deviant program, stored on a computer floppy disk, hard drive, or CD, that can cause unexpected and often undesirable effects, such as destroying or corrupting data. Malware comes in the form of worms, viruses, and Trojan horses, all of which attack computer programs."[1]
- Security audits—a policy should be set and carried out that requires random security audits to monitor access to patients' records. Often, this may be done on a rotating basis by staff members, or it may be done based on a random selection of patients in the database. Of course, the investigation of any rumored or known breaches should include a security audit.
- Off-site access—with the use of current technology, many PMs and EHRs can be accessed via the Internet. Policies must dictate who can access remotely as well as what information can be viewed and/or edited remotely.
- Printing policies—the more information is printed from the EHR or PM software, the more chance there is of unauthorized disclosure. Print only when absolutely necessary.
- Detailed policies and procedures that address privacy or security incidents. Disciplinary action should be addressed in this policy as well.
- Staff education—requirement that all staff (including care providers) participate in continuing education opportunities to reinforce the laws governing privacy and security.
- E-mail—it is a part of everyday life, not just in our personal lives but in our work lives as well. Anything written in an e-mail is protected information. However, it is not a secure means of communication, and the facility should adopt policies related to the sending and receiving of e-mail messages, including what, if any, patient-related information can be sent via e-mail. E-mails, like faxes, can go to the wrong individual, constituting a privacy breach. There must be a policy regarding patient-related e-mails or e-mails to or from patients—are they a part of the patient's health record, and if so, how will the e-mail become part of the record? E-mails should be **encrypted**, which means the words are scrambled and can only be read if the receiver has a special code to decipher it, but encrypting still does not ensure total security. Encryption applies to any information that is electronically transmitted.

[1]Williams, B.K. and Sawyer, S.C. (2010). *Using Information Technology: A Practical Introduction to Computers & Communications*, 9e. New York, NY. McGraw-Hill Companies.

Firewalls should also be used to deter access to the system by unauthorized individuals. Williams and Sawyer define a firewall as "a system of hardware and/or software that protects a computer or a network from intruders."[2]

Hardware also has to be protected, and policies must be written to govern the security of hardware devices. Hardware includes desktop computers, laptop computers, hand-held devices and the like. These devices are always at risk for loss or theft. But to protect the information on a device, follow these simple rules:

- Always lock-down the device and require a password to log on
- Never store the passwords to any of your hardware devices or sites on the computer
- Back up your files onto a CD, external hard drive, or flash drive
- Encrypt PHI if policy allows health records to be stored on it
- Use the portable devices in a secure area—using one in the cafeteria and walking away to freshen your coffee is not secure
- Wipe the hard drive of any computers that are taken out of use before recycling them or placing them in the trash

Privacy and security need to be kept in mind at all times in a healthcare facility. Not doing so, even if unintentionally, may result in fines ranging from $100 for each violation up to $250,000 for multiple violations. Or, if the breach was intentional, the fines start at $50,000 per violation and extend to $1,500,000 for multiple violations.

Healthcare organizations using an EHR must meet the HIPAA standards of privacy and confidentiality. In addition, states may have even more stringent rules. The American Recovery and Reinvestment Act of 2009 (ARRA), through HITECH, made the rules regarding privacy and security of electronic systems more stringent yet. Accounting of disclosures is one area that will affect hospitals and practices alike. Facilities must be able to provide a patient with a listing of disclosures, if requested; this is known as **accounting of disclosures**. Also, facilities with an EHR must be able to provide a patient with a listing of people who had access to their protected health information. This is known as an **access report**. The access report must contain the name of the individuals who accessed that person's record, and also the names of persons who do not work at the facility who had access to the record. For instance, a hospital may grant a local nursing home admissions department the right to view the health record of a patient who is being considered for nursing home placement. This is required to assess whether or not the nursing home has the facilities needed to care for that patient, and is part of the continuum of care; thus, it is a necessary release. The hospital would note, in the access report, that the patient's PHI was released to a certain nursing home, but would not be able to supply the names of the individual(s) who accessed it at the nursing home.

[2]Williams, B.K. and Sawyer, S.C. (2010). *Using Information Technology: A Practical Introduction to Computers & Communications*, 9e. New York, NY. McGraw-Hill Companies.

According to the Office of the National Coordinator for Health Information Technology (ONC) website, "Health information technology (health IT) makes it possible for health care providers to better manage patient care through secure use and sharing of health information." Health IT includes the use of electronic health records (EHRs) instead of paper medical records to maintain people's health information.

To better manage patient care using electronic means, however, it is necessary to comply with certain regulations. The HIPAA rules that address electronic health information are listed in Table 7.1.

Regarding passwords, though longer passwords are more secure than shorter ones, the most secure passwords include a combination of letters (upper and lower case), symbols, and numbers.

TABLE 7.1	Functionality of an EHR as required by HIPAA regulations
Functionality	**Meaning**
Password Protection	Passwords must be assigned to all users of an electronic health record system and the passwords must meet certain criteria: length, properties, expiration intervals, and number of log-in attempts before lock-out.
User Identification	Each user must have a unique identifier to log in. Often consists of the person's first initial and last name. Allows for tracking and reporting of activity within the system by the user.
Access Rights	Policies are written and adhered to regarding access to functionality within the EHR that is dependent on the person's (or position's) need to know.
Accounting of Disclosures	Upon authorized request, an accounting of all disclosures from a patient's health record, going back a minimum of 6 years from the date of request, must be provided. The patient's health record must also be made available to the patient, or to an outside entity at the patient's request.
Security/Back-up/ Storage	A back-up of the EHR database must be kept in a secure location, and restoration of the back-up database must be possible at any given time. Other security requirements include controlled access to the database, use of passwords to access the database, use of firewalls, anti-virus programs, etc.
Auditing	The ability to run reports by user or by patient, that specify the menu, module, or function accessed; the date and time of the access; whether the information was viewed, edited, or deleted; and the user ID of the individual staff member.
Code Sets	The EHR must use ICD-9 codes, CPT codes, and HCPCS codes to store and transmit information.

The password "summerday" is more secure than "summer", for example, yet "summer18$#" is even more secure. Healthcare organizations set their own policies regarding the length and configuration of passwords.

It may be the office administrator who starts the search for EHR software and keeps in mind the requirements of a compliant system. Other individuals who should also be involved in researching, selecting, and implementing the EHR include a representative of care providers, a member of the front office (reception) staff, a clinical staff representative, health information staff, coding/billing staff, and an information technology (IT) professional who is an expert in the technological aspects of the software and hardware, networking, and interoperability of systems. This group should always keep in mind:

- The required components of a compliant EHR
- The needs of the office or facility
- The intended budget for acquiring a system as well as yearly budget requirements
- Staff and training needs
- The intent of the EHR—is it to interface with the existing PM system, or will an entirely new system that accomplishes both be purchased?
- The time line—what is the target date for implementation?

7.3 The Role of Certification in EHR Implementation

There are many agencies that certify EHR software. Both the information technology (IT) and the health information technology (HIT) aspects of an EHR system must be taken into consideration, and during the process of assessing various systems and vendors, looking at certified EHR systems is a good place to start.

Through HITECH, the ONC was given authority to establish a certification program for EHRs. The ONC, through consultation with the Director of the National Institute of Standards and Technology, recognizes programs for this voluntary certification if they are in compliance with certification criteria.[3]

The Healthcare Information and Management Systems Society (HIMSS) is an independent, non-profit organization with the mission "To lead healthcare transformation through the effective use of health information technology."[4] HIIMSS and the American Health Information Management Association (AHIMA) are

---

[3]Department of Health and Human Services. "Proposed Establishment of Certification Programs for Health Information Technology; Proposed Rule." *Federal Register* 75, no. 46 (March 10, 2010): 11327–11373. Retrieved from http://edocket.access.gpo.gov/2010/2010-4991.htm.

[4]HIMSS. (2011) About HIMSS. Retrieved from http://www.himss.org/ASP/aboutHimssHome.asp.

professional associations that are highly respected in the fields of Information Technology (IT) and Health Information Management (HIM). Each has myriad sources, references, guides, best practices, and practice briefs for use in the selection and implementation of an EHR, and both organizations highly value certification.

In 2004, The American Health Information Management Association (AHIMA), the Healthcare Information and Management Systems Society (HIMSS), and the National Alliance for Health Information Technology (NAHIT) organized the Certification Commission for Health Information Technology (CCHIT). Its mission is to create a non-government, non-profit organization that would certify EHR software, and it was called the Certification Commission.

The mission of CCHIT, as found on its website, is to ". . .accelerate the adoption of robust, interoperable health information technology."[5] CCHIT is an independent, non-profit organization that certifies EHR systems.

Other certifying agencies include InfoGard, Drummond Group, Inc., and ICSA Labs, to name just a few. The ONC-certified Health IT Product List can be found at http://onc-chpl.force.com/ehrcert/.

Selecting a product that is certified is good business practice and will save the office administration much of the leg work necessary to ensure selection of a product that not only meets the needs of the organization, but has already been tested and proven to meet regulatory requirements.

It is worth a student's time to view this listing, select one or more products, and view the ONC criteria that has been met by each.

7.4 Applying Security Measures

Assigning passwords, allowing access to only the functions that are necessary to perform a job, and following the other policies outlined in Section 7.1 all play a role in assuring the privacy, confidentiality, and security of the health information stored in your facility's PM and EHR systems.

The next two exercises apply basic security measures in Prime-SUITE. These functions will usually be set up by the office administrator or manager.

Adding Users to PrimeSUITE

EXERCISE 7.1   Go to http://connect.mcgraw-hill.com to complete this exercise.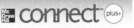

Add a New Clinical User and Assign a Password

In this scenario, the office manager has just hired a new MA, Kevin Goodell, and he is going to set Kevin up as a user in PrimeSUITE. Certain information is needed from Kevin before the office manager begins the

[5]Certification Commision for Health Information Technology. (2011). Retrieved at http://www.cchit.org/

set-up process. You will notice that the password "greenway" is used in the initial set-up of Kevin Goodell. In the examples used throughout the worktext, the default password is "greenway." In an actual work setting, this default password would be changed to a password of the user's choice that meets the practice's password requirements.

Field	Value
Full name	Goodell, Kevin
Username	kgoodell
E-mail	kgoodell@greenwaymedical.com
Sex	Male
Telephone number	(770) 555-1234
DOB	07/08/1958
Soc. Security No.	123-45-6789

Follow these steps to complete the exercise on your own once you have watched the demonstration and tried the steps with helpful prompts in practice mode. Use the information provided in the scenario above to complete the information.

1. Click **User Administration.**
2. Click **Add New.**
3. The ***Username** field is filled out. Press the tab key to confirm your entry.
4. The **Email** field is filled out. Press the tab key to confirm your entry.
5. The **SSN** field is filled out. Press the tab key to confirm your entry.
6. The ***First Name** field is filled out. Press the tab key to confirm your entry.
7. **Tab** is now pressed to bypass the middle name field.
8. The ***Last Name** field is filled out. Press the tab key to confirm your entry.
9. **Tab** is now pressed again to advance past several fields.
10. The **Contact Number** field is filled out. Press the tab key to confirm your entry.
11. The **Date of Birth** field is filled out. Press the tab key to confirm your entry.
12. Click ***Sex.**
13. Clicking the entry **male** selects it.
14. Click **Must Change Password At Next Login.**
15. Click **Save.**
16. The ***New Password** field is filled out. Press the tab key to confirm your entry.
17. The ***Confirm Password** field is filled out. Press the tab key to confirm your entry.
18. Click **OK.**
19. Click **OK.**

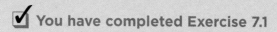 **You have completed Exercise 7.1**

EXERCISE **7.2** (PM) (EHR) (HIM) Go to http://connect.mcgraw-hill.com to complete this exercise. **connect** plus+

Set Up a Care Provider

In our next scenario, there is also a new care provider starting this week, Daisy Logan, M.D. The office manager will set her up in the system, assigning a user ID and user rights.

The information necessary before beginning the set-up process is:

Field	Value
Full name	Logan, Daisy
Sex	Female
Credentials	MD
NPI number	1234567890
State Medical License number	234567
DEA Number	GA123456
On staff at Greensburg Medical Center	Yes
Provides billable services from Greensburg Medical Center	Yes
Assigned User ID	dlogan

PrimeSUITE tip

When a box is checked in the PrimeSUITE exercises, the check mark will not appear until after the information box.

Follow these steps to complete the exercise on your own once you have watched the demonstration and tried the steps with helpful prompts in practice mode. Use the information provided in the scenario above to complete the information.

1. Click **Care Providers.**
2. The ˙**Last Name** field is filled out. Press the tab key to confirm your entry.
3. The ˙**First Name** field is filled out. Press the tab key to confirm your entry.
4. Click **Sex.**
5. Clicking the entry **Female** selects it.
6. Click ˙**Credentials.**
7. **M** is now pressed.
8. **MD** is selected from the drop-down list.
9. The **National Provider Identifier** field is filled out. Press the tab key to confirm your entry.
10. The **State License Number** field is filled out. Press the tab key to confirm your entry.
11. **Tab** is pressed to advance past the State Controlled Substance Number.
12. The **DEA Number** field is filled out. Press the tab key to confirm your entry.
13. Click **On Staff?**
14. Click **Billable?**

15. Click **Set User ID.**
16. The ˙**Username** field is filled out. Press the tab key to confirm your entry.
17. Click **Search.**
18. Click **Daisy.**
19. Click **Select.**
20. Click **Save.**

☑ **You have completed Exercise 7.2**

Setting User Rights for Staff

We will take security functions a step further by adding **user rights.** Log-on rights simply mean that one is assigned a log-in and password to allow access to the computer software, in our case, PrimeSUITE. The user is then assigned user rights, which are privileges that limit access to only the functionality of the software needed by that individual. The position held and job description of each staff member (including care providers) dictate what privileges each person has.

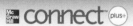   Go to http://connect.mcgraw-hill.com to complete this exercise. **EXERCISE 7.3**

Assign User Rights to an MA

In the scenario that follows, John Greenway is an office manager. He will be setting up the user rights for Kevin Goodell, an MA who is new to the office. We will start by setting up Chart rights from the action bar on the left side of the screen. Chart rights have to do with viewing, adding, editing, or changing documentation within patients' charts. For instance, Kevin will be able to access the Patient Chart page of every patient. He will have access to a very extensive allergy module, which will include setting up a patient's allergy shot schedule, dosage calculations, and similar applications. Of course, *he will do this based only on the physician's orders.* John will be able to delete vital signs from a Facesheet; reasons for this may be that the vitals were incorrectly typed into the Facesheet, or were put on the wrong patient's chart, or that the healthcare professional who entered the blood pressure, for example, did not get an accurate reading. *These privileges are very sensitive and are only given to appropriate staff members with the expertise and position within the practice to warrant such rights.* But even deleted, the original documentation is not lost forever—hidden is actually a better description for it—there is an *audit trail* that shows the original documentation, and then the corrected version. The topic of data integrity and versions of documentation will be covered in more detail later in this chapter.

Custom views of the Facesheet can be set up in many EHR software packages, PrimeSUITE included. The information displayed is consistent, but the way it looks on the screen is different. Some MAs or nurses are granted the right to sign off on lab results; *that right is determined by office policy (and may vary by care provider) as well as level of knowledge of the individual.* An example would be a standard blood test, such as a CBC, that is completely within normal limits on an established patient; the care provider may feel that an experienced MA or nurse is qualified to sign off on those results without

(continued)

sending them through for review by the care provider. The same applies to some prescriptions. The care provider may give a verbal order to an MA or nurse for a prescription renewal to be called in to the patient's pharmacy or refilled by ePrescription. For example, Robyn Berkeley is a long-time patient of Dr. Rodriquez. She has a long-standing prescription for metronidazole for treatment of her rosacea, and she has run out; the MA gives Dr. Rodriguez the request, and he then authorizes her to send through a refill via ePrescirbe. The MA is able to access and print (or electronically transmit) the prescription renewal with Dr. Rodriquez's digital signature.

User rights for all registration functions are also set up; if the healthcare professional works in the reception and registration areas, she would have user rights to any routine daily functions including registering a patient for the first time, editing demographic information, scheduling an appointment, checking a patient in or out, viewing alert flags, and so on.

System rights affect just that—the overall system. The rights you will see in this exercise include importing documents that do not originate within PrimeSUITE and accessing patient tracking.

Follow these steps to complete the exercise on your own once you've watched the demonstration and tried the steps with helpful prompts in practice mode. Use the information provided in the scenario above to complete the information.

1. Click **User Rights.**
2. Click **Current User.**
3. Clicking the entry **Kevin Goodell** selects it.
4. Click **Chart.**
5. Clicking the entry **Chart** selects it.
6. Click **Access the Patient Charts Page.**
7. Click **Allergy Module-Can modify serum sheet status.**
8. Click **Allergy Module-Override EP rules.**
9. Click **Facesheet-Delete vitals.**
10. Click **Facesheet-Manage problem list custom views.**
11. Click **Lab Flowsheet-Initial a lab or revoke initials.**
12. Click **Orders-Add to orders favorite list.**
13. Click **Orders-Edit/delete from orders favorite list.**
14. Click **Prescriptions-Access ePrescribe.**
15. Click **OK.**
16. Click **Prescriptions-Can edit medication alert override.**
17. Click **OK.**
18. Click **Prescriptions-If a digital signature other than this user's is saved with a prescription, allow printing of the signature.**
19. Click **OK.**
20. Click **Save.**
21. Click **Registration.**
22. Click **View Patient or Person Registration Information.**
23. Click **Modify Patient or Person Registration Information.**
24. Click **View Patient List.**
25. Click **Check-In patients**
26. Click **Undo Check-Out.**
27. Click **View and Modify Chart Patient Flags.**
28. Click **View Clinical Alerts Flags.**
29. Click **Save.**

30. Click **System.**
31. Click **Document Import.**
32. Click **Access Document Import.**
33. Click **Save**
34. Click **Patient Tracking.**
35. Click **Access Patient Tracking.**
36. Click **Save.**
37. Click **Close.**

☑ You have completed Exercise 7.3

Setting User Rights for a Manager

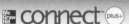 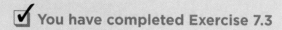 Go to http://connect.mcgraw-hill.com to complete this exercise.   **EXERCISE 7.4**

Assign User Rights to an Office Manager

Office managers or administrators have increased functionality such as setting up files in accounts receivable management, chart configuration and administration, registration screens, research (clinical trial) functionality, reporting, scheduling, and overall system configuration. As you go through the exercise that follows, in which you will assign rights to Jennifer Pierce, take a look at the entire list of rights that are assigned. The research category pertains to participation in clinical trials that are run by the Food and Drug Administration.

Follow these steps to complete the exercise on your own once you have watched the demonstration and tried the steps with helpful prompts in practice mode.

1. Click **User Rights.**
2. Click **Current User.**
3. Clicking the entry **Jennifer Pierce** selects it.
4. Click **A/R Management.**
5. Click **Select All.**
6. Click **Save.**
7. Click **Chart.**
8. Clicking the entry **Chart Admin** selects it.
9. Click **Select All.**
10. Click **Save.**
11. Clicking the entry **Research** selects it.
12. Click **Select All.**
13. Click **Save.**
14. Click **Registration.**
15. Click **Select All.**
16. Click **Save.**
17. Click **Reporting.**
18. Click **Select All.**
19. Click **Save.**

(continued)

20. Click **Scheduling.**
21. Click **Select All.**
22. Click **Save.**
23. Click **System.**
24. Click **Select All.**
25. Click **Save.**
26. Click **Close.**

✔️ **You have completed Exercise 7.4**

Setting Up a Group

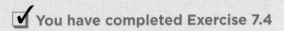 EXERCISE **7.5**   Go to http://connect.mcgraw-hill.com to complete this exercise.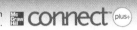

Create a Group

In the previous exercises, we have been working with just one staff member. In this exercise we will set up an entire group within PrimeSUITE. Setting up groups, such as all medical assistants, all receptionists, all care providers, etc., allows the office administrator to give rights by group rather than having to set up each person individually. Of course, if some of the users within the group have higher-level rights, then their profile can be modified by adding rights individually.

In Exercise 7.5 we will be working within the Group Administration module of the Systems Menu. Essentially, a group is formed and the individual staff members are moved into it, and finally the group is named. Or, a group may already exist and staff members are moved into it. The other advantage of groups is that if an e-mail needs to be sent to an entire group, for instance, the health records staff, then just one e-mail needs to be sent rather than to each staff member. An example would be that the health records staff is required to attend an in-service meeting on HITECH regulations at 2:00 p.m. on August 5th. Just one message can be sent to the entire group notifying them of this in-service meeting.

Follow these steps to complete the exercise on your own once you've watched the demonstration and tried the steps with helpful prompts in practice mode.

1. Click **Group Administration.**
2. Click **Allison Tubiak (atubiak).**
3. Click the arrow: **Move highlighted item to selected list.**
4. Click the **scroll button.**
5. Click **Jennifer Brady (jbrady).**
6. Click **Move highlighted item to selected list.**
7. Click **Jared Howerton (jared).**
8. Click **Move highlighted item to selected list.**
9. Click **Kevin Goodell (kgoodell).**
10. Click **Move highlighted item to selected list.**
11. Click **Save Group.**
12. Enter **MAs** in the **Group Name Field.** Press the tab key to confirm your entry.
13. Click **Save.**
14. Click **Enable Messaging.**
15. Click **Save Group.**

✔️ **You have completed Exercise 7.4**

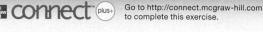
Set General Security

General security settings involve password maintenance. To complete the exercise, you will need the following information regarding Greensburg Medical Center's security policies:

Configuration Setting	Value
Password length	7 characters
Password change occurs	Every 90 days
Maximum inactivity before system automatically logs off	30 minutes
No. of days before password can be re-used	364 days
Log-in banner	Good Morning Greensburg!

for your information

Thirty minutes maximum inactivity before system automatically logs off is a long period of time; many offices set the maximum time limit to 15 minutes or less.

Follow these steps to complete the exercise on your own once you have watched the demonstration and tried the steps with helpful prompts in practice mode. Use the information provided in the scenario above to complete the information. There are already some values that appear in the exercise, so we will not be covering every setting.

1. Click **System Configuration.**
2. The **Min Password Chars** field is filled out. Press the tab key to confirm your entry.
3. The **Days Password Valid** field is filled out. Press the tab key to confirm your entry.
4. **Tab** is now pressed to advance past the Visit Search Max Row Count field.
5. The **Inactivity Limit** field is filled out. Press the tab key to confirm your entry.
6. The **Days Prevent Password Reuse** field is filled out. Press the tab key to confirm your entry.
7. Click **Save.**
8. Click **OK.**

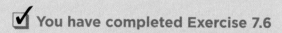 **You have completed Exercise 7.6**

Audit Trails

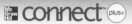
Run an Audit Trail Report

In this exercise, an **audit trail** report will be run. This functionality helps to fulfill the HITECH requirement to provide an accounting of disclosures (or, in this case, accesses to a record), or it may be used to monitor activity of a certain staff member or activity in general in a particular area of the EHR software.

(continued)

Our objective in this exercise is to view the Vitals History accesses over the past month by one of the staff members with the user ID of "greenway."

Follow these steps to complete the exercise on your own once you have watched the demonstration and tried the steps with helpful prompts in practice mode.

1. Click **Report Selection . . . F7.**
2. Click **System.**
3. Click **Audit Log Report.**
4. Click **Report Type.**
5. Click the **scroll button.**
6. Clicking the entry **Vitals History** selects it.
7. Click **User.**
8. **g** is now pressed.
9. Click **greenway.**
10. Click **Date.**
11. Click **Month To Date.**
12. Click **Immediate View.**
13. Click **Print.**
14. Click **Print.**

☑ **You have completed Exercise 7.7**

7.5 Data Integrity

Data integrity refers to the accuracy, timeliness of collection, the consistency of definitions used to collect the data, and, in addition, there is an expectation that there has been no manipulation or tampering with the data once it has been collected and reported. To maintain **data integrity**, the healthcare facility must have strict policies regarding who may access data, the definition of a complete record, accuracy of data, consistent applications of data dictionary definitions, and the timeliness of data entry. Think of it this way: if a patient is seen on Wednesday, but the documentation in the health record is not entered until Friday, how accurate do you think it will be? Or, if one of the staff members instructs a patient to document his past surgical history, but to only include surgeries done under general anesthesia in the past five years, yet the office policy shows a data dictionary definition of surgery as *any* procedure the patient has had while under local, regional, or general anesthetic at any time in the past, then how consistent is the data? What about a healthcare professional who finds a blood pressure reading of 152/80 in a patient, yet enters it as 140/80 and knowingly leaves it as is, figuring it is "close enough." If you were a care provider using the information found in your EHR database, and you knew poor documentation practices were occurring, you wouldn't have much faith in using that data would you? Or, if you were conducting a research study and knew that the data was flawed, how valid would the study be? In other words, any data found within the health record must be accurate, complete, and documented at the time of or as close to the time of occurrence as possible.

Amending a Chart Entry

Integrity also applies to the addition, amendment, or omission of documentation that has already been recorded. Any alteration in the original documentation must be recoverable. With the use of paper records, if an entry in a health record was amended or corrected, it was obvious. See Figure 7.1 for an example of a proper chart correction. You can see readily that the entry was corrected; originally, it read that the patient had sustained a laceration to her right hand, when in fact, it was the left hand. A single line was drawn through the incorrect word, the correct word was inserted, and the correction was initialed and dated by the person who made the correction.

The patient sustained a
4 cm laceration to her
left (mbs 6-10-11)
~~*right hand three days ago.*~~

Figure 7.1 Example of correction to paper documentation

In an electronic record, original documentation that is found to be incorrect or incomplete may be hidden from view, and the amended information becomes part of the health record and is all that is viewable to the healthcare professional or care provider; however, that original hidden documentation can be recovered at any time. Our next exercise illustrates amendment of an entry in PrimeSUITE.

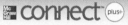

Go to http://connect.mcgraw-hill.com to complete this exercise.

EXERCISE 7.8

Amend a Chart Entry

William Jackson's record contains an error in the progress note. The care provider documented the HPI of William Jackson, but after she completed documenting and saved the note, she noticed a word was misspelled. She accesses the progress note of the chart and makes the correction. Notice, while going through the exercise, that in order to make the correction, the care provider must enter her password in order to change an entry. This additional step allows the care provider to think twice about amending the entry to be certain it is necessary and that the information she is about to add is correct. The original progress note with the error is known as version 1 and the corrected progress note as version 2.

Follow these steps to complete the exercise on your own once you've watched the demonstration and tried the steps with helpful prompts in practice mode.

1. Click **Documents.**
2. Click **Progress Note.**
3. Click **Amend Document.**
4. Click **HPI.**
5. A letter "s" is added to the end of the word "present." Press the tab key to confirm your entry.
6. Click **Save & Sign.**
7. The **Password:** field is filled out with **greenway.** Press the tab key to confirm your entry.
8. Click the **green check mark.**
9. Note the lower left corner of the action bar.

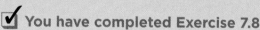 **You have completed Exercise 7.8**

Hiding a Chart Entry

   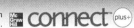

Hide a Chart Entry

There are times when documentation is added to the wrong chart, or when misinformation is given or documented. In these cases, we would need to hide an entry. As noted above, though the entry is hidden, it is still retrievable at a later time. Our next exercise steps us through hiding an entry on William Jackson's chart. In this case, it is a progress note that was intended for another patient's chart. Typically, only certain staff members such as those who are in lead or administrative positions have this user right. This is not a procedure that is done often, nor is it done without a valid reason. Reasons might be that the note was put on the wrong patient's chart, or that the note pertains to that patient but not to that particular visit. Some software vendors use the term *deleting* rather than *hiding*, but regardless, the deleted/hidden entry will *always* be retrievable should the record be needed in a lawsuit, to verify some sort of inconsistency, or for insurance purposes.

Follow these steps to complete the exercise on your own once you have watched the demonstration and tried the steps with helpful prompts in practice mode.

1. Click **Documents.**
2. Click **Manage Chart Documents.**
3. Click **04/11/2011.**
4. Click **Delete.**
5. Click **Yes.**
6. Click **Other.**
7. The **Other** field is filled out with **wrong patient.** Press the tab key to confirm your entry.
8. Click **OK.**

✔ **You have completed Exercise 7.9**

Recovery of a Hidden Entry

   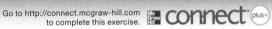

Recover a Hidden Chart Entry

Hiding a document does not mean that it is truly deleted forever. The original documentation can be retrieved by accessing the Documents Menu and then accessing Manage Chart Documents from the action bar.

Follow these steps to complete the exercise on your own once you have watched the demonstration and tried the steps with helpful prompts in practice mode.

1. Click **Documents.**
2. Click **Manage Chart Documents.**
3. Click **View Deleted Docs.**
4. Click **04/11/2011.**
5. Click **Undo Delete.**
6. Click **Yes.**
7. Click **Accidental Delete.**
8. Click **OK.**

✔ **You have completed Exercise 7.10**

Another requirement of Meaningful Use initiatives is to share health information with other healthcare professionals when necessary. For instance, Virginia Hill is a patient of Dr. Ingram's, and he is referring her to a specialist. It is important for the specialist to know her medical history and the reasoning for the referral; therefore, information is released electronically. This reason is known as continuity of care.

Many releases require a written authorization from the patient or legal representative. The specifics of release of information regulations will be covered in another course. For our purposes, we will be accounting for the disclosure. Release of information in the case of this referral would not require an authorization, nor would release of information to an insurance company for purposes of payment of the claim, nor release of information to public health agencies, as required by law. Written authorization is required for all releases of information to physicians' offices or hospitals that are not a result of a direct referral, attorneys, employers (if not a Workers' Compensation claim), spouse, children, and law enforcement agencies. Also, certain records such as those related to drug and alcohol abuse, mental health, and HIV/AIDS have more stringent release of information regulations; those will be discussed in great detail in another course.

Releasing information without a required authorization is known as a **breach of confidentiality**. Offices and healthcare facilities are required to report breaches, as was discussed earlier in this chapter, as part of the HITECH regulations. Not only is the office or facility held liable for any breaches, but individual staff members may be as well.

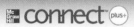 Go to http://connect.mcgraw-hill.com to complete this exercise.   **EXERCISE** **7.11**

Compose a Correspondence Letter to Accompany the Release of a Patient's Immunization Record

Now, let's look at an exercise where a correspondence letter is accompanying the release of immunization records of a patient, Ian Mikeals, to a day care center as requested by the child's mother.

Ian Mikeals has had the following vaccines: Hepatitis B, Pentacel (DTaP – IPV/Hib), PCV13, and ProQuad (MMRV).

Follow these steps to complete the exercise on your own once you've watched the demonstration and tried the steps with helpful prompts in practice mode. Use the information provided in the scenario above to complete the information.

1. Click **Search for Patient.**
2. The *Last Name* field is filled out. Press the tab key to confirm your entry.
3. Click **Search.**
4. Click **Select.**
5. Click **Patient Charts.**

(continued)

6. Click **Create Note.**
7. Click **Correspondence.**
8. Click **Select Template.**
9. Click **Notification of Release of Immunization Record.**
10. Click **WHICH VACCINES WERE GIVEN?**
11. Click **Hepatitis B.**
12. Click **Pentacel (DTaP - IPV / Hib).**
13. Click **Pneumococcal conjugate (PCV13).**
14. Click **ProQuad (MMRV).**
15. Click the **Next** arrow.
16. Click **Sincerely.**
17. Click **Save & Sign.**
18. The **Password:** field is filled out with **greenway.** Press the tab key to confirm your entry.
19. Click the **green check mark.**
20. Click **Print/Fax Document.**

✔️ You have completed Exercise 7.11

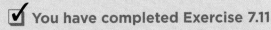

7.7 Accounting of Information Disclosures

An accounting of the releases is also necessary in order to comply with regulations. As noted above, most releases require a written authorization, but to comply with HITECH, *all* releases must be accounted for, whether the disclosure is to internal staff members or external requestors.

EXERCISE 7.12   Go to http://connect.mcgraw-hill.com to complete this exercise.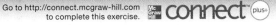

Run a Report of Information Disclosures for a Particular Patient

In this scenario, the office manager needs to run a report of information disclosures (or, in this case, access) of the chart of a patient, Megan Hallertau, whose chart ID is 19927. She is particularly looking for disclosures (accesses) to one of the staff members, Bob Denney, who has a user ID of bdenney, that were made today.

Follow these steps to complete the exercise on your own once you have watched the demonstration and tried the steps with helpful prompts in practice mode. Use the information provided in the scenario above to complete the information.

1. Click **Report Selection. . . F7.**
2. Click **System.**
3. Click **Audit Log Report.**
4. Click **User.**
5. The letter **b** is pressed.
6. The **Patient ID** field is filled out. Press the tab key to confirm your entry.
7. Click **Component.**

8. Clicking the entry **Chart** selects it.

9. Click **Immediate View.**

10. Click **Close.**

11. Click **Close Report.**

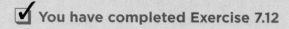 **You have completed Exercise 7.12**

7.8 Information Exchange

Communicating with other healthcare providers is another Meaningful Use requirement. It is known as **Health Information Exchange (HIE)**. An advantage of utilizing an EHR is that patient care improves through the sharing of patient information at the point of care. With this functionality, care providers can access the findings of other physicians or test results immediately. Of course, this sharing is done through a secure environment, and there are regulations that address telecommunications and networking security as well. Secure e-mail is one way that information can be shared between providers, the National Health Information Network (NHIN) Exchange is another, and there are state and private HIE programs as well. The State HIE Cooperative Agreement Program operates through use of ONC funding, and its purpose is to coordinate local HIEs or serve as the HIE for a given area.

for your information **fyi**

Using a search engine, take the time to find your state's HIE on the Internet; each HIE has its own site and includes valuable information for care providers and staff.

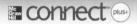 Go to http://connect.mcgraw-hill.com to complete this exercise.   **EXERCISE 7.13**

Exchange of Information for Continuity of Care

In this scenario, Ian Mikeals is a pediatric asthma patient of Dr. Ingram. Dr. Ingram is referring Ian to a pediatric asthma specialist.

Follow these steps to complete the exercise on your own once you've watched the demonstration and tried the steps with helpful prompts in practice mode.

1. Click **Document Import.**

2. Click **Data Submission.**

3. Click **Referral Summary (XDS-MS).**

4. The **Reason for Referral** field is filled out with **asthma.** Press the tab key to confirm your entry.

5. Click **Preview.**

6. Click **Print.**

7. Click **Close.**

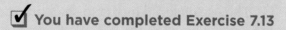 **You have completed Exercise 7.13**

Exchange of Information Outside the Organization

There is another type of information exchange that has nothing to do with continuity of care, business purposes, or insurance purposes. It involves communicating *about* care via **social media**. Social media includes Facebook, YouTube, Twitter, **blogs** (ongoing conversations about a topic that take place on-line), and the like). These outlets are used by patients to share their experience with a healthcare organization or to recount their journey through an illness; they can also be used by the organizations themselves as a means of marketing or public relations. Take a look at the Facebook page of Children's Hospital, Boston, for example, found at http://www.facebook.com/#!/ChildrensHospitalBoston?sk=info. Here you will find videos, testimonials, facts and figures about its patient population, and links to other related sites, as well as support groups and blogs, awards the organization has won, and a link to its social media policy, which is short, to the point and, in summary, states that while all comments are welcome, they should not be offensive, should be on-topic, and should not violate the privacy of patients or their family.

There is some risk in allowing patients to provide comments since not all of them will be positive, but by the same token, they are a vehicle to promote the institution, its accomplishments, and its services. They are also a service to the community by including needed information about the organization as well as links to related sites such as public health, educational sites, and support groups.

Employees of an organization also use social media (Facebook, Twitter, and LinkedIn, for example) and may contribute to blogs about their organization. Since what they say and how they say it can sometimes be misconstrued, it is imperative that healthcare organizations develop a policy to address the use of social media; and it should include this information:

- Circumstances under which an employee may access any social media site during work hours.
- Employees should maintain a positive tone in their posts, and be respectful of the organization and its staff when posting on an organization-sponsored site.
- The PHI of patients should *never* be posted (directly or implied).
- The identity of any patients (directly or implied) should *never* be posted
- No copyrighted materials should be posted.
- No information about the organization may be posted, as this is the responsibility of the marketing or public relations department.
- Penalties or potential disciplinary action for failure to comply with the organization's social media policy.

The use of social media to share information about a particular person, which is set up and maintained by someone authorized by the patient with the objective of keeping family and friends updated on the patient's condition, is gaining popularity. One such site is Caring Bridge (www.caringbridge.org). What the patient or family cares to share on this site is under their control, but healthcare professionals who are or were involved in the patient's care need to be careful. A posting that you intend to be caring and helpful may be misinterpreted and perceived as intrusive by the family, so before posting, you should think twice about what you want to say and how you say it!

7.9 Compliance Plans

Think of all the regulations that affect healthcare—HIPAA, ARRA, HITECH, not to mention Medicare, Medicaid, and managed care plan requirements; it is a daunting task to ensure compliance with all of them. Having a formal compliance plan is key to surviving the regulatory maze. Think of a compliance plan as your office or facility's policies that assure regulations are followed, and use it as a check-sheet to assure that staff and care providers in your office or facility are following your own policies, which in turn ensure the following of rules and regulations. A compliance plan should include:

- A named compliance officer—a staff member who keeps up with new regulations, monitors existing ones, and is the "go-to" person, should an incident occur that is not in compliance.
- Written policies that cover, at a minimum:
  - Routine daily operations (registration, scheduling, human resources, etc.)
  - File back-up
  - Computer access (both physical access as well as access to software and databases)
  - Release of patient information
  - Breach of confidentiality, including unauthorized disclosure
  - Security breaches, internal and external
  - Coding and billing (including anti-fraud and -abuse practices)

Policies should be kept in a location accessible to all office staff. All policies should also include the disciplinary process, should policies not be followed, intentionally or unintentionally.

An example of a Policy Statement regarding computer access and use of passwords may read:

> *Access to computer software, databases, and equipment shall be restricted to employees (including care providers) of Greensburg Medical Center. The extent to which access and rights are given is based on position description in order to carry out their job duties. Employees (including care providers) are required to keep their log-in user ID and password confidential; sharing with others is grounds for immediate disciplinary action, up to and including dismissal.*

Reporting of compliance with Meaningful Use is also required; specific compliance strategies to conform with Meaningful Use will be covered in Chapter 9.

The use of formal internal audits, which should be performed on every staff member (including care providers) on a periodic basis, not only allows the administrative staff to be proactive in finding and correcting problems, it also serves as a reminder and an educational tool for staff.

7.10 Safeguarding Your System and Contingency Planning

Protecting computer hardware and software is as important as protecting the information within the systems. Computer crime, unauthorized access to information, and natural disasters are all security concerns that must be addressed within any healthcare organization that processes or stores digital data.

Written policies as noted in Section 7.9 are deterrents at a very basic level, in particular, regarding controlling access. Restricting access in offices or areas where computers are present to employees only, turning computer screens away from public view, and shredding printed documents that include patient information are all examples. **Encryption** of data is necessary to deter unauthorized access to what is documented. Tracking the computer accesses of all employees on a periodic basis helps ensure that access is only on a need-to-know basis. Carefully screening job applicants and verifying previous employment are additional important screening mechanisms, since people are the greatest threat to computer security.

Backing up data on a daily basis is crucial. Back-up can be made to online secondary storage, hard disk, optical disk, magnetic tape, and/or flash memory. A key component of back-up is that the backed-up files sholud be stored at an off-site location. Should a fire or flood occur in your office, and the back-up files are also damaged by the flood, they do little good.

Recent worldwide disasters have shown the need for having a **disaster recovery plan**. The plan must be written and staff must know what to do in the event of a disaster that affects the computer systems within the facility.[6]

At a minimum, the plan should include:

* An accounting of all functions that are performed electronically within the office
* A listing of all computer hardware, software, and data related to each of those functions
* The specific location of the back-up files and the format used for the back-up
* Step by step procedures for restoring the backed-up data
* An alert system to notify personnel of the disaster
* Required security training for all personnel

Unfortunately, many facilities lack a disaster recovery plan and may not realize its importance until a data loss, security breach, or other disaster occurs. Not only should the facility have a plan, they should actually carry out the plan periodically as any other disaster plan would be practiced.

The importance of keeping *all* computerized functions safe, confidential, and secure cannot be overstated.

[6]Williams, B.K. and Sawyer, S.C. (2010). *Using Information Technology: A Practical Introduction to Computers & Communications*, 9e. New York, NY. McGraw-Hill Companies.

chapter 7 **summary**

LEARNING OUTCOME	CONCEPTS FOR REVIEW

7.1 Identify the HIPAA privacy and security standards. pp. 129–133	– HIPAA passed in 1996
	– Contains, privacy and security rules, among others
	– HITECH made HIPAA rules more stringent and gave government authorities the power to enforce the privacy and security rules
	– The intent is to ensure protected health information (PHI) is private and secure
	– Covered entities include any healthcare facilities, health plans, clearinghouse, or other businesses that handle PHI
	– Only minimum necessary information may be released
	– Standards include:
	  • Define directory information
	  • Use of authorization to release PHI
	  • Enforce minimum necessary information release
	– Password configuration and protection
	– Appointment of a privacy and/or security officer
	– System configured to minimize number of log in attempts
	– Protection from viruses and malware
	– Use of security audits to monitor access
	– Policy to address remote access to the system
	– Policy on use and protection of hardware, particularly wireless devices
	– Written policy and procedures on breach notification
	– Staff education

7.2 Evaluate an EHR system for HIPAA compliance. pp. 134–135	**HIPAA Regulations and the EHR** – Password protection – Use of unique identifier for each user – Access to PHI only for those who have a need to know – Accounting of all disclosures (internal and external) – Security policy that addresses back-up of data, storage, and restoration of backed-up data – Ability to audit by user or by patient who has accessed a record, and which area(s) of the record were viewed, edited, or deleted – Use of code sets—ICD-9-CM, CPT, and HCPCS to store and transmit information
7.3 Describe the role of certification in EHR implementation. pp. 135–136	– CCHIT organized by AHIMA, HIMSS, and NAHIT in 2004 – Mission is to accelerate the use of an interoperable health information technology – Role is to certify EHR systems that meet all requirements of HIPAA and HITECH

LEARNING OUTCOME	CONCEPTS FOR REVIEW
7.4 Apply procedures to set up security measures in PrimeSUITE. pp. 136–144	– Add new clinical users – Assign password to new clinical users – Set up a care provider's user rights – Assign user rights to a healthcare professional (medical assistant) – Assign user rights to an office manager – Create a group – Set general system-wide security requirements – Run an audit trail report
7.5 Apply procedures to ensure data integrity. pp. 144–146	– The integrity of data can be ensured only if it is complete, accurate, consistent, timely, and has not been altered, destroyed or accessed by unauthorized individuals – Strict organization-wide policies that are adhered to must be in place – Amendments and deletions to entries must be obvious, and the original format must remain – Amend a chart entry – Hide a chart entry – Recover a hidden chart entry
7.6 Apply procedures to release health information using PrimeSUITE. pp. 147–148	– Release of information is necessary for a multitude of reasons, including continuation of care – Authorization to release information may be required, and must be addressed in written organization policies – Must account for all disclosures to comply with HITECH – Compose correspondence and release immunization record using PrimeSUITE
7.7 Account for data disclosures using PrimeSUITE. pp. 148–149	– Internal and external disclosures of PHI must be accounted for – Run a report of information disclosures from a patient's chart
7.8 Exchange information with outside healthcare providers for continuity of care using PrimeSUITE. pp. 149–150	– Meaningful Use standards require exchange of information between providers for smooth continuation of care – Sharing of electronic information must be through secure means – Exchange information for continuity of care using PrimeSUITE
7.9 Outline the content of compliance plans. p. 151	– Healthcare organizations must have written compliance plans that address how the organization ensures compliance with all regulations governing operation of the organization as well as privacy, security, Meaningful Use, and general health information regulations – Written policies must be kept and available to all staff at all times
7.10 Appraise the importance of contingency planning. pp. 151–152	– Contingency plan is equivalent to a back-up plan, should the system fail or a natural or other disaster occur – All potential security concerns should be addressed with a detailed back-up plan – A written Disaster Recovery Plan should be in effect

chapter **review**

MATCHING QUESTIONS

Match the terms on the left with the definitions on the right.

_____ 1. **[LO 7.4]** breach

_____ 2. **[LO 7.1]** confidentiality

_____ 3. **[LO 7.1]** hardware

_____ 4. **[LO 7.4]** audit trail

_____ 5. **[LO 7.1]** virus

_____ 6. **[LO 7.1]** covered entity

_____ 7. **[LO 7.1]** password

_____ 8. **[LO 7.10]** disaster recovery

_____ 9. **[LO 7.1]** directory

_____ 10. **[LO 7.1]** encryption

a. person or group who has legal right to access protected health information by virtue of being a healthcare provider, clearinghouse, or health insurance plan

b. private, secure code that allows a user access to computer systems and software

c. security measure in which words are scrambled and can only be read if the receiving computer has the code to read the message

d. listing of patient information, such as hospital room number

e. plan for addressing critical issues in the event of a crisis

f. permanent record of the changes made to various documents; available even after files are deleted

g. a break or failure of security measures that results in information being compromised

h. devices such as laptops, PDAs, and desktop computers that are at risk for theft

i. keeping information about a patient to oneself

j. deviant program, stored on a computer floppy disk, hard drive, or CD, that can destroy or corrupt data.

MULTIPLE-CHOICE QUESTIONS

Select the letter that best completes the statement or answers the question:

1. **[LO 7.6]** In the event of a breach, who may be held responsible?
   a. Providers
   b. Office staff
   c. The facility
   d. All of the above

2. **[LO 7.1]** Which of the following would be considered a covered entity?
   a. Healthcare provider
   b. Friend
   c. Significant other
   d. Teacher

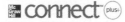 Enhance your learning by completing these exercises and more at http://**connect.mcgraw-hill.com**!

3. **[LO 7.4]** Of the following, which factor contributes to the access rights allowed a user?
   a. Annual job performance
   b. Job description
   c. Level of education
   d. Number of patients seen

4. **[LO 7.10]** It is critical that back-up files be stored:
   a. in paper form.
   b. offsite.
   c. onsite.
   d. with the originals.

5. **[LO 7.7]** HITECH regulations require that _____ information releases are accounted for.
   a. all
   b. external
   c. internal
   d. no

6. **[LO 7.2]** According to HIPAA regulations, healthcare providers must use _____ as opposed to written diagnoses to store and transmit information to insurance carriers.
   a. CPT codes
   b. ICD-9 codes
   c. HCPCS codes
   d. all of the above

7. **[LO 7.3]** Meaningful Use standards require offices to select an EHR that is:
   a. certified.
   b. cheap.
   c. fast.
   d. simple.

8. **[LO 7.6]** Releasing information without proper authorization is called a/an:
   a. breach of confidentiality.
   b. breach of trust.
   c. information breach.
   d. security breach.

9. **[LO 7.5]** When a document is amended or changed in an EHR, the original documentation is:
   a. deleted.
   b. hidden.
   c. printed.
   d. visible.

10. **[LO 7.9]** An office's compliance manual should be kept in a/an _____ location.
    a. accessible
    b. external
    c. electronic
    d. protected

11. **[LO 7.8]** The sharing of health information must be done in a _____ environment.
    a. healthcare
    b. private
    c. public
    d. secure

12. **[LO 7.4]** Under a care provider's order, medical assistants and nurses _____ allowed to send an ePrescription or call in a refill prescription to a pharmacy.
    a. are
    b. are not
    c. might be
    d. should not be

13. **[LO 7.1]** To help guard against security breaches, e-mails containing protected health information should be:
    a. deleted.
    b. encrypted.
    c. forbidden.
    d. sent.

14. **[LO 7.3]** The mission of CCHIT is to:
    a. actively promote the use of smartphones.
    b. ensure information security.
    c. increase the implementation of EHR systems.
    d. train facilities on HIPAA regulations.

SHORT ANSWER QUESTIONS

1. **[LO 7.2]** According to the ONC website, how does health information technology help care providers manage patient care better?

2. **[LO 7.6]** Define continuity of care.

3. **[LO 7.1]** List at least four ways to keep information stored on your computers and hardware safe.

4. **[LO 7.5]** Why must a user enter her password in order to change a chart entry in PrimeSUITE?

5. **[LO 7.9]** List at least six pieces of information that must be included in an office's compliance plan

6. **[LO 7.10]** List the six pieces of information that form the minimum requirements of a disaster recovery plan.

7. **[LO 7.4]** List three responsibilities that fall into the office manager's or office administrator's job description.

8. **[LO 7.3]** What does it mean if an EHR system has been certified by the Office of the National Coordinator?

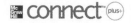 Enhance your learning by completing these exercises and more at http://connect.mcgraw-hill.com!

9. **[LO 7.1]** Explain what a security audit is, and list one example of when a security audit might need to take place.

10. **[LO 7.8]** Explain one advantage of using an EHR for communicating with other health-care providers as discussed in the text.

11. **[LO 7.9]** What is the best way to ensure that your office is following all the different regulatory bodies governing healthcare?

12. **[LO 7.7]** Why must an office manager account for all information released, including those released internally?

13. **[LO 7.4]** Would a care provider and a medical assistant be assigned the same rights in PrimeSUITE? Why or why not?

14. **[LO 7.2]** List six things that an office's EHR team should keep in mind when rolling out a new system.

15. **[LO 7.10]** List three methods to safeguard computer hardware and software systems.

APPLYING YOUR KNOWLEDGE

1. **[LOs 7.1, 7.8]** Discuss two advantages and two disadvantages of using e-mail to send information between providers.

2. **[LOs 7.1, 7.2, 7.4, 7.9, 7.10]** Discuss why many practices require users to change their passwords after a specified period, and why they do not allow users to reuse the same passwords over and over again.

3. **[LO 7.3]** Imagine that you are working in a small healthcare practice. Your supervisor has asked you to spearhead the adoption of an EHR program. Follow the link provided in the text to find the website listing certified EHRs. After browsing the site and looking at the sheer number of products listed, discuss some methods your healthcare office could use to choose the best EHR option.

4. **[LOs 7.5, 7.6]** Provide an example of both an internal and an external Breach of Confidentiality that might occur in a healthcare setting, and list a possible consequence of each breach. (For example, letting a temporary employee access a patient's chart with your username would be an internal breach; a consequence could be that a patient's health information is compromised when the temp accidentally sends the patient's chart information out in an accidental "reply all" e-mail.)

5. **[LOs 7.1, 7.4, 7.5, 7.9, 7.10]** You are in the office cafeteria getting some water. One of your colleagues is at her desk, working on a laptop. She gets up to join you at the water cooler. As the two of you are talking, another staff member sits down in your colleague's chair and begins using the laptop to check her e-mail. What is wrong with this scenario?

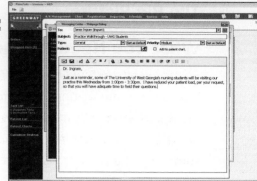

Management of Information and Communication

Learning Outcomes

At the end of this chapter, the student should be able to:

8.1 Use software as an internal communication tool.

8.2 Differentiate the steps used to import documents using scanning technology.

8.3 Build master files and templates using PrimeSUITE.

8.4 Create custom screens within PrimeSUITE.

8.5 Develop a task list within PrimeSUITE.

8.6 Set up system flags within PrimeSUITE.

Key Terms

Default values
Flags
Internet
Intranet
Live

Master file
Optical character recognition (OCR)
Resolution
Scanner
Templates

The Big Picture

What You Need to Know and Why You Need to Know It

So far in this text, we have mainly looked at information being collected. In this chapter we will look at communicating that information. The information collected in a healthcare environment is shared with external sources such as public health agencies, Medicare, insurance companies, and professional organizations. The information included may be in the form of a summary of a patient's chart, a report that answers a question, such as the local public health office asking how many cases of flu-related illnesses were seen during a given time period, or a piece of correspondence from one care provider to another. Additionally, the communication may be internal—within the facility. With PM and EHR software, communicating internally through use of an internal e-mail system is efficient. Information is key to almost everything we do, personally and professionally, so having the information we need at our fingertips and communicating that information accurately and in a timely fashion are key a to a well-run organization. Taking it a step further, patients who receive timely, accurate information and who experience good communication within the practice will have more confidence in the practice as a whole.

8.1 | Internal Communications

The **Internet** is a series of networks that allows instant access to information from around the world. Internet sites may be private, requiring a user ID and password to gain access, or they may be public sites that are viewable by anyone. Within an organization, however, the **intranet** exists. An intranet is a secure environment or private internal network that is available only to a select group, e.g., the staff, within an organization. Examples of what might be shared on an intranet site include:

Facility's mission and value statements	Directory of staff and care providers	Compliance officer's name and contact information
Policies and procedures	FAQs	Forms, publications, newsletters
Organization charts	Office meeting minutes	Calendar of events
Link to the IT department	Calendar of upcoming events	Internal webmail link

The intranet is a one-stop-shop of all the information needed to stay informed about a company and a way to send and receive messages from colleagues. Of course, someone (usually a webmaster) has to keep the information up-to-date; otherwise, the outdated information is not information at all, and there is no benefit to having an intranet. When staff starts noticing that the site is not being kept current, they will stop accessing it and information will no longer be shared. If your current employer does have an intranet, take some time to really navigate it—look for the information stated above, and see if you can find other useful information there.

The use of internal messaging improves communication within an office. It is particularly helpful in avoiding the "no one ever told me" syndrome. When internal e-mail is used to communicate work-related information, and is not cluttered with personal communications, it is even more valuable. Many organizations have policies regarding work e-mail for personal use, and though they may not mandate that it cannot be used as a personal means of communication, such use is most likely frowned upon and may lead to more stringent policies. Some offices use a priority rating on their work-related e-mails. This is particularly helpful to the care providers in sifting out what needs to be done immediately versus what can wait for a later time. High-priority messages would include patient care matters, medium priority would include changes in meeting dates or time-sensitive information, and low priority might be information such as lunch is ready in the lounge or FYI messages. When establishing rules for the priority system, everyone should at least be clear on what is and *is not* considered high priority.

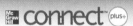 Go to http://connect.mcgraw-hill.com to complete this exercise.   **EXERCISE 8.1**

Send an Electronic Message Using PrimeSUITE Messaging

In this exercise we will look at carrying out an internal communication using PrimeSUITE. In the exercise that follows, Dr. Ingram is to attend an EMR meeting, but the date and time have been changed. In this instance, the message would only be sent to Dr. Ingram; if the message were for all of the care providers, then it would be sent using a group rather than typing in one name.

This function is accessible from the desktop screen.

Follow these steps to complete the exercise on your own once you have watched the demonstration and tried the steps with helpful prompts in practice mode. Use the information provided in the scenario above to complete the information.

1. Click **No unread messages.**
2. Click **Compose Message.**
3. The **To:** field is filled out with **jingram.** Press the tab key to confirm your entry.
4. Press **Tab** again to advance to the next field.
5. The **Subject:** field is filled out with **EMR Meeting.** Press the tab key to confirm your entry.
6. Click **Priority:.**
7. Click **Medium.**
8. The **Salutation** (Dr. Ingram) is added. Press the tab key to confirm your entry.

 for your information

You learned earlier in this text that the terms *electronic medical record (EMR)* and *electronic health record (EHR)* are often used interchangeably. At Greensburg Medical Center, EMR is the preferred terminology.

(continued)

9. The message body (Just as a reminder, the EMR meeting this week has been moved to Thursday at 3:30 p.m.) is filled out. Press the tab key to confirm your entry.
10. Click **Send message.**
11. Click the "x" to **Close.**

☑ **You have completed Exercise 8.1**

8.2 Importing Documents to the EHR

Communication involves many forms other than e-mail messages. Reports, test results, or verifications of insurance coverage, just to name a few, are communicated many times throughout the day. These reports may be sent to the practice in digital or hard–copy format but in the end must be merged into the appropriate patient's record.

For example, Dr. Ingram sent Max Shaw to Memorial Hospital for a chest x-ray. The x-ray is completed and the report of the radiologist's findings is sent electronically to Greensburg Medical Center. It then needs to be merged (attached) to the patient's chart—the flow of this is depicted in Figure 8.1.

Not all documents can be sent electronically, however. Case in point—let's say a patient, David Malone, had his chest x-ray at Duffields Hospital, which does not have electronic capability yet. Instead, the report of the x-ray findings is in hard–copy form only. It can be faxed, mailed, or picked up from the hospital by a staff member. Since the goal of Greensburg Medical Center is a paperless office with a unit record for all patients, a hard–copy image would need to be manually scanned into the EHR once it arrives at the office (Figure 8.2).

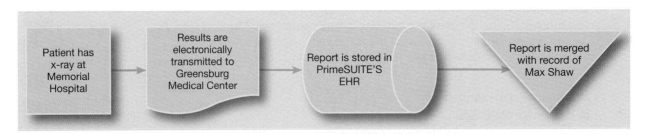

Figure 8.1 Flow of report from hospital to merging with appropriate record in PrimeSUITE

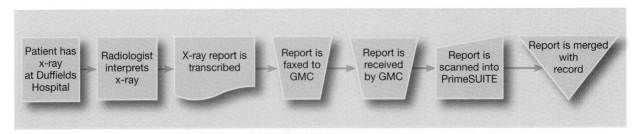

Figure 8.2 Flow of faxed report from hospital to PrimeSUITE

When a hard–copy document needs to be scanned, the health-care professional simply feeds the document through the scanner (or lays the document flat on a screen) (see Figure 8.3), follows the prompts that appear on the computer screen, and finally merges (attaches) the document with the proper patient's record within PrimeSUITE. The process of scanning is much like the process of making a photocopy. Just as a hard-copy document can be misfiled, so can a scanned image. Before a scanned image is attached to a patient's health record, the healthcare professional verifies that the correct patient and the correct visit are selected. Also, the type of document (correspondence, authorization, history or physical exam, for example) may be bar-coded so that the document is easily retrievable electronically.

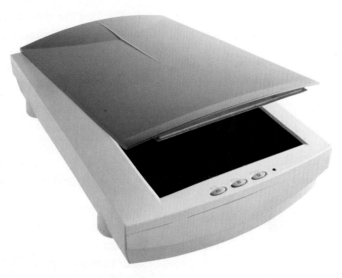

Scanners digitize documents into a format that is readable by the computer. The scanning of documents utilizes **optical character recognition** technology to convert the document into a format that is computer readable. There are other scanning functions that you may be aware of and may not even realize it—in a grocery store, the cashier passes the bar code from a can of green beans across a small light source;

Figure 8.3   Scanner used to import a document

he has just scanned the bar code so that the computer reads it as a 15.5-ounce can of green beans with a price of $1.25. In that case, the optical reader has read a bar code rather than words. This process not only results in a price for the item, it is also part of an inventory control system—the person(s) responsible for re-order now know that there is one less can of beans on the shelf!

Mc Graw Hill **connect** plus+   Go to http://connect.mcgraw-hill.com to complete this exercise.   **Exercise**   **8.2**

Scan an Insurance Card into a Patient's Record

In the scenario that follows, Jessie Hamilton's insurance card is scanned using a desktop scanner at the time he checks in. Once it is scanned, the document is merged (attached) with Jessie's chart in PrimeSUITE. If your doctor's office is automated, the next time you arrive for an appointment and present your insurance card, watch this process. In all, it only takes a minute. In the exercise that follows, you are asked to enter the **resolution**, that is, the quality of the image as it will appear in the record. Obviously, in a legal record, the highest resolution would be selected.

Follow these steps to complete the exercise on your own once you have watched the demonstration and tried the steps with helpful prompts in practice mode. Use the information provided in the scenario above to complete the information.

(continued)

1. Click **Document Import.**
2. The ˙**Last Name** field is filled out. Press the tab key to confirm your entry.
3. Click **Search.**
4. Click **Select.**
5. Click **Quick Scan using existing scanner settings.**
6. Press **Click to move all pages to Selected list** (double arrows).
7. Click **Select Document Type:.**
8. Clicking the entry **Insurance Card** selects it.
9. Click **Save Resolution.**
10. Click **Quality (High).**
11. Click **Save.**

✓ **You have completed Exercise 8.2**

8.3 **Master Files and Templates**

Care providers and all healthcare professionals are extremely busy. Their first concern is the patient, not documentation. So, to make documenting easier and faster, **master files** (datasets that provide structure and are the building blocks for parts of the chart notes) and **templates** (preformatted documents built into the PM and EHR systems) are used. If you think back to the exercises in Chapter 4, you saw many master files. Figure 8.4 is an example of a master file for selecting conditions in a patient's past medical history.

At Greensburg Medical Center, before the EHR went **live** (in use in real time), members of the staff built these master files with input from care providers. Master files list common conditions and diagnoses that patients at Greensburg Medical Center have had. Diagnoses can be added to an individual's record, or to the master file itself. Other master files in PrimeSUITE include PE, ROS, orders, diagnosis favorites, and HPI.

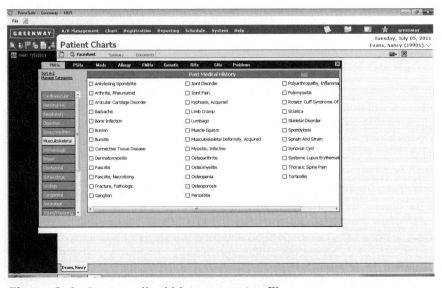

Figure 8.4 **Past medical history master file**

Building templates within the system is an administrative task that is done prior to going live, but they can be added to as necessary. Templates are preformatted documents that allow screenshots to be built, letters to be written, and progress notes to appear out of individual selections from master files. Care providers may prefer their documentation to look a certain way, so a practice that has five care providers may have five templates for written progress notes.

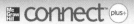
   EXERCISE 8.3

Build a Master File in PrimeSUITE

To build a master file in PrimeSUITE, the Desktop will be accessed and then Review of Systems Admin will be selected from the Chart menu. In the exercise that follows, we will build the master file for Review of Systems (ROS). The end product will be indicative of what this care provider wants as the **default values** (the value that automatically appears in a field) on the ROS screen and appears each time he sees a patient. For instance, the care provider wants the default value for weight loss to be a negative response; in other words, if a patient is asked if she has experienced unexplained weight loss, most of the time the answer will be no; therefore, this response will show as (-) weight loss on the ROS screen.

Setting up these default values is done from the System Set-Up module on the Chart menu.

Follow these steps to complete the exercise on your own once you have watched the demonstration and tried the steps with helpful prompts in practice mode.

1. Click **Review of Systems Admin.**
2. Click **Constitutional.**
3. Clicking the entry **fatigue** selects it.
4. Clicking the entry **weight loss** selects it.
5. Click **Genitourinary.**
6. Click **urgency.**
7. Click **frequency.**
8. Click **dysuria.**
9. Click **Save.**

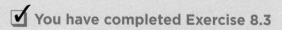 You have completed Exercise 8.3

8.4 Customization

Care providers, registration staff, medical assistants, nurses, therapists, billers, and coders all use the information in the PM and EHR software. But not all of the users "see" things the same way. The way information and subsets of information display in relation to one another on a computer screen is often most effective when the user is satisfied with how the information appears. Much PM and EHR software includes flexibility to allow customization of screen configurations, and PrimeSUITE is no exception. Care providers and healthcare professionals in general will be more accepting of an EHR if they know they have some say in the appearance of the information.

EXERCISE 8.4   Go to http://connect.mcgraw-hill.com to complete this exercise.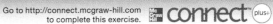

Customize a Facesheet Screen

We will now look at a couple of exercises where customization is possible. The first task is to customize a Facesheet screen. In this scenario, the healthcare professional is going to customize a Facesheet. He starts by entering the User Settings Admin within the System Setup module that is in the Chart menu. Watch as he chooses the elements that will show on the Facesheet, and then how he changes the order in which they appear.

Follow these steps to complete the exercise on your own once you have watched the demonstration and tried the steps with helpful prompts in practice mode.

1. Click **User Settings Admin.**
2. Clicking the **Facesheet & History** tab selects it.
3. Click **History Sections.**
4. Click **Facesheet Sections.**
5. Click **Save User Preferences.**
6. Click **Patient Charts.**
7. Click **Customize Facesheet.**
8. Click **Reason For Visit.**
9. Click **Allergy List.**
10. Click **Clinical Alerts.**
11. Click **Confidential.**
12. Click **Family Medical History.**
13. Click **Flowsheets.**
14. Click **Medication List.**
15. Click **Orders Tracking History.**
16. Click **Past Medical History.**
17. Click **Past Surgical History.**
18. Click **Problem List.**
19. Click **Social History.**
20. Click **Task List.**
21. Click **Visit History.**
22. Click **Vital Signs.**
23. Click anywhere to the left of the **Customize Facesheet** menu to close it.
24. Drag **Medication List.**
25. Drop on **Confidential.**

In addition to the Facesheet, the desktop can also be customized to meet the individual user's preferences.

 You have completed Exercise 8.4

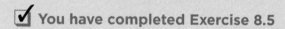

Customize a Clinical Desktop

Watch as this user sets up the Desktop (the first screen that appears when a user logs on) to meet her needs and preferences.

Follow these steps to complete the exercise on your own once you have watched the demonstration and tried the steps with helpful prompts in practice mode.

1. Click **Customize Desktop.**
2. Click **Patient List.**
3. Click **Use Clinician Desktop.**
4. Click **Show Orders Tracking.**
5. Click **Show Unsigned Documents List.**
6. Click **Show Task List.**
7. Click **Section First.**
8. Clicking the down-arrow opens a drop-down list.
9. Click **Patient List.**
10. Click **Save.**

☑ **You have completed Exercise 8.5**

8.5 Using Software to Organize Your Work—Task Lists

With all the requirements we deal with in healthcare, having help with organizational skills is certainly an advantage! In PrimeSUITE, there is a functionality called a Task List or Tasks, where a care provider or other healthcare professional assigns tasks to another staff member or to an entire group. For instance, Dianna Pike, a care provider, wants a particular report to be run by the office administrator, Jon Viria. The request is simply put into Jon's task list so that he is aware that he has a task that needs to be completed. Or, if it is a task to be completed by an entire group, for instance, the health information department staff, the task—completion of a computerized in-service—can be assigned to the group rather than to each individual, saving the office administrator much time and ensuring that everyone gets the *same* message!

Some examples of tasks include:

- Renewing magazine subscriptions for the reception area
- Registering for an upcoming seminar
- Calling a patient regarding the need for a follow-up laboratory test
- Making reservations for the office holiday party

As you can see, the tasks may not be clinical in nature; they can be anything that needs to be done by an individual or individuals in the practice.

Copyright © 2012 The McGraw-Hill Companies

Create a Task for the Receptionist

In the scenario that follows, a task is set up for Charlotte Baker to schedule a training session on ePrescribing. The message is "Charlotte, will you please contact Greenway and arrange a training session covering ePrescribe? I would like to have this done between April 15th and May 30th. Thanks!" (without the quotes).

This function also allows the user to select the priority of the task—high, medium, or low. Practice policy may dictate what circumstances dictate each, and whether prioritization is used at all.

Follow these steps to complete the exercise on your own once you have watched the demonstration and tried the steps with helpful prompts in practice mode. Use the information provided in the scenario above to complete the information.

1. Click **Tasks.**
2. Click **Add New Task.**
3. Click **Type:.**
4. Clicking the entry **General Task** selects it.
5. Click **Send To:.**
6. Click **scroll button.**
7. Click **Baker, Charlotte (cbaker).**
8. Click **OK.**
9. Click **Subject:.**
10. The **Subject:** field is filled out with eRX training. Press the tab key to confirm your entry.
11. Click **Due Date**
12. Click **15.**
13. Click **Status.**
14. Clicking the entry **New** selects it.
15. Click **Add Comment:.**
16. The **Comment:** field is filled out. Press the tab key to confirm your entry.
17. Click **OK.**
18. Click **Save & Return.**
19. Click **Close.**

☑ **You have completed Exercise 8.6**

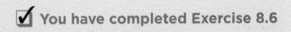

8.6 Using Software as a Reminder

If you work in healthcare you have a lot to remember, as you have already seen. It would be next to impossible to remember every situation about every patient. Using the functionality of PM or EHR software, including PrimeSUITE, makes keeping on top of everything easier, though, by including alerts or reminders in a patient's chart, through a series of flag alerts (reminders), or icons, each of which has a particular meaning.

Flags can be added in the system and can be used for any and all patients.

Examples of common flags include:

- Frequently cancels appointments
- Phone number on file is no longer in service
- Confidentiality messages (such as do not leave message on home phone)
- Co-pay required (and can include amount)
- Patient is noncompliant
- Account in collections
- Do not charge late fee
- Payment plan set up
- Allergic to penicillin (can have several different medications)
- Environmental allergy to _____
- Sensitive information contained in chart
- Clinical alerts
  - Bone density scan due
  - Diabetic patient
  - Requires patient education
  - Pap smear due

A flag can be set up in the system for just about anything the office sees a need for. A word of caution though; do not set up so many flags that it is difficult to remember their meaning, or so that the alert becomes the rule rather than the exception and therefore is ignored!

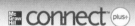 Go to http://connect.mcgraw-hill.com to complete this exercise.   **EXERCISE** **8.7**

Assign a Flag to a Patient's Chart

In our final exercise, you will set up a system flag for a patient. In this case, Jessie Hamilton is allergic to bee stings, so the healthcare professional will add that flag to Jessie's chart.

Follow these steps to complete the exercise on your own once you have watched the demonstration and tried the steps with helpful prompts in practice mode. Use the information provided in the scenario above to complete the information.

1. Click **Search for Patient.**
2. The `Last Name` field is filled out. Press the tab key to confirm your entry.
3. Click **Search.**
4. Click **Select.**

(continued)

5. Click **View/Edit Patient Flags.**
6. Click **Allergic to Bee Stings.**
7. Click **Save.**

So as you can see, computerization of the practice management and health record functions has many other benefits to care providers and staff than just maintenance of the information they collect. The use of software streamlines the processes and increases efficiency as well.

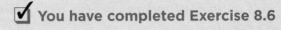 **You have completed Exercise 8.6**

chapter 8 **summary**

LEARNING OUTCOME	CONCEPTS FOR REVIEW
8.1 Use software as an internal communication tool. pp. 160–162	– Difference between Internet and intranet – Examples of information commonly shared on an intranet – Send a message using PrimeSUITE
8.2 Differentiate the steps used to import documents using scanning technology. pp. 162–164	– Reports within a chart are a type of communication – Documents may be imported from within PrimeSUITE or from an external source – Scanning a document involves a process of feeding (or laying flat) the document in the scanner, then attaching the document to the appropriate patient's chart – Scanning digitizes documentation into readable format – Optical character recognition (OCR) allows scanned images to be edited – Scan an insurance card and import it into the record of Jessie Hamilton
8.3 Build master files and templates using PrimeSUITE. pp. 164–165	– A master file is a listing of possible choices, e.g., a list of allergies, list of conditions, list of surgeries – Templates allow for building an end–product such as a progress note, a piece of correspondence, or a screen view – Build a master file for an ROS
8.4 Create custom screens within PrimeSUITE. pp. 165–167	– Allow flexibility and personalization for individual users – Design a Facesheet view for a user
8.5 Develop a task list within PrimeSUITE. pp. 167–168	– Tasks are reminders that a job has been assigned – Can be made by any user – Can be a task set for a single user or a group – Assign a task to a user in PrimeSUITE
8.6 Set up system flags within PrimeSUITE. pp. 168–170	– Flags are alerts or reminders – Use them sparingly; otherwise, they no longer point out the exception to the rule, but rather become the rule – Set up a flag on a patient's record in PrimeSUITE

chapter **review**

MATCHING QUESTIONS

Match the terms on the left with the definitions on the right.

_____ 1. **[LO 8.6]** flag

_____ 2. **[LO 8.5]** task list

_____ 3. **[LO 8.3]** master file

_____ 4. **[LO 8.3]** templates

_____ 5. **[LO 8.1]** intranet

_____ 6. **[LO 8.3]** live

_____ 7. **[LO 8.2]** scanner

_____ 8. **[LO 8.2]** optical character recognition (OCR)

a. secure internal environment available only to a select group

b. device that digitizes documents into a format readable by computers

c. an alert or reminder that appears in a patient's chart

d. dataset that provides structure and is the building block for parts of the chart notes

e. software that allows a saved document to be edited

f. using something in real time

g. area where work can be assigned to staff members and progress can be monitored

h. preformatted documents built into an EHR or PM system

MULTIPLE–CHOICE QUESTIONS

Select the letter that best completes the statement or answers the question:

1. **[LO 8.1]** The Internet is _____ and an intranet is _____.
   a. public; private
   b. private; public
   c. private; private
   d. public; public

2. **[LO 8.2]** A hard–copy document is attached to a patient's electronic chart by:
   a. copying.
   b. e–mailing.
   c. scanning.
   d. shredding.

3. **[LO 8.3]** Using templates makes it easier for care providers to focus on their first priority, which is:
   a. documentation.
   b. patient care.
   c. office staff.
   d. training.

4. **[LO 8.4]** PrimeSUITE allows each user to _____ certain features to their liking.
   a. access
   b. customize
   c. delete
   d. revise

5. **[LO 8.1]** A facility needs to make sure that the information on their intranet does not become:
   a. outdated.
   b. overused.
   c. private.
   d. secure.

6. **[LO 8.6]** It is _____ to have too many flags set up in PrimeSUITE.
   a. impossible
   b. possible
   c. necessary
   d. required

7. **[LO 8.3]** The Review of Systems menu choices in PrimeSUITE is an example of a/an:
   a. index.
   b. master file.
   c. real–time menu.
   d. template.

8. **[LO 8.5]** A healthcare professional may assign work to another user with Prime-SUITE's _____ functionality.
   a. assignment
   b. groups
   c. tasks
   d. workload

9. **[LO 8.6]** Which of the following is another term for "flag"?
   a. Alert
   b. Avatar
   c. Decal
   d. Symbol

10. **[LO 8.4]** Which of the following PrimeSUITE functions may be customized by a user?
    a. Access rights
    b. Insurance policies
    c. Patient information
    d. Screen layout

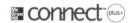 Enhance your learning by completing these exercises and more at http://**connect.mcgraw-hill.com**!

SHORT ANSWER QUESTIONS:

1. **[LO 8.1]** List four things that might be found on an organization's intranet.

2. **[LO 8.3]** Could one medical office have more than one template for a referral letter? Explain.

3. **[LO 8.2]** Explain the process of scanning.

4. **[LO 8.1]** What will happen if an office's intranet is not kept current?

5. **[LO 8.3]** List four advantages of using master files and templates in a healthcare office.

6. **[LO 8.6]** List at least eight common flags used in PrimeSUITE.

7. **[LO 8.6]** Why might it be good to have a "Sensitive information contained in chart" alert pop-up when users access specific patient charts?

8. **[LO 8.5]** Explain how using the Task List function in PrimeSUITE helps to organize work.

9. **[LO 8.4]** Why might healthcare professionals be more accepting of an EHR if they are able to customize it in some way?

APPLYING YOUR KNOWLEDGE

1. **[LO 8.4]** How might a care provider "see" the information display in PrimeSUITE in the same way a patient registration staff member would?

2. **[LOs 8.1, 8.2, 8.6]** As office manager, what are some ways for you to ensure that staff members remember to attach hard–copy documents to the patient charts they are working on?

3. **[LO 8.3]** Discuss two advantages and any potential disadvantages to using templates for communication documents.

4. **[LOs 8.5, 8.6]** You are the office manager for a small practice. Since your office recently implemented an EHR system, you would like to have a staff training session to set forth guidelines and best practices for using system flags. Explain how you would use PrimeSUITE to assist you in your task, and come up with four talking points about proper use of flags and alerts.

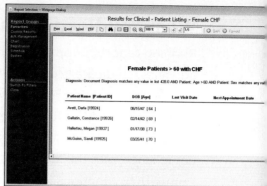

chapter **nine**

Decision and Compliance Support: Utilizing the Database

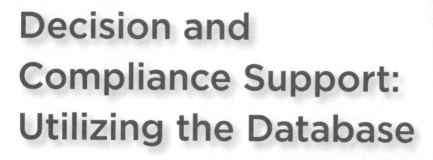

Learning Outcomes

At the end of this chapter, the student should be able to:

9.1 Describe the uses of the dashboard in PrimeSUITE to meet Meaningful Use standards.

9.2 Explain how data and information are used in decision support.

9.3 Set up system reports using PrimeSUITE.

9.4 Set up custom reports using PrimeSUITE.

9.5 Illustrate uses for an index.

9.6 Describe uses for a registry.

9.7 Explain how data gathered in PrimeSUITE is used in the credentialing process.

Key Terms

Aggregate
Benchmarking
Center for Medicare and Medicaid Services (CMS)
Clinical Decision Support (CDS)
Core objectives
Credentialing
Custom report
Dashboard
Detail report
Drug formulary
Healthcare Integrity and Protection Data Bank (HIPDB)

Index
In-network
Meaningful use
Menu objectives
Master Patiet Index (MPI)
National Practitioner Data Bank (NPDB)
Physicians' Quality Reporting Initiative (PQRI)
Query
Registry
Summary report
Variable

Copyright © 2012 The McGraw-Hill Companies

175

What You Need to Know and Why You Need to Know It

Running reports, supplying information to agencies, and ensuring compliance with licensing agencies, Medicare/Medicaid rules, managed care plans, and accrediting agencies are all responsibilities of administrative personnel. This person may be an MA who is an office manager, a health information professional, or a healthcare administrator. Participation in the Meaningful Use incentive program, in particular, will require submission of data that shows compliance with the standards in order to receive incentive grants. In this chapter, we will cover PrimeSUITE functionality that allows us to prove compliance with Meaningful Use, licensing agency, insurance providers, and state and federal reporting requirements.

9.1 Using the Dashboard in PrimeSUITE to Meet Meaningful Use Standards

In order for eligible professionals and hospitals to receive stimulus money, they must successfully show **meaningful use** of electronic health data. In other words, eligible professionals and hospitals that implement (or upgrade) certified electronic health record systems and comply with the core and menu objectives (covered below) will be eligible for monetary grants. The **Center for Medicare and Medicaid Services (CMS)** will administer the program. An agency of the Department of Health and Human Services, CMS is responsible for administering the Medicare program. The **core objectives** that show meaningful use of electronic health information include those listed in

TABLE 9.1	Medicare Core Objectives, 2011
Core Objective	**Explanation**
Use of computerized physician order entry (CPOE)	Medication orders made by care providers are done electronically rather than in writing in a paper record
Drug-drug and drug-allergy checks	An alert system exists, based on the medications and allergies entered for a patient, for potential drug to drug, or drug to allergy effects
ePrescribing	Care providers place prescriptions electronically rather than by paper
Recording of patient demographic information	The following demographics must be collected on all records: – Preferred language – Gender – Race – Ethnicity – Date of birth
Recording of a problem list	A listing of all current and active diagnoses for which the patient is being treated must be maintained

Recording of a medication list	A listing of all current and active medications being taken by the patient; if the patient is on no medications, the record must reflect that as well
Recording of a medication allergy list	A listing of medication(s) to which the patient is allergic
Recording of vital signs	On each visit, the following must be recorded: – Height – Weight – Blood pressure – Body Mass Index (BMI) – Maintenance of a growth chart (for children 2–20 years, including BMI)
Recording of smoking status	For patients 13 years of age and older, smoking status must be recorded
Clinical decision support functionality	At least one clinical decision support rule must be implemented. Example: A patient with a fasting blood sugar above 120 mg/dL may trigger an alert for diabetes mellitus, type 2
Reporting clinical quality measures	Each provider must specify the Reporting Numerators, Denominators, and Exclusions for each quality measure reported
Ability to exchange key clinical information between/among care providers	The capability to share among care providers such information as problem list, medication list, allergies, and diagnostic test results
Ability to provide an electronic copy of health information	Patients must be provided with electronic health information upon request; includes test results, problem list, medication list, and medication allergies
Ability to provide clinical summaries	For each office visit, a clinical summary should be provided to each patient
Privacy and Security provisions	The software in use meets or exceeds standards set forth by the ONC Meaningful Use standards and includes technical specifications that ensure the privacy and confidentiality of information found in the database

Table 9.1. For 2011, meeting the 15 core objectives listed in Table 9.1 is required.

Core objectives are the basic functions that should be completed on a patient's visit or hospitalization.

For hospitals, the core objectives include all of those listed in the table *except* ePrescribing.

The 2011 **Menu Objectives** for Medicare include those listed in Table 9.2. Of the 10 listed, five must be met.

Menu objectives are additional functions that allow for greater use of EHR functionality, for instance running statistical reports, registries, or lists; checking for drug interactions; providing patients with educational materials about their illness; and the like.

TABLE 9.2   Medicare Menu Objectives, 2011

Menu Objective	Explanation
Drug-Formulary Checks	The office or hospital has access to at least one internal or external **drug formulary** (a list of provider-preferred generic and brand-name drugs covered under various insurance plans)
Lab test Results Documented in the EHR	Results of laboratory tests ordered must be entered into the patient's EHR rather than being filed in paper format; results may be entered electronically through electronic data interchange, scanned into the record via manual scanning methods, or manually keyed in to the record from the paper results
Keeping of Patient Lists	The ability to generate a list of patients with a specific condition in order to satisfy quality improvement initiatives, reduce disparities, for research, or for outreach to patients with that diagnosis
Patient Reminders Generated	The ability to send reminder letters (or electronic reminders) for preventive and/or follow-up care
Timely Electronic Access	The ability to provide patients with their electronic record within four business days of the information being available in electronic form
Patient Education	Access to educational resources using EHR technology and providing the resources to patients, if appropriate
Medication Reconciliation	Documentation of medications the patient is taking as prescribed by other care providers
Summary of Care	The care provider submits a summary of care to physicians or another healthcare facility that is assessing the patient or taking over the care of the patient
Immunization Registries	The capability to submit electronic data to immunization registries or other immunization information systems in accordance with applicable law
Syndromatic Surveillance	The capability to submit electronic data to public health agencies in accordance with applicable law

See Figure 9.1 for a Clinical Visit Summary given to a patient at the conclusion of the visit, which would satisfy the Summary of Care objective.

Hospitals must incorporate five of the 10 menu objectives listed in Table 9.2 to be eligible for incentive grants in 2011.

Medicaid–eligible providers (physicians, dentists, nurse midwives, nurse practitioners, or physicians' assistants in rural health clinics), with some restrictions based on percentage of patients who are covered by Medicaid, will qualify for the full stimulus amount in the first year if a practice shows they have adopted, upgraded, or implemented EHR.

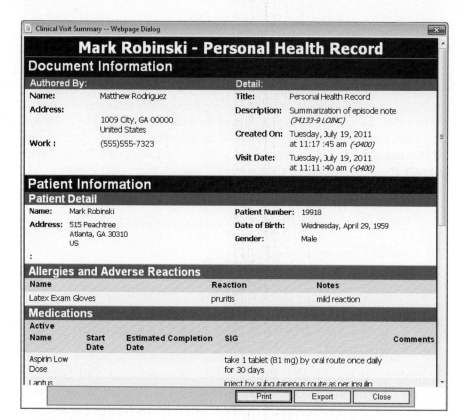

Figure 9.1 Clinical visit summary

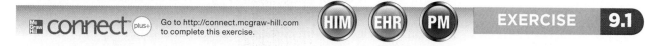

Go to http://connect.mcgraw-hill.com to complete this exercise.

HIM EHR PM **EXERCISE 9.1**

View a Practice's Dashboard

In the scenario that follows, we are going to view the **dashboard** (a visual comparison of actual performance to required performance) of a particular physician, Dr. William Childs. Notice that for each core and menu objective, the provider's performance is compared to the required performance. The office manager, health information professional, or other designated individual should keep close watch on the dashboard to ensure compliance with meaningful use requirements. He or she would then take appropriate action should the percentage of participation fall or should it be apparent that a care provider is in jeopardy of not meeting the threshold. Appropriate action would start with education of the care providers to ensure they all understand the importance of compliance with meaningful use and understand that not complying will put the practice in jeopardy for receiving stimulus funding.

Follow these steps to complete the exercise on your own once you have watched the demonstration and tried the steps with helpful prompts in practice mode.

1. Click **MU Dashboard.**
2. Click **Provider.**
3. The **Search** field is filled out with **Childs.** Press the tab key to confirm your entry.
4. Click **William H. Childs MD.**
5. Click **View.**

Take a few moments to review this dashboard. Notice that 15 of the 15 required core objectives were met. This means that this physician used the

(continued)

PrimeSUITE tip

PrimeSUITE refers to the core objectives as core requirements.

EHR in his practice to fulfill all of the core objectives. Let's look at one of the core objectives—keeping a medication list. The requirement is that more than 80% of all patients seen by the care provider need to have at least one entry (or documentation that the patient is not currently prescribed any medication) as a documented data item. Dr. Childs met this requirement 96.9% of the time—he documented the medication(s) each patient is taking (or that they are not taking any) 96.9% of the time. For charting vital signs, Dr. Childs met that objective in 96.1% of his patients, while the requirement for that objective is that for more than 50% of all patients (age 2 and over), records show documentation of the height, weight, and blood pressure recorded as structured data.

☑ **You have completed Exercise 9.1**

9.2 Data and Information Used in Decision Support

According to the Health Information Management and Systems Society, "**Clinical Decision Support** (CDS) is defined broadly as a clinical system, application, or process that helps health professionals make clinical decisions to enhance patient care. Clinical knowledge of interest could range from simple facts and relationships to best practices for managing patients with specific disease states, new medical knowledge from clinical research, and other types of information" (HIMSS, 2011).

CDS includes reminders and alerts, diagnostic and therapeutic guidance, links to expert resources (CDC, Mayo Clinic, and clinical trials, for example), and results of best practices. Many EHR vendors link directly to one of these expert sites. The trigger that a clinical alert or support should be displayed comes from the data that has already been captured in the patient's record. This is where the data dictionary and structured data that we covered in Chapter 2 apply. In the exercise that follows, the trigger for the alert flag will be the patient's age (calculated by the system), the CPT codes for colonoscopy, and whether or not one of those codes has been assigned to any visit for a patient over the past 5 years (derived from calculating five years prior to the date of the visit). Decision support, or clinical decision support, is a functionality of an EHR whose value cannot be overestimated. Use of CDS tools improves patient safety, decreases duplication of procedures, reduces the performance of unnecessary testing, and as a result reduces the cost of healthcare, while improving patient outcomes, efficiency of care, and provision of clinically relevant, evidence-based care. Clinical decision support tools are built into most EHRs, including PrimeSUITE.

Recall that for 2011, meaningful use requires that at least one clinical support rule be implemented through the use of an EHR, and that there is a means to track compliance. An alert that pops up to ask a patient if he or she has had a colonoscopy does not meet the requirement unless that alert appears based on certain information found in the EHR about *that* patient compared to evidence-based criteria that has been embedded in the EHR software. For instance, an alert for colonoscopy would appear when a patient is 50 years of age and older, and/or there is an entry in the patient's problem list showing a history of rectal bleeding, or a family history of colon cancer is documented in the history section of his chart, and no CPT procedure codes for colonoscopy have appeared in the patient's visit history in the past 5 years.

Of course, if a care provider has this functionality available through the practice's EHR software and does not use it, then it is not beneficial to the patient, to the care provider, to the practice, or to satisfy meaningful use standards. There are still care providers who view CDS systems as "cookbook medicine"; those who find it too time consuming or who are annoyed by the pop-up reminders. One incentive to encourage the use of a CDS is pay-for-performance programs available in certain managed-care plans. In other words, if the practice's fiscal position is improved by using CDS technology, then the care providers are more accepting of CDS systems.

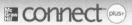 Go to http://connect.mcgraw-hill.com to complete this exercise.   EXERCISE 9.2

Build a Clinical Alert, Part A

In our next scenario, we are going to build a clinical alert in PrimeSUITE. This is a lengthy process for the alert we have chosen, so this will be done in two parts—Exercise 9.2 (Part A) and Exercise 9.3 (Part B).

We are going to build a clinical alert for all patients who are 50 years of age or older who have not had a colonoscopy in the past 5 years. To do this, we will use CPT codes for colonoscopy, of which there are eight. There are many CPT codes for colonoscopy because the codes differ based on the reason for doing the procedure as well as the extent of the procedure. (You will enter these codes in the order code fields in numerical order during the exercise.) The colonoscopy codes are:

45378	45382
45379	45383
45380	45384
45381	45385

These are called "filters," which will select (or exclude) patients from the database who do (or in this case do not) meet certain criteria. In this particular alert we will **query** the database for patients who are 50 years of age or older and who do not have one of the colonoscopy codes listed above attached to any of their visits for the past 5 years; once the alert is set up, their electronic record will then have the red ribbon icon attached to show that a colonoscopy is needed. To query means that we are going to search or "ask" the database for records that meet (or do not meet) the criteria noted in the filters. In our example we are querying the database for patients who are 50 years of age or older and who *do not* have one of the eight colonoscopy codes listed above attached to any of their visits over the past 5 years.

(continued)

Follow these steps to complete the exercise on your own once you have watched the demonstration and tried the steps with helpful prompts in practice mode. Use the information provided in the scenario above to complete the information.

1. Click **Clinical Alerts.**
2. The **Clinical Alert Description** field is filled out with **Pt due for colonoscopy.** Press the tab key to confirm your entry.
3. Click **Clinical Alert Filters.**
4. Under the **Include patients that meet All of the following criteria:** section, click **Field Name.**
5. Click **scroll button.**
6. Click **Patient: Age.**
7. Click **Operator.**
8. Clicking the entry **is greater than or equal to** selects it.
9. The **Match Value** field is filled out with **50.** Press the tab key to confirm your entry.
10. Under the **Include the patients that have NOT had or do NOT meet All of the following criteria:** section, click **Field Name.**
11. Click **scroll button.**
12. Click **Order: Order Code.**
13. Click **Operator.**
14. Click **matches any value in list.**
15. Clicking the entry **Create Match List** selects it.
16. The **Order: Order Code** field is filled out. Press the tab key to confirm your entry. (This is where you will start entering the codes, beginning with **45378.**)
17. Click **Add.**
18. The **Order: Order Code** field is filled out. Press the tab key to confirm your entry.
19. Click **Add.**
20. The **Order: Order Code** field is filled out. Press the tab key to confirm your entry.
21. Click **Add.**
22. The **Order: Order Code** field is filled out. Press the tab key to confirm your entry.
23. Click **Add.**
24. The **Order: Order Code** field is filled out. Press the tab key to confirm your entry.
25. Click **Add.**
26. The **Order: Order Code** field is filled out. Press the tab key to confirm your entry.
27. Click **Add.**
28. The **Order: Order Code** field is filled out. Press the tab key to confirm your entry.
29. Click **Add.**
30. The **Order: Order Code** field is filled out. Press the tab key to confirm your entry.
31. Click **Add.**
32. Click **OK.**

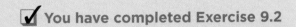 **You have completed Exercise 9.2**

Build a Clinical Alert, Part B

In Part B we will continue adding filters, and you will need the following information:

The URL needed for the Clinical Alert URL is: http://www.cdc.gov/cancer/colorectal/basic_info/screening/guidelines.htm. This practice has chosen to use the Centers for Disease Control and Prevention (CDC) as the organization from which they base their expert advice.

This alert will be named "Colonoscopy Needed" (without the quotes).

Follow these steps to complete the exercise on your own once you have watched the demonstration and tried the steps with helpful prompts in practice mode. Use the information provided in the scenario above to complete the information.

1. In the second row from the top, click **Field Name.**
2. Click **scroll button.**
3. Click **Order: Order Date.**
4. In the second row from the top, click **Operator.**
5. Clicking the entry **in the past** selects it.
6. Click **#.**
7. Click **5.**
8. Click **year(s).**
9. Clicking the entry **OK** selects it.
10. Click **OK.**
11. Click **Clinical Alert Flag.**
12. Click **Colonoscopy Needed.**
13. Click **OK.**
14. The **Clinical Alert URL** field is filled out. Press the tab key to confirm your entry.
15. Click **Save.**
16. The **Enter Alert Name** field is filled out. Press the tab key to confirm your entry.
17. Click **Save.**

✔ **You have completed Exercise 9.3**

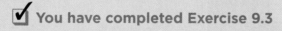

9.3   Use of Report-Writer for System Reports

PrimeSUITE and other PM/EMR software offer a multitude of standard reports that are set to run at certain times (end of month, for example) or on demand, as the information is needed. Some of the standard reports available in PrimeSUITE are:

- Payment analysis
- Procedure code analysis
- Provider revenue summary
- Patient balances

- Referring provider
- Appointment analysis report

The standard reports listed above and others in the reports library are necessary for efficient running of the office. Not keeping a close watch over revenue, balances, and constantly battling scheduling conflicts is not good business practice. Surprises in any of these areas can negatively impact the bottom line and cause unhappy staff, providers, and patients.

Running standard reports is as easy as a click of a button. It is always important to know the date ranges you want to include and if it is a report you run on a routine basis, you should always use the same parameters. In other words, if you run a report routinely that includes all of the care providers, do not make the mistake of running it next time with just a few of the providers; otherwise, you are not comparing apples to apples! Figure 9.2 shows the A/R Management Report Selection screen. This is the screen from which you would choose to run a Procedure Code Analysis Report, for example. This is a report that shows all procedures, and the volume of each, that are performed in the office. They are listed by CPT code. If you work for a dermatologist, the CPT code 42400, biopsy of salivary gland, should not appear on your Procedure Code Analysis Report, for example. If it does, then someone has made a coding error, since dermatologists typically do not excise salivary glands. If this does happen, then the affected account should be found and the code corrected. Another use for this type of report is cost justification. If one of the providers wants to purchase a newer model of a particular piece of equipment, and it will cost approximately $200,000, the managing partners in the practice most likely would not approve the

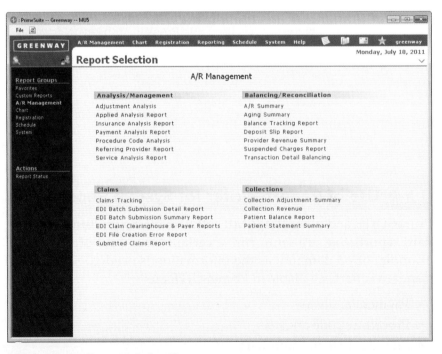

Figure 9.2   Report Selection screen

purchase if only a small number of procedures it will be used for are performed each year.

Major decisions, especially those that involve funding, should always be analyzed, and standard reports are a good starting point for the analysis. The findings from these reports give information—either baseline findings or changes over time. If information found in these reports is not analyzed, decisions will be made arbitrarily rather than based on facts.

Standard clinical reports are used as well. Examples include a listing of all active patients in the practice with a particular diagnosis, or a listing of all patients with an alert flag of smoker. You may want to run this type of report to answer a survey, where just the number of active smokers is requested. In this case, a **summary report** that includes only the total number (**aggregate**) of active smokers for a specific time period would be included rather than their name, address, etc. Reports that do include patient identifying information and list each case individually are known as **detail reports**.

Figure 9.3 depicts a Provider Revenue Summary report in PrimeSUITE.

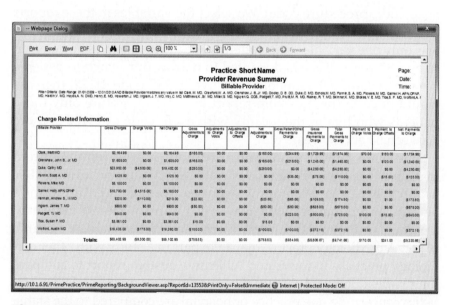

Figure 9.3   Provider Revenue Summary

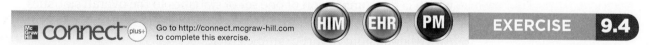

Go to http://connect.mcgraw-hill.com to complete this exercise.

EXERCISE   9.4

Run a Report of All Patients between the Ages of 60 and 80 Years Old

The first report we will run is a detail report of all patients in the practice between the ages of 60 and 80 years old. You may need to run this report because one of the managed care plans that your practice participates in has sent you a survey asking for the **aggregate** (sum total) of your patient population between the ages of 60 and 80, for example.

(continued)

Follow these steps to complete the exercise on your own once you have watched the demonstration and tried the steps with helpful prompts in practice mode.

1. Click **Report Selection. . . F7.**
2. Click **Custom Reports.**
3. Click **Patient Demographics.**
4. Click **Patients in the Practice 60–80.**
5. Click **Immediate.**
6. Click **Close.**

✓ **You have completed Exercise 9.4**

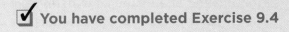

9.4 Custom Report Writing

Custom reports are built to include **variables**. Variables are the factors that vary from one patient to the next (e.g., age, ZIP code, diagnosis code, procedure code). We select the variables in these reports that we want our patients to meet or not meet. In Exercise 9.4 there was only one variable—the patient's age—which had to be between 60 and 80 years. If we had wanted to narrow our search to patients between 60 and 80 years old who live in ZIP code 21122, then we would have to run a custom report in order to capture only those patients who live in the locality with a ZIP code of 21122 and are between 60 and 80 years old.

We often run these custom reports to answer inquiries from managed care agencies, federal or state departments of health, public health agencies, or accrediting agencies. We may even do so for a newspaper reporter or a student who just wants aggregate data about a particular diagnosis in order to write an article or write a research paper. A cardiology practice may take part in a study with other cardiology practices in town, and will run a custom report to compare their patient demographics to those of the other practices. When statistics concerning one practice or hospital are compared to the statistics of other practices or hospitals, this is referred to as **benchmarking,** which is the comparison of one set of statistics to the overall statistics (using the same variables).

Other custom report examples include:

- The number of patients treated in the practice with a particular diagnosis, for example, congestive heart failure sorted by care provider
- The number of patients treated in your practice who live in a particular ZIP code, are smokers, and have diabetes
- The number of patients in a practice who have Medicaid as their primary source of payment and are between the ages of 30 and 60 years.
- The number of patients who have allergies to penicillin, are Hispanic, and live in ZIP code 12345

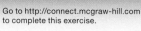
Build a Custom Report of All Patients with a Diagnosis of 428.0 Who Are Female and over the Age of 60, Part A

In this custom report, we are going to choose female patients *over* the age of 60 who have a diagnosis documented in their chart of congestive heart failure (CHF), which is ICD-9-CM code 428.0. (You will need to enter this code in the exercise.) There are other more specific CHF codes; however, for our purposes we will just look at the unspecified CHF cases. This exercise is split into two parts because of its length—Exercise 9.5 (Part A) and Exercise 9.6 (Part B).

Follow these steps to complete the exercise on your own once you have watched the demonstration and tried the steps with helpful prompts in practice mode.

1. Click **Report Designer.**
2. Click **Clinical—Patient Listing.**
3. Click **Import.**
4. Clicking the folder **Chart** opens it.
5. Clicking the folder **Clinical—Patient Listing** opens it.
6. Clicking the folder **Reports** opens it.
7. Click **Patients with Diagnosis X (v2).**
8. Click **Start Import.**
9. Click **Clinical—Patient Listing.**
10. Click **Patients with Diagnosis X (v2).**
11. Click **Filter.**
12. Click **Current Report Filter.**
13. Click **Edit Match List.**
14. Click **Clear.**
15. The **Diagnosis: Document Diagnosis** field is filled out. Press the tab key to confirm your entry.
16. Click **Add.**
17. Click **OK.**

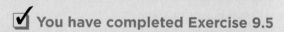 **You have completed Exercise 9.5**

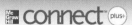

Build a Custom Report of All Patients with a Diagnosis of 428.0 Who Are Female and over the Age of 60, Part B

Now, continue on to Part B of building this custom report. The name of the report is Female patients > 60 with a diagnosis of CHF. The description is "A listing of female patients older than 60 years with a document diagnosis of 428.0" (without the quotes).

(continued)

1. In the second row from the top, click **Field Name.**
2. Click **scroll button.**
3. The entry **Patient: Age** is selected.
4. In the second row from the top, click **Operator.**
5. Clicking the entry **is greater than** selects it.
6. The **Match Value** field is filled out with **60.** Press the tab key to confirm your entry.
7. In the third row from the top, click **Field Name.**
8. Click **scroll.**
9. The entry **Patient: Sex** is clicked on.
10. Click **Operator.**
11. Click **matches any value in list.**
12. Clicking the entry **Create Match List** selects it.
13. Clicking the entry **Female** selects it.
14. Click **OK.**
15. Click **OK.**
16. Click **Properties.**
17. Use the Delete key or the Backspace key to clear the entry. (If one key doesn't work in your browser, use the other key.) The **Name:** field is filled out. Press the tab key to confirm your entry.
18. Use the Delete key or the Backspace key to clear the entry. (If one key doesn't work in your browser, use the other key.) The **Description:** field is filled out. Press the tab key to confirm your entry.
19. Click **Save.**
20. Click **Save.**
21. Under Actions, **Immediate** is clicked on.

☑ **You have completed Exercise 9.6**

9.5 Uses of Indexes

An **index** is a listing. Indexes are generally used to find basic information; a disease index is run and is sorted by ICD-9-CM diagnosis code and under each code lists each patient by name and health record number (dates of admission/discharge, attending physician, discharge disposition may also be included). Hospitals run the disease index to get a grasp of the types of patients being seen in the facility. This is also a good way to check for inaccuracies in coding. Another example would be a listing of all patients who are assigned to each care provider individually. In inpatient and outpatient settings, the Disease, Operation (procedure), and Physicians' Indexes are commonly run reports.

Managed care insurance plans often want to see the Physicians' Index or Diagnosis Index to get a profile of the type of patients treated by a practice before considering it for **in-network** status (meaning there is a contract between a managed care plan and the provider to offer services to members of the managed care plan at a pre-negotiated rate). Another reason to see this index is to provide proof that a physician has cared for a certain number of patients when he or she is seeking board certification, such as a board-certified urologist, a board-certified obstetrician, etc. Disease indexes are also used for case finding for such entities as the cancer registry, trauma registry, birth defect registries, and so on. Registries will be discussed in the next section.

A common index in a hospital setting is the **Master Patient Index (MPI)** (the listing of all patients seen in a hospital), which includes basic identifying information. Running the entire MPI may be done to look for missing information, to look for duplicate patients, or to look for names entered outside the practice's defined specifications (i.e., making sure that names are formatted according to data dictionary specifications).

9.6 Uses of Registries

Whereas an index is a listing of information, a **registry** is also a listing, but it is in chronological order. Examples in a hospital are admission and discharge registries, since they are run on a daily basis and include the names of all patients admitted and all patients discharged on a certain date. Another example is a birth registry—it is kept by date and time of birth, but it is sorted by the name of the newborn and also includes the name of the mother, the time of birth, and the name of the attending physician. And death registries, which are kept by date and time of death, include the patient's name, cause of death, and the signature of the person pronouncing the death, among other data elements.

Cancer registries are required by law. These are registries of all patients diagnosed or treated for cancer. The registry of these patients is then sent to the state cancer registry where statewide statistics are compiled regarding the incidence of each type of cancer as well as survival rates by type of cancer within that state. The state registry is responsible for reporting to the Centers for Disease Control and Prevention (CDC). Hospitals, physicians' offices, outpatient radiation therapy facilities, and ambulatory care centers may keep and report a registry of cancer patients on a yearly basis. Take the time to look for the top 10 cancers in the United States during 2007 by following the link to the United States Cancer Statistics found at http://www.cdc.gov/cancer/npcr/. Cancer registries will be covered in more detail in another course.

Trauma registries are one of the newer registries, created in the early 1990s; as the name implies, this is a registry of all patients diagnosed or treated with traumatic injuries, and includes fractures, burns, open wounds, and the like. The 2010 Annual Report of the American College of Surgeons' National Trauma Databank can be found at http://www.facs.org/trauma/ntdb/pdf/ntdbannualreport2010.pdf. It is interesting to page through the report; you will see the enormous amount of data reported by hospitals throughout the country. In Table 16 on page 29 of the report, you will see a breakdown by mechanism of injury (fall, burn, suffocation, transport vehicles, motor vehicle accidents, etc.). From there, the data gets more specific, for instance, incidence of falls by age or incidents by region of the country (Table 42, page 60). As you can see, the southern part of the country has the highest incidence of traumatic incidents at 34.76%. The Northeast has the lowest at 17.15%. State and local health and safety officials can then use this information to analyze reasons for a higher–than–average incidence (in the case of the South), or a lower–than–average incidence (as is the case in the Northeast).

Immunization registries are of particular importance to public health. Some private physician offices keep a registry of immunizations by patient; however, not all medical practices keep this registry; it may just be a public health department that does so. Some states require reporting of immunizations by law. For instance, a West Virginia state law requires all providers to report all immunizations they administer to children under age 18 within 2 weeks of administering the immunization.

Other registries include birth defect, diabetes, implant (any material implanted into the body), transplant, and HIV/AIDS registries. The requirements for these vary from state to state as well as by managed care plan or other third-party requirements, and for quality reporting purposes.

Prime SUITE, like most other EHR systems, makes the process of running an index or registry very fast. Its accuracy depends on whether the entry of the data was correct in the first place! This is another reason why accuracy is so important.

The **Center for Medicare and Medicaid Services** (CMS) receives registry information directly from PrimeSUITE. This information satisfies the **Physician Quality Reporting Initiative (PQRI)** measures. Participation in PQRI is voluntary and is a pay–for–performance incentive program. Participating care providers submit data on any of the 100 designated quality measures, which include diabetes, hypertension, stroke, and glaucoma, just to name a few. The full list is accessible at http://www.cms.gov/PQRS/Downloads/2011_PhysQualRptg_MeasuresList_033111.pdf.

PrimeSUITE includes an option to receive an alert at the point of care if the information entered for a patient qualifies for one or more of the PQRI Measure Groups.

There are times when hospitals, medical practices, or other healthcare entities contribute to outside registries. Of note is the **National Practitioner Data Bank (NPDB)**, which came about as part of the Health Care Quality Improvement Act of 1986. This is a database of malpractice payments, revocation of privileges, licensure denial or suspension, denial of medical staff privileges, and the like. Reporting any of these adverse actions to the NPDB is required by law. Hospitals or offices considering granting privileges to or hiring of care providers, state boards of medical examiners or licensing boards, state boards of medicine, or the care providers themselves can query the databank when necessary. Healthcare entities that are considering granting privileges to a physician must query the NPDB during the hiring/privileging process.

Hospitals, care providers, and all other healthcare organizations must report adverse actions related to fraud and abuse to the **Healthcare Integrity and Protection Data Bank** (HIPDB). Reporting to either the NPDB or the HIPDB can be done on one site rather than attempting to determine which specific data bank to report incidences to. More information about both of these can be found at http://www.npdb-hipdb.com/.

9.7 The Credentialing Process

Credentialing does not involve a database, nor does the process necessarily require the use of a database. It is mentioned here because information is captured and maintained for reporting purposes when a healthcare professional files for renewal of a medical license, applies for board certification (and continuing board certification), applies for hospital privileges (or maintaining such privileges), and reports to managed care entities.

Credentialing is the process of ensuring a care provider has the proper qualifications to practice medicine. In other words, if a physician claims to be a cardiac surgeon, then the practice or hospital must verify that he has the educational background and experience (medical residency) necessary to perform surgeries typically carried out by a cardiac surgeon. It must verify that he has shown verification that he is a qualified medical professional in that specialty. Also, it means that he is in compliance with specific policies (called bylaws) for that organization, and that he has purchased sufficient malpractice insurance coverage. Some insurance carriers will not reimburse providers who perform medical care for which they are not qualified. Further, some will not invite physicians to be participating providers in an insurance plan unless they are board-certified. Board certification involves successfully completing a test that is directly related to the specialty area, and which goes above and beyond state medical licensure. Physicians must be Medicare-credentialed in order to submit claims to Medicare for payment. When a medical practice hires a new care provider, information regarding education, experience, state license number, DEA number, NPI number, proof of malpractice insurance, and documentation of any pending or settled claims against the care provider are all on file, usually within the PM software. And, as noted above, the NPDB and HIPDB must also be queried prior to granting privileges, hiring, or including him as a participating provider by insurance carriers.

chapter 9 **summary**

LEARNING OUTCOME	CONCEPTS FOR REVIEW
9.1 Describe the uses of the dashboard in PrimeSUITE to meet Meaningful Use Standards. pp. 176–180	– List core objectives for providers and hospitals – List menu objectives for providers and hospitals – Use the dashboard in PrimeSUITE to assess performance
9.2 Explain how data and information are used in decision support. pp. 180–183	– Define clinical decision support – Use improves patient safety, decreases duplication, reduces unnecessary testing, reduces cost of healthcare – Use improves patient outcomes, improves efficiency – Some care providers are not accepting of CDS technology
9.3 Set up system reports using PrimeSUITE. pp. 183–186	– Standard reports are commonly used by most medical practices – Standard reports are system built – Administrative as well as clinical standard reports are available – Differentiate between summary and detail reports
9.4 Set up custom reports using PrimeSUITE pp. 186–188	– Custom reports are run based on specific parameters or variables – Custom reports are used when standard reports do not provide the level of detail necessary
9.5 Illustrate uses for an index. pp. 188–189	– Index is a list – Typically used to find all patients who meet a certain criteria – Examples: Master Patient Index, Diagnosis Index, Procedure Index, Physician Index
9.6 Describe uses for a registry. pp. 189–191	– A listing of information in chronological order – Examples: birth registry, cancer registry, trauma registry, PQRI Measures registry – Submissions required by National Practitioner Data Bank (NPDB) – Submissions required by Healthcare Integrity and Protection Data Bank (HIPDB)

9.7 Explain how data gathered in PrimeSUITE is used in the credentialing process. p. 191	– Verification that care provider holds certain credentials
	 – Included in the credentials are:
	   • education (undergrad as well as medical school)
	   • residency(ies) dates and institution(s)
	   • pending or settled malpractice cases
	   • proof of purchase of malpractice insurance

chapter **review**

MATCHING QUESTIONS

Match the terms on the left with the definitions on the right.

_____ 1. **[LO 9.1]** dashboard

_____ 2. **[LO 9.5]** in-network

_____ 3. **[LO 9.1]** meaningful use

_____ 4. **[LO 9.6]** CMS

_____ 5. **[LO 9.6]** registry

_____ 6. **[LO 9.5]** index

_____ 7. **[LO 9.2]** decision support

_____ 8. **[LO 9.3]** detail report

_____ 9. **[LO 9.3]** summary report

_____ 10. **[LO 9.1]** core objectives

_____ 11. **[LO 9.6]** PQRI Measures Group

_____ 12. **[LO 9.1]** drug formulary

_____ 13. **[LO 9.7]** credentialing

a. list of provider-preferred generic and brand–name drugs covered under various insurance plans

b. consolidated clinical data that removes any patient information in the printout

c. tool built into most EHRs that provides staff with results of research and best practices to enhance patient care

d. a chronologically ordered list used in calculating statistics and record-keeping

e. subgroup of common or similar conditions pulled from registry data

f. consolidated clinical data that includes specific, demographic, or patient–identifying information in the printout

g. verification process that ensures a care provider is legally authorized through education and experience to practice medicine

h. care provider or practice that contracts with insurance companies to provide care to their subscribers at a reduced rate

i. feature of PrimeSUITE that allows a provider to visually track their fulfillment of core objectives

j. requirements that must be met for a professional to receive Medicare stimulus money to purchase or upgrade an EHR

k. benchmark tasks that demonstrate meaningful use of electronic health information

l. agency to which quality reporting measures are reported

m. a listing of specified information, such as all patients covered by one care provider

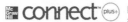 Enhance your learning by completing these exercises and more at http://connect.mcgraw-hill.com!

MULTIPLE-CHOICE QUESTIONS

Select the letter that best completes the statement or answers the question:

1. **[LO 9.7]** A credentialing requirement is:
   a. being hired by a professional organization.
   b. gaining additional medical degrees.
   c. having malpractice insurance.
   d. knowing procedures outside of one's specialty.

2. **[LO 9.1]** Hospitals are exempt from the core objective of:
   a. drug-allergy checks.
   b. ePrescribing.
   c. privacy and security provisions.
   d. recording smoking status.

3. **[LO 9.2]** When an alert is created, specifying a detail such as "search for patients 30 years or older" is an example of using a/an:
   a. decision.
   b. filter.
   c. outlier.
   d. trend.

4. **[LO 9.5]** A healthcare professional will typically use an index to locate _____ information.
   a. basic
   b. encrypted
   c. statistical
   d. virtual

5. **[LO 9.1]** Healthcare facilities have _____ year[s] after the adoption of an EHR to prove meaningful use.
   a. 1
   b. 2
   c. 3
   d. 4

6. **[LO 9.3]** PrimeSUITE's reports can be used to:
   a. justify the cost of new equipment.
   b. perform quality checks.
   c. track care provider data.
   d. All of the above.

7. **[LO 9.2]** Meaningful use requires that a practice not only implement at least one clinical support rule, but also:
   a. reduce alerts.
   b. prove use.
   c. track compliance.
   d. use evidence.

8. **[LO 9.4]** Custom reports have at least _____ variable(s) that is/are not available through a standard report.
   a. one
   b. two
   c. three
   d. four

9. **[LO 9.6]** _____ are listed in chronological order.
   a. Dashboards
   b. Indices
   c. Registries
   d. Reports

10. **[LO 9.3]** PrimeSUITE's Referring Provider report is an example of a _____ report.
    a. clinical
    b. custom
    c. special
    d. standard

11. **[LO 9.5]** Care providers who contract with insurance carriers typically agree to a _____ rate of reimbursement for those services.
    a. higher
    b. lower
    c. special
    d. standard

12. **[LO 9.6]** Currently, participation in the Physician Quality Reporting Initiative is:
    a. discouraged.
    b. mandatory.
    c. standard.
    d. voluntary.

SHORT ANSWER QUESTIONS

1. **[LO 9.1]** What does it mean for a healthcare setting to report clinical quality measures?

2. **[LO 9.5]** Why might a hospital need to periodically run an entire Master Patient Index?

3. **[LO 9.3]** Contrast a summary report and a detail report.

4. **[LO 9.1]** Discuss what will happen if a provider does not achieve her core menu/objective percentages?

5. **[LO 9.2]** Explain the purpose of using filters.

6. **[LO 9.7]** What information is included in a provider's credentials?

7. **[LO 9.4]** If you needed to run a report of all the patients in your practice who were diagnosed with asthma, were African American, and were under the age of 15, what type of report would you be running? Explain your answer.

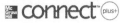 Enhance your learning by completing these exercises and more at http://connect.mcgraw-hill.com!

8. **[LO 9.3]** What is a Procedure Code Analysis Report?

9. **[LO 9.2]** List the benefits of clinical decision support.

10. **[LO 9.6]** List three things a registry might be used for.

APPLYING YOUR KNOWLEDGE

1. **[LO 9.1]** Why might hospitals be exempt from the ePrescribing core objective?

2. **[LOs 9.1, 9.3, 9.4, 9.5, 9.6]** As a healthcare professional, part of your job is answering patient questions. One day, a patient comes in very concerned. When you ask what's wrong, she says, "I read about this term called Syndromatic Surveillance, and it really worries me! I don't want the government keeping tabs on me when I'm sick!" What would you say to her to alleviate her fears?

3. **[LO 9.6]** Why are registries kept in chronological order?

4. **[LO 9.2]** How could PrimeSUITE assist a practice in the fight against cancer?

5. **[LOs 9.2, 9.3, 9.4, 9.6]** Imagine that the state you reside in recently passed a measure requiring that a report of all immunizations administered at your practice be submitted to the state office of public health. How would you go about fulfilling this request while maintaining patient confidentiality? How could your office use the data to improve patient care?

6. **[LO 9.7]** Dr. Smith is a new provider in your office. Currently, he does not have board certification. Is it imperative that he obtain this credential? Why or why not?

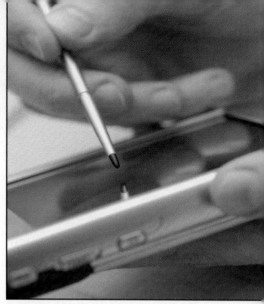

10

Looking Ahead— The Future of Health Information and Informatics

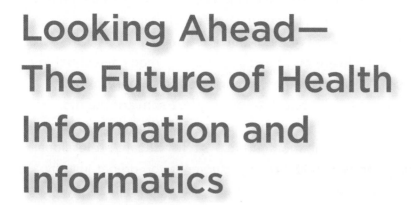

Learning Outcomes

At the end of this chapter, the student should be able to:

10.1 Compare information management to health informatics.

10.2 Discuss barriers to the adoption of electronic health records.

10.3 Describe three emerging technologies or models that are improving the care of patients through information technology.

10.4 Illustrate three mobile devices that will make the collection and sharing of health information more timely and efficient.

10.5 Describe how virtual private networks (VPNs) are advancing the use of EHRs.

Key Terms

Decryption
Encryption
Evidence-based medicine
Firewall
Health Information Management
Health informatics
Local area network (LAN)
Patient-Centered Medical Home (PCMH)
Patient portal
Personal digital assistant (PDA)

Personal health record (PHR)
Picture Archiving and Communications
  Systems (PACS)
Smart Phone
Tablet computer
Telemedicine
Telehealth
Virtual private network (VPN)
Wide area network (WAN)
Wi-Fi

What You Need to Know and Why You Need to Know It

Technology is part of the healthcare world, whether you are a clinician or hold an administrative role. It was mentioned in Chapter 1 that healthcare as a whole has been reluctant to embrace the digital age. That is not so when it comes to computerization of medical technology such as diagnostic and treatment procedures, however. Newer technologies are less invasive, require shorter recovery time, require less (or no) hospitalization, and are safer overall than previous procedures. Though we are far ahead in the use of medical technology for diagnostic and treatment purposes, we lag far behind other industries where computerization of *information* is concerned. In this final chapter we will explore some of the more common methods to access electronic records and will discuss newer (at least to healthcare) technologies that are in limited use, but gaining in momentum. As a healthcare professional, it is imperative that you stay abreast of emerging technologies. Even if you do not initially hold a position where you are involved in selection or implementation, you will definitely *use* technology in all of the positions you will hold throughout your career. And, since you have chosen healthcare as a profession, you have also chosen to become a lifelong learner—do not get too comfortable with how something is done today, as it will surely change in the blink of an eye!

10.1 Health Information versus Health Informatics

The American Health Information Management Association (AHIMA) Committee on Professional Development defined **Health Information Management** as follows:

> *Health Information Management improves the quality of healthcare by ensuring that the best information is available to make any healthcare decision. Health information management professionals manage healthcare data and information resources. The profession encompasses services in planning, collecting, aggregating, analyzing, and disseminating individual patient and aggregate clinical data. It serves the following healthcare stakeholders: patient care organizations, payers, research and policy agencies, and other healthcare-related industries.*[1]

Where health information management pertains to both paper and automated capture, retrieval, storage and use of health information, **health informatics** is the management of automated health information in particular. Health information professionals whose work is geared more toward informatics focus on

[1]American Health Information Management Association. (2003). *A Vision of the e-HIM Future: A Report from the AHIMA e-HIM Task Force.* Supplement to the *Journal of AHIMA.*

structure of data, interoperability, design of input and output tools, security controls, development of data dictionaries, workflow configuration in an automated environment, and classification systems and terminologies used in a computerized healthcare system.

In short, health informatics is the technological side of managing health information—the design, development, structure, implementation, integration, and management of the technical aspects of electronic record-keeping. HIM professionals have historically ensured accurate, complete, readily available health information for use by care providers, administrators, researchers, public health officials, and insurers. Their focus is the content of the record, as well as integration of systems, and the ability to share electronic information. They manage health information regardless of the media on which it is kept. The HIM professional and the IT professional within a facility have always worked very closely together to ensure that standards are met and information is available, yet private and secure. In health informatics there is a melding of the two disciplines—IT expertise with HIM expertise, and this may be one and the same person in many cases.

For years, Health Information Management programs at all levels have included coursework in information-related software as well as electronic record-keeping in their curriculums, and now colleges and universities have begun including in-depth coverage of the electronic health record in their medical assisting, medical billing and coding, medical office management, and healthcare administration programs as well.

In a physician's office, as well as other outpatient facilities, there may not be degreed health information professionals per se, but there is an individual within the facility who should know the requirements of a legal electronic health record, documentation requirements, and privacy and security regulations. Vendors also have support staff who are active participants in the installation and training of a PM or EHR system. They advise practices on using the software efficiently and effectively to ensure security and privacy of the information collected, and to ensure that documentation requirements are being met. If the practice does not have a full- or part-time technology position staffed, the office will contract with either a consultant or the vendor's team.

Check Your Understanding

1. Between health information management and health informatics, which discipline is most closely associated with IT and which with information itself?

2. How could a practice management software vendor assist an office or facility that does not have a degreed HIM professional on staff?

In Chapter 1, resistance to an electronic system was discussed. But this subject is worth revisiting before discussing even newer technologies that, though in use, are still the exception rather than the rule.

For years, care providers have been documenting the health records of patients by writing orders, progress notes, and chart notes, or by dictating History & Physicals (H&Ps), discharge summaries, operative reports, consultation reports, and correspondence. They are used to it; it is the way it has always been done. Providers know that if a laboratory test result is needed during a patient's visit, they need only flip to the laboratory tab of the patient's folder and it will be there (well, hopefully it will be). Paper and folders are inexpensive, relatively speaking. If it was impossible to complete the record at the time the patient was seen, the record would be sent to the health information department for completion at a later time, or if a patient was seen, in the office and the provider needed to dictate the chart note, it was easy enough to take the record back to her private office to complete later. Many care providers see this paper system as being easier, and it may seem more efficient; however, the quality of documentation that is written or dictated days (or even weeks) after the care was provided is questionable, paper records are often illegible if they are handwritten, and if dictation and transcription are used there is lag time before the typed report is filed in the record. Additionally, from a security perspective, a paper record can easily be picked up by someone with no need to have or see it and, if a paper record gets lost, hours of staff time can be spent searching for it.

Implementing and maintaining an electronic record is expensive, that is true. But, the argument for patient safety, higher quality medical care, point of care documentation, faster results of diagnostic tests, and ability to both share information with other care providers when necessary and access a patient's chart from any location, not to mention access clinical decision support, should outweigh the "high cost" argument. Financial incentives through HITECH have been the driving force for many practices that have now decided to convert to a paperless (or almost paperless) system. Recall that beginning in 2011, hospitals and physicians' practices that adopt meaningful use of EHRs will receive incentive payments. Those hospitals and practices that hold out will be penalized if they have not adopted meaningful use of an EHR by 2015.

Converting from a paper system to an electronic system can be a lengthy, sometimes chaotic process. It can no doubt cause loss of productivity for both staff and care providers. When procedures within the office that are seemingly efficient in the manual form are computerized, there are bound to be errors in conversion, steps that are overlooked, and general frustration for all involved. However, proper planning, heeding the advice of the software vendor's installation team, and accepting the fact that the conversion, training of staff, and use of the system will all take longer than expected should make the whole process more tolerable. It does take time and effort to convert to and use an electronic system, but the same can be said for any change in procedure in any profession.

Check Your Understanding

1. Healthcare facilities that do not adopt electronic record technology will begin facing penalties in the year _____.
2. Up to this point, what has been the driving force behind facilities adopting EHRs?

10.3 Emerging Technologies and Models

Patient Portals

Patients today are becoming more interested and involved in their own healthcare. They are taking a more active role, and thanks to the Internet, arrive at their appointments knowing what their care provider may ask and why, and what treatment options exist. They have a list of questions ready for the care provider, which allows for a more productive visit. **Patient portals** are another means to better, more meaningful communication with a care provider, and are a functionality of EHRs that satisfy Meaningful Use regulation. A patient portal is a method of accessing portions of one's own office health record. These portals are secure and can only be accessed with a user ID and password. In PrimeSUITE the portal is known as PrimePRACTICE. Through it, the patient can:

- E-mail the practice with questions about concerns they may have regarding their care
- Make appointments
- Complete history forms and authorizations online
- Request prescription refills
- Get results of tests

More information is available about PrimePATIENT at http://www.greenwaymedical.com/dynamicData/pdf/products/2011/Greenway_PrimePATIENT.pdf.

By using the secure portal, the office staff spends less time answering phone calls, calling patients back (or playing phone-tag), and entering data in the record; patients are more satisfied because their questions are answered more promptly, and they feel that they are more in control of their care. You may not realize that your care provider offers patient portals; if the office is automated, and an EHR is in use, ask about it!

Many insurance plans have similar options for their subscribers, including communicating with a nurse or care provider to answer questions about symptoms, treatment options, coverage, and the like. Take a few moments to look at the website for your health insurance—does it have patient portal capability?

Personal Health Records (PHRs)

The **Personal Health Record (PHR)** is maintained and kept with the patient, and is a record of his or her past and current health information including drug allergies or reactions, immunization dates, past and present medical conditions, surgical procedures, family history, list of current medications, and insurance information. The PHR is not a legal record because it is just that—personal; there are no safeguards to ensure it is complete, it is not written by a medical professional, much of it may have been compiled from memory, and it does not meet the legal requirement of "being compiled during the normal course of business." However, it is a valuable tool when a patient seeks medical care, particularly if emergency care is required or if there has been a change in care providers. The PHR is only as good as the information in it—*all* of the information should be up-to-date and accurate. It also needs to be available when needed. If patients expect their PHR to be a useful document, family members should know where the PHR is kept, and it should be taken to office visits or to the emergency department when such visits occur. Patients may keep the PHR in a paper format or online (or may print it from the online portal). There are many options for doing so, including the PHR websites of many major insurance carriers and the AHIMA PHR website found at http://www.myphr.com/. Other free online PHRs include Microsoft Health Vault, iHealthRecord, Telemedical.com, and MedsFile.com, just to name a few. The AHIMA website provides a full list. PHRs are not a new technology, but their use is becoming more prevalent.

Telemedicine

Telehealth and **Telemedicine** are of great benefit to patients who do not have the means to travel to a doctor's appointment or who live in remote, medically underserved areas. Telehealth is more associated with preventive care. With the use of audiovisual equipment, the patient and the care provider or healthcare professional can connect through teleconferencing technology, allowing each to see and hear the other. Through telemedicine technology, a patient's blood pressure, heart rate, respiratory rate, EKG tracing, or medical imaging can be monitored remotely. Should the care provider find something that is not within normal limits, the patient would then need to seek on-site care (or emergency care dispatched). The imaging technology of **Picture Archiving and Communications Systems (PACS)**, whereby radiologic images are viewed remotely, is one of the original uses of telemedicine.

Through the use of telemedicine there is cost savings to both the insurance carrier and the patient; patients who would not otherwise be able to make visits to their care providers now have better access to care, which in turn improves outcomes and in general is more convenient for patients, particularly those who do not have transportation or who live a distance away from their care provider.

Take time to investigate telemedicine further by reading the Institute of Medicine report *Telemedicine: A Guide to Assessing Telecommunications for Health Care* found at http://www.nap.edu/openbook.php?record_id=5296&page=137.

Many Veterans Affairs Medical Centers provide telemedicine or telehealth to assist in the care of veterans. The Department of Veterans Affairs telehealth website can be found at http://www.telehealth.va.gov/index.asp.

Patient-Centered Medical Homes (PCMH)

Patient Centered Medical Home (PCMH) is a model that was developed to care for patients with chronic conditions by the American Academy of Family Practitioners. The premise encourages and facilitates the patient's (and family's) involvement in his or her own care. It is mentioned in this chapter because it ties in with the concept of a patient-centric health model. The PCMH also encourages a primary care physician approach to patient care, which is also the premise of many managed care insurance plans that require a "gatekeeper" to reduce redundancy and overutilization of testing and services, and provide overall more efficient and effective healthcare.

The use of health information technology is paramount to the PCMH model because the use of quality measures, including registries, referral tracking, results tracking, medication alerts, performance measures, use of evidence-based medicine, an updated problem list and current medication list, are all part of the PCMH model—all of the elements that are requirements of Meaningful use as well.

Evidence-Based Medicine

Meaningful use of data requires decision support capability as part of the EHR. This is also known as **evidence-based medicine** because the diagnostic and treatment protocols are based on proven research and best practices. Through evidence-based medicine, a patient's plan of care is based on current, proven practice. Alerts or reminders automatically appear in a patient's chart based on data captured about that patient. An example would be a female patient who has just passed her fortieth birthday. The FDA Office of Women's Health recommends a screening mammogram be performed at the age of 40 and every 1 to 2 years thereafter.[2] Current EHR software makes it possible for physicians to be alerted to the latest diagnostic and treatment recommendations and modalities, which in

[2]FDA Office of Women's Health. (2011). Mammograms. Retrieved from http://www.fda.gov/downloads/ForConsumers/ByAudience/ForWomen/UCM121896.pdf.

turn improves efficiency, patient care, and clinical outcomes. It is clear why the use of evidence-based medicine is part of the Meaningful Use regulations.

Check Your Understanding

1. What are the diagnostic and treatment protocols of evidence-based medicine based on?
2. Is a patient's Personal Health Record a legal document? Explain your answer.
3. If a patient is being monitored using telemedicine, what would happen if an abnormal reading was found?
4. How does a PCMH make a patient's experience more positive?

10.4 Making the World of Health Informatics User-Friendly and Convenient

In order for an electronic health record system to be successful, the care providers need to be satisfied with the product. They typically look for portability, mobility, flexibility and convenience—all qualities of products used in the twenty-first century and all requirements of the healthcare team if they are to work efficiently.

Portable devices allow for flexibility and portability. They are advantageous because they are convenient (the provider does not have to find a computer to use); are cost effective (the provider can use an inexpensive device and there is no need to rework because notes and procedure codes are entered at the point of care, which reduces the number of lost or missing charges); improve accuracy (the care provider does not have to jot down notes that would need to be transferred into the record at a later time); and, in general, create overall satisfaction since the information needed to care for patients is available at any time from any location. The connection to the EHR may be through a **local area network (LAN)** or **wide area network (WAN)**. LANs link computers and related devices that are physically close to one another such as within a building; WANs connect computer networks together that are not physically close (see Figure 10.1). And, of course, access can be via the Internet. The types of portable devices used include **personal digital assistants (PDAs)**; they are small enough to fit in one's hand, yet allow access to LANs, WANs, and the Internet and may also have phone capability. **Smart Phones** are telephones that also allow Internet browsing as well as, audio, video, and camera functionality; and **tablet computers** are larger than PDAs or Smart Phones, yet smaller than a laptop computer—they too provide access to LANs, WANs, and the Internet.

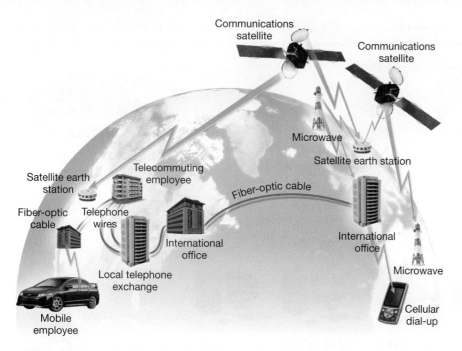

Figure 10.1   Depiction of a wide area network (WAN)

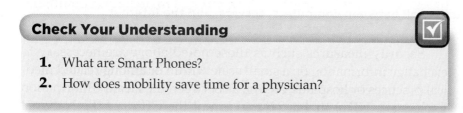

Check Your Understanding

1. What are Smart Phones?
2. How does mobility save time for a physician?

10.5   Virtual Private Networks—Advancing the Use of EHRs Remotely Yet Securely

To use mobile functionality, a wireless connection is necessary. This is known as **Wi-Fi**, which sends data via high radio frequency. Of course, utilizing mobile technology does require high levels of security. The use of a **virtual private network (VPN)** is one way to ensure the security of the information flowing between the mobile device and the EHR. A VPN uses the Internet as its path, but built into the VPN is software that **encrypts** (codes) the data being sent and interprets the data being received **(decryption)**. A VPN also verifies the identity of the user through his or her user ID and password, and only allows users access who have been granted permission to sign on to the network. The use of a VPN provides for the secure environment to allow sharing of health information with users at remote locations. In addition to the VPN, a **firewall** is another security method (see Figure 10.2). Firewalls prevent unauthorized access into or out of the network through use of both hardware and software devices that filter activity over the network. Based on predefined rules, the firewall acts as a barrier—activity that passes the rules may continue in or out of the network; activity that does not pass the rules may not.

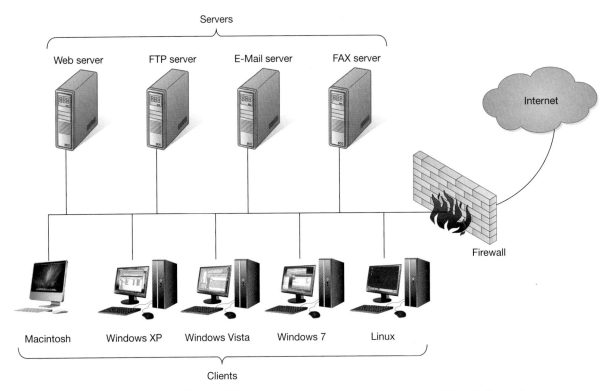

Figure 10.2 Placement of a firewall between computers, servers, and the Internet

Security measures such as those noted above are necessary to exchange information on a small scale within or among related medical practices or hospitals, as well as between the Health Information Exchanges (HIEs) that are the vision of the Office of the National Coordinator (ONC).

Pulling It All Together

The intent of this worktext has been to introduce students to the automation of health information with emphasis on those of you who have chosen to study health information management, medical assisting, and medical billing and coding. Having chosen one of these professions, you will work closely with automated systems; many of you will be lucky enough to be involved in choosing a system from the very first steps, others will use the systems on a daily basis, and yet others will climb the ladder into implementation, training, and developing computer programs and systems that will enhance the automated exchange of information.

Medicine and healthcare are not static; changes occur daily. Those changes need to be communicated, implemented, and tracked to determine their impact on patient care. As a healthcare professional, you will not be observing from the sidelines; instead, you will be an active participant in improving access to, quality and utilization of readily available, complete, accurate, and secure health information.

Check Your Understanding

1. How does a VPN verify a user's identity?
2. What role does encryption play in using VPNs?

chapter 10 **summary**

LEARNING OUTCOME	CONCEPTS FOR REVIEW
10.1 Compare Health Information Management to health informatics. pp. 198–199	– Define Health Information Management – Define health informatics – Role of HIM professional in each
10.2 Discuss barriers to the adoption of electronic health records. pp. 200–201	– Written records and dictation have been the norm – Paper and dictation are fairly inexpensive – Lengthy process to convert to electronic records – Training time is extensive – Loss of productivity – High frustration level
10.3 Describe three emerging technologies or models that are improving the care of patients through information technology. pp. 201–204	– Patient portals—means of communication between patient and medical practice – Personal Health Record—patient keeps own record of history, immunizations, allergies, surgeries, past conditions, and family history – Telemedicine—allows patient to be "seen" without leaving the home – Patient-Centered Medical Home (PCMH)—primary care physician is leader of a team that cares for the patient; patient is more involved than in traditional approach; use of technology inherent in the process – Evidence-based medicine—technology "researches" best practices and decision support to assure that patient is receiving most up-to-date diagnostic and treatment options
10.4 Illustrate three mobile devices that will make the collection and sharing of health information more timely and efficient. pp. 204–205	– Use of EHR can be more convenient by making it mobile; use of personal digital assistants (PDAs), Smart Phones, and tablet computers allow for portability – Wireless (Wi-Fi) connections are required to use portable devices
10.5 Describe how virtual private networks (VPNs) are advancing the use of EHRs. pp. 205–206	– Though portability is necessary, so is security – Virtual Private Networks encrypt and interpret information that is sent and received via wireless networks – Use of firewalls as a security device

chapter review

MATCHING QUESTIONS

Match the terms on the left with the definitions on the right.

_____ 1. **[LO 10.5]** encryption

_____ 2. **[LO 10.1]** Health Information Management

_____ 3. **[LO 10.3]** patient portal

_____ 4. **[LO 10.3]** evidence-based medicine

_____ 5. **[LO 10.3]** Personal Health Record (PHR)

_____ 6. **[LO 10.3]** telemedicine

_____ 7. **[LO 10.5]** VPN

_____ 8. **[LO 10.4]** Wi-Fi

_____ 9. **[LO 10.1]** health informatics

a. clinical decision support based on research and best practices

b. science that deals with health information, its structure, acquisition, and uses

c. improving healthcare through working with data and ensuring that the best information is available for decision making

d. coding data to make it more secure

e. high radio frequency wireless connection used by Smart Phones and PDAs

f. the monitoring or exchange of health information remotely

g. secure method of accessing individual health records and information through an EHR

h. secure Internet environment that encrypts data and allows remote access to health information

i. medical history maintained and kept by an individual patient

MULTIPLE-CHOICE QUESTIONS

Select the letter that best completes the statement or answers the question:

1. **[LO 10.1]** Health informatics is basically the _____ part of managing health information.
   a. critical
   b. structural
   c. technological
   d. usable

2. **[LO 10.4]** One benefit of accessing the EHR through mobile devices is a reduction in:
   a. cost.
   b. errors.
   c. satisfaction.
   d. both A and B are correct

3. **[LO 10.2]** Incentives are being offered to EHR adopters through _____ legislation.
    a. CCHIP
    b. HIPAA
    c. HITECH
    d. ONC

4. **[LO 10.3]** Care providers use _____ as a way to support their decisions and diagnoses.
    a. current medical trends
    b. evidence-based medicine
    c. Meaningful Use
    d. patient-centric care

5. **[LO 10.1]** Which of the following stakeholders are served by the health information management profession?
    a. Patient care organizations
    b. Payers
    c. Research agencies
    d. All of the above

6. **[LO 10.2]** According to the text, which of the following is a way to make the transition to EHRs easier?
    a. Allowing staff members to be frustrated and anxious about the change
    b. Following the advice and suggestions of the EHR vendor's installation team
    c. Providing immediate training so that ramp-up is quicker
    d. Saving money for EHR costs by eliminating staff

7. **[LO 10.3]** A PCMH focuses on _____ communication between patients and providers.
    a. decreased
    b. increased
    c. random
    d. structured

8. **[LO 10.1]** There _____ be a degreed health information professional on staff in a healthcare office.
    a. might
    b. must
    c. will
    d. will not

9. **[LO 10.4]** There must be a _____ available for providers to use portable devices to access health information.
    a. computer terminal
    b. Internet hookup
    c. wireless connection
    d. wireless router

Enhance your learning by completing these exercises and more at http://connect.mcgraw-hill.com!

10. **[LO 10.3]** Who is in charge of a Personal Health Record?
    a. HIM professional
    b. Patient
    c. Provider
    d. Medical staff

11. **[LO 10.2]** Penalties for facilities not adopting electronic health records will begin in
    _____.
    a. 2011
    b. 2013
    c. 2015
    d. 2018

12. **[LO 10.3]** Videoconferencing and remote vital sign monitoring are part of:
    a. patient-centric care.
    b. a patient portal.
    c. telemedicine.
    d. virtual health networks.

13. **[LO 10.5]** What does VPN stand for?
    a. Verifying Provider Network
    b. Verified Protocol Network
    c. Virtual Private Network
    d. Virtual Provider Network

14. **[LO 10.3]** Recent advances in healthcare rely increasingly on:
    a. change.
    b. precedent.
    c. technology.
    d. tradition.

SHORT ANSWER QUESTIONS

1. **[LO 10.1]** Explain the difference between health information and health informatics.

2. **[LO 10.3]** What are some advantages to a healthcare facility using the Patient Portal function?

3. **[LO 10.4]** What is meant by mobile device?

4. **[LO 10.5]** How does a VPN ensure data integrity and security?

5. **[LO 10.2]** Explain why many care providers view a paper-based system as easier than an electronic one.

6. **[LO 10.1]** What does an HIM professional do?

7. **[LO 10.2]** How can healthcare facilities make the adoption of EHRs as easy and painless as possible?

8. **[LO 10.4]** How do mobile applications reduce costs and errors?

9. **[LO 10.3]** Describe a Patient Centered Medical Home [PCMH].

10. **[LO 10.5]** What is Wi-Fi?

APPLYING YOUR KNOWLEDGE

1. **[LO 10.3]** After reading about the patient portal in your text, are there any disadvantages to using a system like PrimePRACTICE? Justify your answer.

2. **[LO 10.2]** What is your opinion on the use of incentives to encourage healthcare facilities to adopt EHRs? Explain your answer.

3. **[LOs 10.4, 10.5]** You are a healthcare professional who has the ability to work from home on certain days. How would you go about accessing the work you need to do on a given day from your home?

4. **[LOs 10.1, 10.2, 10.3, 10.4, 10.5]** Your healthcare office is beginning to discuss adopting an EHR system, mobile accessibility, and other new capabilities such as telemedicine. Your supervisor has asked you to come up with some brief talking points for the staff discussing the new technologies, their advantages, and ways in which each staff member will be impacted by the new systems. Come up with a short outline for your presentation.

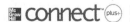 Enhance your learning by completing these exercises and more at http://connect.mcgraw-hill.com!

glossary

a

Abuse   Coding and billing that is inconsistent with typical coding and billing practices.

Access report   A report of all persons (within the facility) who have had access to a patient's protected health information.

Accounting of Disclosures   Providing the patient, upon request, with a listing of all disclosures of his/her health information.

Accounts payable   Monies being paid from the medical practice, for instance, to pay for supplies, rent, utilities, payroll, etc.

Accounts receivable   Monies coming into a medical practice, for instance, insurance payments or payments made by patients.

Administrative information   Identifying information, insurance-related information, authorizations, and business correspondence found in a patient's health record.

Aggregate   The sum total; for instance, the sum total of patients between the ages of 60 and 100 in a practice.

American Association of Medical Assistants (AAMA)   Association of medical assisting professionals that offers certifying exams and provides members with up-to-date, relevant information about clinical and administrative medical practices, continuing education opportunities, networking opportunities, publications, and career assistance.

American Health Information Management Association (AHIMA)   Association of health information management professionals that offers certifying exams and provides members with up-to-date, relevant information about health information and healthcare in general, continuing education opportunities, networking opportunities, publications, and career assistance.

American Medical Technologist Association (AMT)   Association of allied health professionals that offers certifying exams and provides members with up-to-date, relevant information about health information and healthcare in general, continuing education opportunities, networking opportunities, publications, and career assistance.

American Recovery and Reinvestment Act of 2009 (ARRA)   Signed into law by President Obama on February 17, 2009, and otherwise known as the "stimulus plan," it is an economic stimulus plan that includes provisions for the Health Information Technology for Economic and Clinical Health Act (HITECH).

Application   Software that has a special purpose, such as word processing, spreadsheet, or for a particular industry such as practice management or electronic health record software.

Audit trail   A permanent record or accounting of accesses, additions, amendments, or deletions to a health record.

Also, a report that shows accesses by a user to each function of the software.

b

Benchmarking   Comparison of one set of statistics to the overall statistics (using the same variables).

Blog   Ongoing conversations about a topic that take place online via the Internet.

Breach of confidentiality   Releasing information without a required, properly executed authorization.

c

Care provider   Term used to refer to physicians, physicians' assistants, dentists, psychologists, nurse practitioners, or midwives.

Centers for Medicare and Medicaid Services (CMS)   An agency of the Department of Health and Human Services, CMS is responsible for administering the Medicare program.

Certifying Commission for Health Information Technology (CCHIT)   A non-profit, non-governmental agency whose purpose is to certify electronic health records for functionality, interoperability, and security.

Clearinghouse   A clearinghouse is a service that processes data into a standardized billing format and checks for inconsistencies or other errors in the data.

Clinical Decision Support   Allows access to current treatment options for a disease, through electronic or remote methods. Alerts the care provider to possible medication interactions, gives treatment options based on results of clinical trials or research and alerts provider that a patient may have a particular diagnosis based on the data found in the patient's electronic record.

Clinical information   Documentation that includes the patient's medical history, current condition(s), treatment rendered, results of treatment, prognosis, plan of care, diagnosis, and any instructions given by the provider.

CMS-1500 form   Form used by physicians' offices to submit insurance claims.

Compliance plan   A formal, written document that describes how the hospital or physician's practice ensures rules, regulations, and standards are being adhered to.

Confidentiality   The patient's right to expect that his/her health information will be kept confidential.

Co-payment (co-pay)   The amount due from the patient at the time of the office visit; typically a requirement of managed care plans.

Core Objectives   Related to meaningful use of electronic health records (EHR), these are the basic functions that an EHR would include. Examples include recording of a problem list, recording of a medication list, electronic prescribing.

Covered entity   Any healthcare entity that captures or utilizes health information. These include healthcare plans (insurance companies), clearinghouses that process healthcare claims, individual physicians and physicians' practices, any type of therapist (mental health, physical, speech, occupational), dentists, the staffs of hospitals, ambulatory facilities, nursing homes, home health agencies, pharmacies, and employers.

Credentialing   The process of ensuring a care provider has the proper qualifications (educational, experience, malpractice coverage, where applicable) to practice medicine.

Current Procedural Terminology (CPT)   Coding system used to convert narrative procedures and services into numeric form. CPT is used to code procedures and services in a physician's office. In a hospital setting, they are used for outpatient coding (emergency room, outpatient diagnostic testing, or ambulatory surgery, for example).

d

Dashboard   A visual comparison of actual performance to required performance.

Data   A single fact such as a patient's name, height, weight, or other raw fact. Often used interchangeably with *information*, though they are not synonymous terms.

Decryption   Interprets data being received in encrypted (scrambled) form.

Default value   The value that automatically appears in a field each time it appears on a screen. For instance, a default date may be the current date, or a default area code may be the local area code.

Demographic information   Administrative data that identifies the patient. Consists of name, date of birth, sex, social security number (may vary by facility policy).

Detail reports   Reports that do include patient identifying information and list each case individually rather than as sum totals.

Directory information   Information denoting that a patient is an inpatient (or being treated as an outpatient) as well as his/her location within the facility.

Disaster Recovery Plan   A written document that details an inventory of hardware and software, back-up procedure, including location of back-up files, the system used to alert users of the disaster, required security training for personnel, and procedure for restoring back-up files.

Drug formulary   A list of provider-preferred generic and brand name drugs covered under various insurance plans.

e

Electronic claims submission   Submitting insurance claims via wire to a clearinghouse or directly to the insurance carrier.

Electronic health record (EHR)   Comprehensive record of all health records for a patient that is able to be shared electronically with other healthcare providers as necessary.

Electronic medical record (EMR)   The legal patient record that is created within any healthcare facility (hospital, nursing home, ambulatory surgery facility, physician's office, etc.). The EMR is the data source for the electronic health record (EHR).

Encounter   A visit to a healthcare facility for diagnostic or therapeutic services. Examples include physician's office visit, outpatient laboratory or radiology, or emergency department visit.

ePrescribing   Submitting prescriptions via wire to the pharmacy of the patient's choice.

Encounter form   Synonymous with Superbill. A document (paper or electronic) that is used in medical offices to capture the diagnoses and services or procedures performed and from which the CMS-1500 billing form is completed.

Encryption   A security method in which words are scrambled and can only be read if the receiver has a special code to decipher the scrambled message.

Evaluation and Management (E&M) code   The CPT codes used to capture the face-to-face time between a patient and the care provider; takes into consideration the extent of the history, extent of the physical exam, and level of medical decision making required.

Evidence-based medicine   Diagnostic and treatment protocols that are based upon proven research and documented best practices.

Explanation of Benefits (EOB)   An explanation of the charges for services, the amount paid by the insurance company, and the amount due by the subscriber, which is sent to the subscriber (and also to the provider, in some instances).

f

Federal Register   Published daily by the federal government, it includes all actions (proposed and final) taken by the government on that date.

Fee schedule   The amount charged for services rendered in a physician's office by Current Procedural Terminology (CPT) code.

Firewall   A system of hardware and/or software that protects a computer or a network from intruders by filtering activity over the network.

Flag   A message that appears on a screen in written form or as an icon that is a reminder to staff and care providers. Flag examples include: co-payment due; patient due for a screening test; patient is on a payment plan, etc.

Fraud   Intentional or unintentional deception, which in healthcare takes advantage of a patient, an insurance company, Medicare, or Medicaid.

h

Hardware   The tangible items that are used in automation; hardware includes the processing unit, screen, keyboard, screen, mouse, laptops, hand-held devices, etc.

Healthcare administrator   A leadership position within a healthcare facility, including chief executive officer, chief operating officer, chief financial officer, chief information officer, or other higher level management positions. May also be referred to as healthcare manager or health systems manager.

Healthcare Common Procedure Coding System (HCPCS) Coding system required by Medicare and Medicaid to document services and procedures (Level 1–Current Procedural Terminology (CPT) and equipment, supplies, and transport (HCPCS level 2).

Healthcare Information and Management Systems and Society (HIMSS) A non-profit organization that focuses on the use of information technology (IT) and management systems needed to improve healthcare and provides important information regarding the electronic health record.

Health informatics The management of automated health information; the technological side of managing health information—the design, development, structure, implementation, integration and management of the technical aspects of electronic (automated) health record keeping.

Healthcare Integrity and Protection Data Bank (HIPDB) A database of adverse actions related to fraud and abuse; care providers and other healthcare facilities are required to submit to and make inquiries from the HIPDB.

Healthcare manager See healthcare administrator.

Health Information Exchange (HIE) The movement or sharing of information between healthcare entities in a secure manner and in keeping with nationally recognized standards.

Health Information Technology for Economic and Clinical Health Act (HITECH) A portion of the American Recovery and Reinvestment Act (ARRA) that is meant to increase the use of an electronic health records by hospitals and physicians through a monetary incentive program.

Health Insurance Portability and Accountability Act (HIPAA) Passed in 1996, this Act included regulations that afford people who leave their employment the ability to keep their insurance or obtain new health insurance even if they have had a pre-existing medical condition. Also set standards for storing, maintaining, and sharing electronic health information while ensuring the privacy and security of health information.

Health systems administrator See Healthcare administrator

Help A function or menu item that takes the user to a user's guide or gives step-by-step instructions.

Index A listing, as in a listing of all patients who have received care in a hospital, or all patients who have received care in a physician's practice, or all patients listed by diagnosis code. An index is filed alphabetically or numerically.

i

Information Raw facts that have meaning when looked at as a whole.

In-network Care providers who contract with a managed care plan to offer services to members of the managed care plan at a pre-negotiated rate.

Institute of Medicine (IOM) An independent, nonprofit, non-governmental organization that works to provide unbiased and authoritative advice to decision makers and the public.

Insurance plan The medical insurance contract under which a patient is covered; the extent to which services are covered.

Insurance verification The process of contacting the insurance carrier and receiving validation of coverage for that patient, deductible status, and co-pay amount.

International Classification of Diseases, 9th revision, Clinical Modification (ICD-9-CM) The classification system used to convert narrative diagnoses into numeric codes.

Internet A series of networks that allow instant access to information from around the world.

Interoperability Through a single database, many different functions can take place and information can be shared.

Intranet An intranet is a secure environment or private internal network that is available only to a select group, e.g., the staff, within an organization.

l

Library In computer software, a listing of entities from which to choose, for instance, employers, insurance plans, ICD-9-CM codes, or CPT codes.

Live The point at which computer software is put into use in real-time.

Local area network (LAN) Links computers and related devices that are physically close to one another such as within a building.

m

Malware Includes examples such as worms, viruses, and Trojan horses, all of which attack computer programs.

Managed care plans Insurance plans that promote quality, cost-effective healthcare through monitoring of patients, preventive care, and performance measures of providers. Physicians contract with managed care plans to provide care at a pre-determined rate.

Master files Datasets that provide structure and are the building blocks for parts of chart notes.

Master Patient (Person) Index (MPI) A permanent listing of all patients who have received care in a hospital (inpatient or outpatient).

Meaningful Use Part of the requirements of the Health Information Technology for Economic and Clinical Health (HITECH) Act that is meant to increase the use of an electronic health record through monetary incentives provided that the electronic health record is used in a meaningful way to improve patient care.

Medical necessity The fact that there is a medical reason to perform a procedure or service. Documentation exists in the patient's record to show there are sufficient signs, symptoms, or history to warrant the services provided.

Menu objectives Related to meaningful use of electronic health records (EHR), these are additional functions that allow for greater use of EHR functionality. Examples include running statistical reports, registries, or lists; checking for drug interactions; etc.

Minimum necessary As required by the Health Insurance Portability and Accountability Act (HIPAA), releasing the minimum information to satisfy the reason the information is needed or the minimum necessary to perform a job function.

n

National Health Information Network (NHIN) A set of standards, services, and policies that enable the secure exchange of health information over the Internet.

National Practitioner Data Bank (NPDB) Required by law, a database of malpractice payments, revocation of privileges, licensure denial or suspension, denial of medical staff privileges, and similar actions. Care providers and other healthcare facilities are required to submit to and make inquiries from the NPDB.

National Provider Identifier (NPI) number A unique identifier that must be used on insurance claims to identify the care provider and/or group practice that rendered care to the patient.

Notice of Privacy Practices A requirement of the Health Insurance Portability and Accountability Act (HIPAA) that patients be made aware (in writing) of their rights under HIPAA including the fact that they have the right to view/receive a copy of their own record and that amendment to the documentation may be requested; it also documents the ways in which their health information will be used and released to outside entities and the procedure used to file a complaint with the Department of Health and Human Services.

o

Office Administrator Administrative position within an outpatient setting (physician's office practice).

Office of the National Coordinator of Health Information Technology (ONC) The principal federal entity charged with coordination, implementation, and use of health information technology and the electronic exchange of health information.

Optical character recognition (OCR) Technology that converts a document into a format that is computer readable, i.e., into an electronic file.

p

Password A unique code, known only to the user, which is used to gain access to computer applications.

Patient-Centered Medical Home A model that was developed to care for patients with chronic conditions by the American Academy of Family Practitioners to encourage and facilitate a patient's (and family's) involvement in the patient's own care.

Patient flow The step-by-step process of a patient's encounter from check-in (registration) through check-out at the completion of the visit.

Patient list A list of all patients seen by a medical practice, typically filed by patient's last name.

Personal digital assistant (PDA) Mobile device that is small enough to fit in one's hand, yet allows access to local area networks (LANs), wide area networks (WANs), and the Internet; may also have telephone capability.

Personal Health Record (PHR) A record, kept by the patient, that contains a person's health history, immunization status, current and past medications, allergies, and instructions given by a care provider; it often includes patient education materials as well.

Physician Quality Reporting Initiative (PQRI) A voluntary pay-for-performance incentive program. Participating care providers submit data on any of the 100 designated quality measures and receive monetary incentives for doing so.

Picture Archiving and Communications Systems (PACS) Computerized system for enhanced viewing and sharing of images such as x-rays, scans, ultrasounds, mammograms, etc.

Point of care Documentation, dictation, ordering of tests and procedures that occur at the same time the patient is being seen.

Practice management Software used in physicians' offices to gather data on every patient and perform administrative functions from the time an appointment is made through the time the bill for each visit is paid.

Privacy The right to be left alone; the right to expect that one's personal space is respected while undergoing healthcare.

Protected Health Information (PHI) Any piece of information that identifies a patient—includes a patient's name, date of birth, address, e-mail address, telephone number, employer, relatives' names, social security number, medical record number, account numbers tied to the patient, fingerprints, photographs, and characteristics about the patient that would automatically disclose his or her identity. PHI also includes any clinical information about an identified patient.

q

Query Searching a database for patients who meet (or do not meet) certain criteria.

r

Regional Extension Centers (REC) Lend technical assistance and guidance regarding best practices in the selection, implementation, and maintenance of an electronic health record that will satisfy the meaningful use requirements.

Registry A listing that is filed in chronological order based on when something occurred. Examples include a cancer registry, birth registry, or death registry.

Regional Health Information Organization   Healthcare organizations in a geographic area that exchange health information with the goal of improving patient care, reducing duplication, and reducing unnecessary costs.

Registration   The process of being checked in (accounted for) at the time of an appointment in a physician's office or for services in a hospital or other healthcare facility.

Remittance Advice (RA)   A detailed accounting of the claims for which payment is being made by an insurance company. The remittance advice accompanies the payment from the insurance company.

Resolution   The quality of a scanned image as it will appear in the record.

s

Scanner   A piece of equipment that digitizes documents into a format that is readable by a computer.

Smart Phones   Telephones that allow Internet browsing, audio, video, and camera functionality.

Social media   Interactive communication sites via the Internet. Examples are Facebook, MySpace, and Twitter.

Speech (voice) Recognition Technology   Software that recognizes the words being said by the person dictating, and converts the speech to text.

Subscriber   The primary person covered by an insurance plan.

Summary report   Statistical report that includes totals rather than data for individual patients.

Superbill   A document (paper or electronic) that is used in medical offices to capture the diagnoses and services or procedures performed on a patient and from which the CMS-1500 billing form is completed.

t

Tablet computers   Computers that are larger than PDAs or Smart Phones, yet smaller than a laptop computer; allow access to local area networks (LANs), wide area networks (WANs), and the Internet.

Telehealth   Associated with preventive care, telehealth is the use of audiovisual equipment through which the patient and the care provider or healthcare professional can connect remotely.

Telemedicine   The use of technology to remotely monitor a patient's vital signs and perform tests such as an EKG, or to forward radiologic images.

Templates   Preformatted documents built into practice management and electronic health record systems.

Transaction   Posting of charges and the payment of claims in the Practice Management system to update patients' accounts.

u

UB-04 form   Form used to submit insurance claims for hospital patients.

User rights   Privileges that limit access to the functionality of the software needed by that individual.

v

Variable   In relation to a statistical report, the factors that vary from one patient to the next; examples include ZIP code, age, or certain diagnosis codes, and include (or exclude) certain patients from appearing on a report. For example, a report of all patients between 60 and 100 includes every patient within that age range; however, a report of patients between the ages of 60 and 100 who live in ZIP code 12345 excludes all patients from the original report who do not live in ZIP code 12345.

Virtual Private Network (VPN)   Software that encrypts (codes) the data being sent as well as interprets the data being received.

Virus   A deviant program, stored on a computer floppy disk, hard drive, or CD, that can cause unexpected and often undesirable effects, such as destroying or corrupting data.

w

Wide area network (WAN)   Connects computer networks together that are not physically close.

Wi-fi   Data exchange via high radio frequency.

chapter 1

Greenway Medical Solutions. (2009). *Integrated Electronic Health Record Solution (EHR) Fundamentals Training Manual v14.6.* Atlanta, GA. Greenway Medical Technologies.

Greenway Medical Solutions. (2011). Retrieved from http://www.greenwaymedical.com/solutions/.

PrimeSuite: *Integrated Electronic Health Record (EHR), Practice Management and Interoperability Solution: PrimeEnterprise.* Retrieved from http://www.greenwaymedical.com/dynamic/pdf/products/primesuiteproductbrochure.pdf.

PrimeSuite: *The Power of One.* (2011). Retrieved from http://www.greenwaymedical.com/dynamicData/pdf/products/2011/Greenway_PrimeSUITE.pdf.

chapter 2

About the Certification Commission for Health Information Technology. (n.d.). Retrieved from http://www.cchit.org/about.

About the Institute of Medicine. (2011). Retrieved from http://iom.edu/About-IOM.aspx.

Evidence Based Information Cycle (2004). Retrieved from Centre for Health Evidence: http://www.cche.net/info.asp.

Garets, D. and Davis, M. (2005, October). Electronic Patient Records: EMRs and EHRs. *Healthcare Informatics.* Retrieved from http://www.providersedge.com/ehdocs/ehr_articles/Electronic_Patient_Records-EMRs_and_EHRs.pdf.

Health Care Administrator (2004). Retrieved from http://www.mshealthcareers.com/careers/healthcareadmin.htm.

Key Capabilities of an Electronic Health Record System. Retrieved from http://www.iom.edu/Reports/2003/Key-Capabilities-of-an-Electronic-Health-Record-System.aspx.

Newby, C. (2009). *HIPAA for Allied Health Careers.* New York, NY: McGraw-Hill Companies.

U.S. Department of Health and Human Services, Centers for Medicare and Medicaid Services. Medicare Learning Network. (2011). *The National Provider Identifier (NPI): What You Need to Know.* Retrieved from http://www.cms.gov/MLNProducts/downloads/NPIBooklet.pdf.

U.S. Department of Health and Human Services, Centers for Medicare and Medicaid Services. (2010). *HIPAA Privacy and Security Standards.* Retrieved from http://www.cms.gov/HIPAAGenInfo/04_PrivacyandSecurityStandards.asp#TopOfPage.

U.S. Department of Health and Human Services. (2011). HHS Region Map. Retrieved from http://www.hhs.gov/about/regionmap.html.

U.S. Department of Health and Human Services, The Office of the National Coordinator for Health Information Technology. (2011). Retrieved from http://healthit.hhs.gov/portal/server.pt/community/healthit_hhs_gov__home/1204.

U.S. Department of Health and Human Services, The Office of the National Coordinator for Health Information Technology. (2011). *HITECH and Funding Opportunities.* Retrieved from http://healthit.hhs.gov/portal/server.pt/community/healthit_hhs_gov__hitech_and_funding_opportunities/1310.

U.S. Department of Health and Human Services, The Office of the National Coordinator for Health Information Technology. (2011). *National Health Information Network: Overview.* Retrieved from http://healthit.hhs.gov/portal/server.pt?open=512&objID=1142&parentname=CommunityPage&parentid=25&mode=2&in_hi_userid=11113&cached=true.

chapter 3

AHIMA. "Fundamentals for Building a Master Patient Index/Enterprise Master Patient Index (Updated). Appendix A: Recommended Core Data Elements for EMPIs." *Journal of AHIMA.*

Centers for Medicare and Medicaid Services. Eligible Professional Meaningful Use Table of Contents Core and Menu Set Measures. Retrieved from http://www.cms.gov/EHRIncentivePrograms/Downloads/EP-MU-TOC.pdf.

Core Health Data Elements: Report of the National Committee on Vital and Health Statistics, 1996. http://ncvhs.hhs.gov/ncvhsr1.htm.

Newby, Cynthia (2010). *From Patient to Payment: Insurance Procedures for the Medical Office,* 6e. New York. McGraw-Hill.

chapter 4

Booth, K.A., Whicker, L.G., Wyman, Terri D., Moany Wright, Sandra (2011). *Administrative Procedures for Medical Assisting,* 4e. New York, NY: McGraw-Hill Companies.

Green, M.A., Bowie, M.J. (2011). *Essentials of Health Information Management: Principles and Practices,* 2e. Clifton Park, NY: Delmar, Cengage Learning.

Newby, C. (2010). *From Patient to Payment: Insurance Procedures for the Medical Office,* 6e. New York: McGraw-Hill Companies.

chapter 5

NCH Software: Dial Dictate Telephone Dictation System. Retrieved from http://www.nch.com.au/dialdictate/index.html.

Recording History: The History of Recording Technology. Retrieved at http://www.recording-history.org/HTML/dicta_tech5.php.

Recording History: *Edison and Columbia Establish the Business.* Retrieved from http://www.recording-history.org/HTML/dicta_biz2.php.

Recording History: The History of Recording Technology. *The 1970s and the Decline of Dictation.* Retrieved from http://www.recording-history.org/HTML/dicta_biz7.php.

Greenway Medical Technologies. (2011). ePrescribing. Retrieved from http://www.greenwaymedical.com/solutions/eprescribing/.

Wiedemann, Lou Ann. "CPOE Lessons Learned." *Journal of AHIMA* 81, no.10 (October 2010): 54-55.

chapter 6

Booth, K.A., Whicker, L.G., Wyman, Terri D., Moany Wright, Sandra (2011). *Administrative Procedures for Medical Assisting,* 4e. New York, NY: McGraw-Hill Companies.

Current Procedural Terminology (2010). Chicago. American Medical Association.

Greenway Medical Technologies. (2011). *Prime RCM.* Retrieved from http://www.greenwaymedical.com/dynamicData/pdf/products/2011/Greenway_PrimeRCM.pdf.

ICD-9-CM Volumes I, II, & 3. (2010). Ingenix.

ICD-10-CM Integrated Codebook. (2011). 3M Corporation.

Newby, C. (2010). *From Patient to Payment: Insurance Procedures for the Medical Office,* 6/e. New York, NY. McGraw-Hill.

The Qui Tam Online Network. *Common Types of Qui Tam Fraud.* Retrieved from http://www.quitamonline.com/fraud.html.

World Health Organization. (2011) International Classification of Diseases. Retrieved from http://www.who.int/classifications/icd/en/.

chapter 7

Abdelhak, M., Grostick, S., Hanken, M.A., Jacobs, E. (2007). *Health Information: Management of a Strategic Resource*, 3e. Philadelphia, PA: Elsevier.

Centers for Medicare and Medicaid Services, Office for Civil Rights. "Collection Use and Disclosure Limitation." The HIPAA Privacy Rule in Electronic Health Information Exchange in a Networked Environment. Retrieved from www.hhs.gov/ocr/privacy/hipaa/understanding/special/healthit/collectionusedisclosure.pdf.

Certification Commission for Health Information Technology. (2011). Retrieved from http://www.cchit.org/.

Dimick, Chris. "Empowered Patient: Preparing for a New Patient Interaction." *Journal of AHIMA* 81, no.2 (February 2010): 26-31.

Hamilton, Byron R. (2011). *Electronic Health Records*, 2e. New York, NY. McGraw-Hill Companies.

Heubusch, Kevin. "Access Report: OCR Tries Subtraction through Addition in Accounting of Disclosure Rule." *Journal of AHIMA* 82, no.7 (July 2011): 38-39.

HIMSS. (2011) About HIMSS. Retrieved from http://www.himss.org/ASP/aboutHimssHome.asp.

Miaoulis, William M. "Access, Use, and Disclosure: HITECH's Impact on the HIPAA Touchstones." *Journal of AHIMA* 81, no.3 (March 2010): 38-39; 64.

National Alliance for Health Information Technology. "Defining Key Health Information Technology Terms." April 28, 2008. www.hhs.gov/healthit/documents/m20080603/10_2_hit_terms.pdf.

U.S. Department of Health and Human Services. *Health Information Privacy*. Retrieved from: http://www.hhs.gov/ocr/privacy/hipaa/understanding/index.html.

U.S. Department of Health and Human Services. Office of the National Coordinator for Health Information Technology. (2011). *Health IT Home*. Retrieved from http://healthit.hhs.gov/portal/server.pt/community/healthit_hhs_gov__home/1204.

U. S. Department of Health and Human Services. "Proposed Establishment of Certification Programs for Health Information Technology; Proposed Rule." *Federal Register* 75, no. 46 (March 10, 2010): 11327–11373. Retrieved from http://edocket.access.gpo.gov/2010/2010-4991.htm.

Williams, B.K., Sawyer, S.C. (2010). *Using Information Technology: A Practical Introduction to Computers & Communications*, 9e. New York, NY. McGraw-Hill Companies.

chapter 8

Greenway Medical Technologies. (2011). *PrimeSUITE® The Power of One™ Ambulatory Solution™* Instruction Manual: PrimeSUITE 2011.

Williams, B.K. and Sawyer, S. C. (2011). *Using Information Technology: A Practical Introduction to Computers & Communications*, 9e. New York, NY: McGraw-Hill Companies.

chapter 9

Centers for Medicare and Medicaid Services. Medicare & Medicaid EHR Incentive Program: Meaningful Use Stage 1 Requirements. Retrieved from https://www.cms.gov/EHRIncentivePrograms/Downloads/MU_Stage1_ReqOverview.pdf.

HIMSS (2011). *Clinical Decision Support*. Retrieved from http://www.himss.org/ASP/topics_clinicalDecision.asp.

PrimeSUITE 2011 Users' Manual. (2011). *PrimeSUITE 2011 EHR: Introducing Meaningful Use*.

U. S. Department of Health and Human Services (2011). *The DataBank*. Retrieved from http://www.npdb-hipdb.com/.

chapter 10

Abdelhak, M., Grostick, S., Hanken, M.A., Jacobs, E. (2007). *Health Information: Management of a Strategic Resource*. Philadelphia, PA: Saunders.

American Health Information Management Association (AHIMA) Body of Knowledge, *A Vision of the e-HIM Future: A Report from the AHIMA e-HIM Task Force*. (2003) Supplement to the *Journal of AHIMA*.

American Telemedicine Association. "Telemedicine Defined." Retrieved from www.americantelemed.org/i4a/pages/index.cfm?pageid=3333.

Association for Medical Ethics. (2011). *History of Evidence-Based Medicine*. Retrieved from http://www.ethicaldoctor.org/History.html.

Cantrell, S. (2010). Reference and Information Services in the 21st Century: An Introduction. 2/e. *Journal of the Medical Library Association*, 98(3), 264-265. doi:10.3163/1536-5050.98.3.019

Institute of Medicine. (1996). *Telemedicine: A Guide to Assessing Telecommunications for Health Care*. Retrieved from http://www.nap.edu/openbook.php?record_id=5296&page=R1.

LaTour, K.M., Eichenwald-Maki, S. (2010). *Health Information Management: Concepts, Principles and Practice*, 3e. Chicago, IL: AHIMA.

Menachemi, N., Powers, T. L., Brooks, R. G. (2011). Physician and Practice Characteristics Associated with Longitudinal Increases in Electronic Health Records Adoption. *Journal of Healthcare Management*, 56(3), 183-197. Retrieved from EBSCO*host*.

Shi, L., Sing, D.A. (2010). *Essentials of the U.S. Health Care System*, 2e. Sudbury, MA: Jones and Bartlett Publishers.

index

EASY ITALIAN
RECIPES

Publications International, Ltd.

Favorite Brand Name Recipes at www.fbnr.com

Illustrated by Julie Ecklund.

Front cover photography by Stephen Hamilton Photographics, Inc.

Pictured on the front cover: Greens and Gemelli *(page 64).*

Pictured on the back cover *(clockwise from left):* Savory Onion Focaccia *(page 4),* Swordfish Messina Style *(page 96)* and Polenta Apricot Pudding Cake *(page 174).*

ISBN: 0-7853-9682-9

Library of Congress Control Number: 2003109984

Manufactured in China.

8 7 6 5 4 3 2 1

Microwave Cooking: Microwave ovens vary in wattage. Use the cooking times as guidelines and check for doneness before adding more time.

Preparation/Cooking Times: Preparation times are based on the approximate amount of time required to assemble the recipe before cooking, baking, chilling or serving. These times include preparation steps such as measuring, chopping and mixing. The fact that some preparations and cooking can be done simultaneously is taken into account. Preparation of optional ingredients and serving suggestions is not included.

Contents

Appetizers

Savory Onion Focaccia

1 pound frozen pizza or
   bread dough*

1 tablespoon olive oil

1 clove garlic, minced

1⅓ cups *French's*® French Fried
   Onions, divided

1 cup (4 ounces) shredded
   mozzarella cheese

½ pound plum tomatoes
   (4 small), thinly sliced

2 teaspoons fresh chopped
   rosemary *or* ½ teaspoon
   dried rosemary

3 tablespoons grated
   Parmesan cheese

*Pizza dough can be found in frozen section
of supermarket. Thaw in refrigerator before
using.*

Bring pizza dough to room temperature. Grease 15×10-inch jelly-roll pan. Roll or pat dough into rectangle same size as pan on floured board.** Transfer dough to pan.

Combine oil and garlic in small bowl; brush onto surface of dough. Cover loosely with kitchen towel. Let dough rise at room temperature 25 minutes. Prick dough with fork.

Preheat oven to 450°F. Bake dough 20 minutes or until edges and bottom of crust are golden. Sprinkle 1 *cup* French Fried Onions and mozzarella cheese over dough. Arrange tomatoes over cheese; sprinkle with rosemary. Bake 5 minutes or until cheese melts.

Sprinkle with remaining ⅓ *cup* onions and Parmesan cheese. Bake 2 minutes or until onions are golden. To serve, cut into rectangles. *Makes 8 appetizer servings*

**If dough is too hard to roll, allow to rest on floured board.*

Prep Time: 30 minutes
Cook Time: 27 minutes

Savory Onion Focaccia

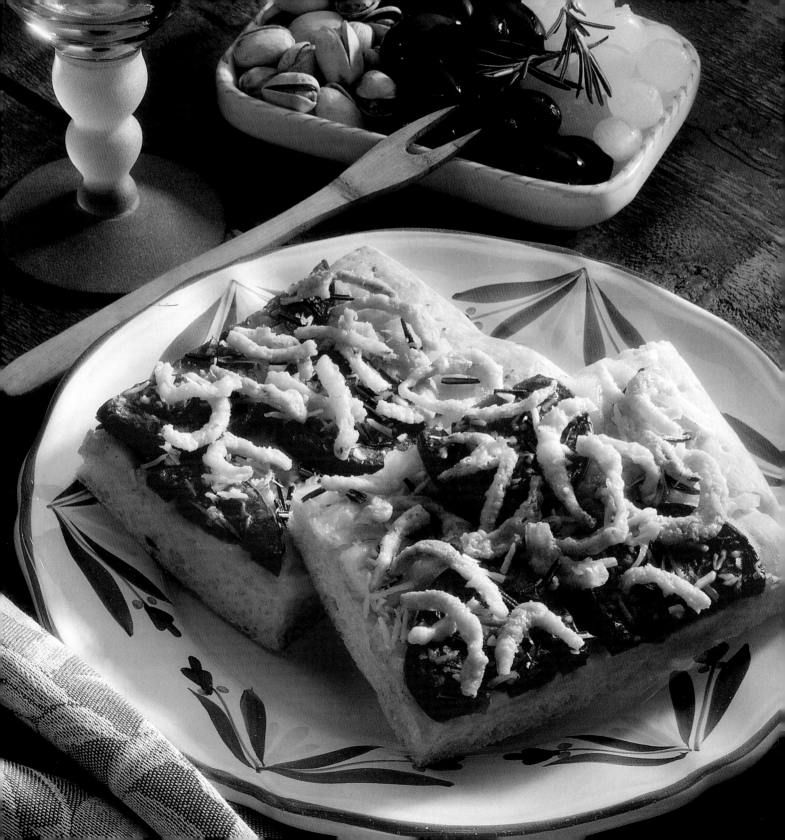

Skewered Antipasto

1 jar (8 ounces) SONOMA®
   marinated dried tomatoes

1 pound (3 medium) new
   potatoes, cooked until
   tender

1 cup drained cooked egg
   tortellini and/or spinach
   tortellini

1 tablespoon chopped fresh
   chives *or* 1 teaspoon dried
   chives

1 tablespoon chopped fresh
   rosemary *or* 1 teaspoon
   dried rosemary

2 cups bite-sized vegetable
   pieces (such as celery, bell
   peppers, radishes, carrots,
   cucumber, green onions)

Drain oil from tomatoes into medium bowl. Place tomatoes in small bowl; set aside. Cut potatoes into 1-inch cubes. Add potatoes, tortellini, chives and rosemary to oil in medium bowl. Stir to coat with oil; cover and marinate 1 hour at room temperature. To assemble, alternately thread tomatoes, potatoes, tortellini and vegetables onto 6-inch skewers.

Makes 12 to 14 skewers

Garlic Cheese Bread

2 tablespoons I CAN'T BELIEVE
   IT'S NOT BUTTER!®
   Spread-tub or stick

1 clove garlic, finely chopped

1 loaf French or Italian bread
   (about 12 inches long),
   halved lengthwise

¼ cup shredded mozzarella
   cheese (about 2 ounces)

2 tablespoons grated
   Parmesan cheese

Preheat oven to 350°F.

In small bowl, blend I Can't Believe It's Not Butter!® Spread and garlic. Evenly spread bread with garlic mixture, then sprinkle with cheeses.

On baking sheet, arrange bread and bake 10 minutes or until bread is golden and cheeses are melted. Slice and serve.

Makes 2 servings

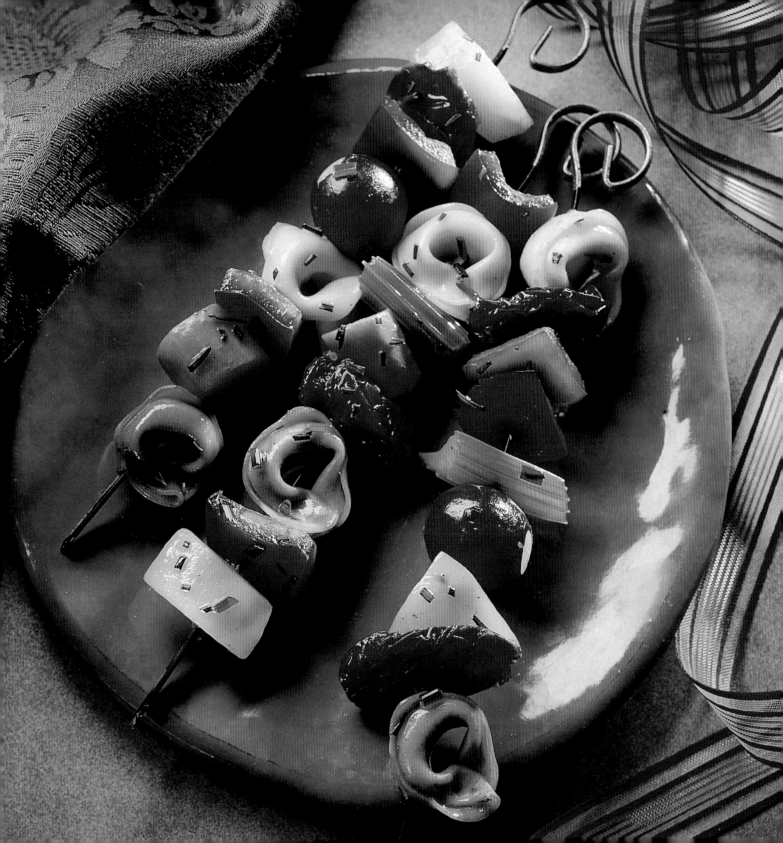

Zesty Bruschetta

1 envelope LIPTON® RECIPE
   SECRETS® Savory Herb
   with Garlic Soup Mix

6 tablespoons BERTOLLI®
   Olive Oil*

1 loaf French or Italian bread
   (about 18 inches long),
   sliced lengthwise

2 tablespoons shredded or
   grated Parmesan cheese

*Substitution: Use ½ cup margarine or butter,
melted.

Preheat oven to 350°F. Blend savory herb with garlic soup mix and oil. Brush onto bread, then sprinkle with cheese.

Bake 12 minutes or until golden. Slice, then serve.

Makes 1 loaf, about 18 pieces

Caponata Spread

1½ tablespoons BERTOLLI®
   Olive Oil

1 medium eggplant, diced
   (about 4 cups)

1 medium onion, chopped

1½ cups water

1 envelope LIPTON® RECIPE
   SECRETS® Savory Herb
   with Garlic Soup Mix

2 tablespoons chopped fresh
   parsley (optional)

Salt and ground black
   pepper to taste

Pita chips or thinly sliced
   Italian or French bread

In 10-inch nonstick skillet, heat oil over medium heat and cook eggplant with onion 3 minutes. Add ½ cup water. Reduce heat to low and simmer covered 3 minutes. Stir in soup mix blended with remaining 1 cup water. Bring to a boil over high heat. Reduce heat to low and simmer uncovered, stirring occasionally, 20 minutes. Stir in parsley, salt and pepper. Serve with pita chips.

Makes about 4 cups spread

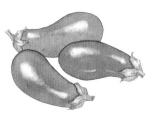

*Left to right: Zesty Bruschetta and
Caponata Spread*

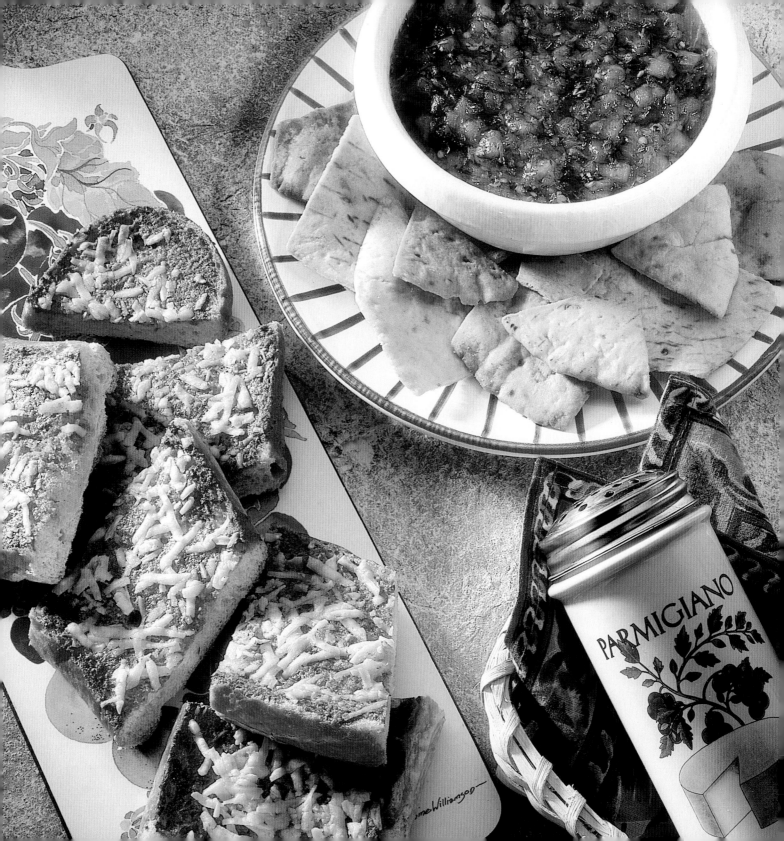

Mushroom Parmesan Crostini

1 tablespoon BERTOLLI®
   Olive Oil

1 clove garlic, finely chopped

1 cup chopped mushrooms

1 loaf Italian or French bread
   (about 12 inches long), cut
   into 12 slices and toasted

¾ cup RAGÚ® Pizza Quick®
   Sauce

¼ cup grated Parmesan cheese

1 tablespoon finely chopped
   fresh basil leaves *or*
   1 teaspoon dried basil
   leaves

Preheat oven to 375°F. In 8-inch nonstick skillet, heat oil over medium heat and cook garlic 30 seconds. Add mushrooms and cook, stirring occasionally, 2 minutes or until liquid evaporates.

On baking sheet, arrange bread slices. Evenly spread Ragú Pizza Quick Sauce on bread slices, then top with mushroom mixture, cheese and basil. Bake 15 minutes or until heated through.   *Makes 12 crostini*

Recipe Tip: Many varieties of mushrooms are available in supermarkets and specialty grocery stores. Shiitake, portobello and cremini mushrooms all have excellent flavor.

French Bread Florentine

¾ pound hot or sweet Italian
   sausage links, removed
   from casing and crumbled

⅓ cup chopped onion

1 loaf French bread (about
   12 inches long), halved
   lengthwise

1 cup RAGÚ® Pizza Quick®
   Sauce

1 box (10 ounces) frozen
   chopped spinach, thawed
   and squeezed dry

1 cup shredded mozzarella
   cheese (about 4 ounces)

Preheat oven to 375°F.

In 10-inch nonstick skillet, brown sausage with onion over medium-high heat until sausage is no longer pink.

On baking sheet, arrange bread halves. Evenly spread Ragú Pizza Quick Sauce on bread halves, then top with sausage mixture, then spinach and cheese. Bake 20 minutes or until cheese is melted.   *Makes 4 servings*

Recipe Tip: These sausage-spinach pizzas are great for parties and after-school snacks. Cut them into 2-inch pieces to fit kid-size mouths.

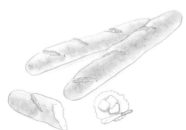

Mushroom Parmesan Crostini

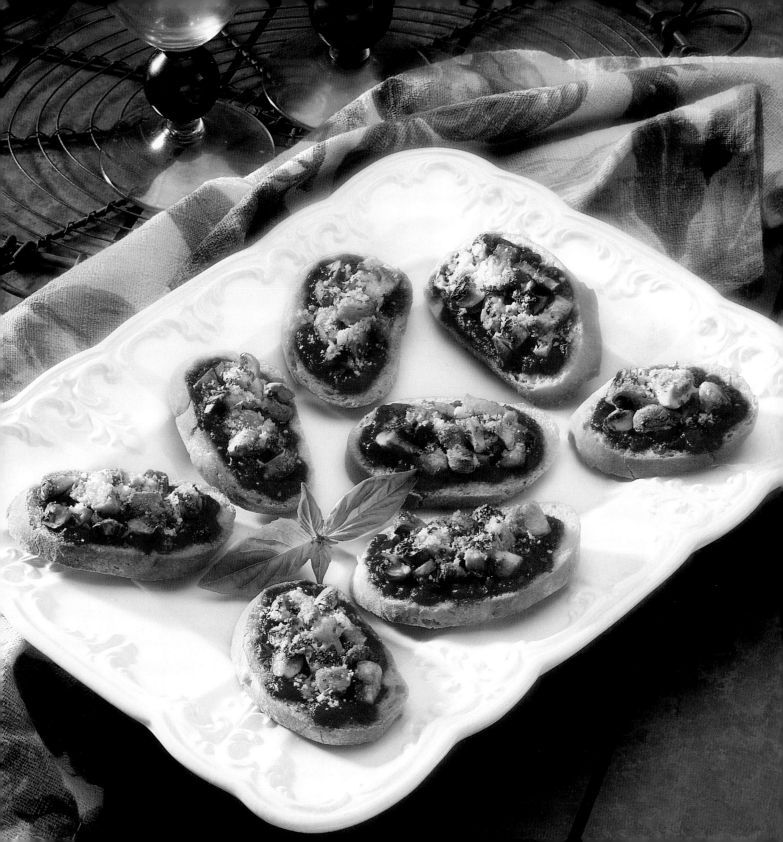

Chicken Pesto Pizza

1 loaf (1 pound) frozen bread dough, thawed

8 ounces chicken tenders, cut into ½-inch pieces

½ red onion, cut into quarters and thinly sliced

¼ cup prepared pesto

2 large plum tomatoes, seeded and diced

1 cup (4 ounces) shredded pizza cheese blend or mozzarella cheese

Preheat oven to 375°F. Roll out bread dough on floured surface to 14×8-inch rectangle. Transfer to baking sheet sprinkled with cornmeal. Cover loosely with plastic wrap and let rise 20 to 30 minutes.

Meanwhile, spray large skillet with nonstick cooking spray; heat over medium heat. Add chicken; cook and stir 2 minutes. Add onion and pesto; cook and stir 3 to 4 minutes or until chicken is cooked through. Stir in tomatoes; remove from heat and let cool slightly.

Spread chicken mixture evenly over bread dough within 1 inch of edges. Sprinkle with cheese.

Bake on bottom rack of oven about 20 minutes or until crust is golden brown. Cut into 2-inch squares. *Makes about 20 appetizer pieces*

Pizza-Stuffed Mushrooms

12 large or 24 medium fresh mushrooms

¼ cup chopped green bell pepper

¼ cup chopped pepperoni or cooked, crumbled Italian sausage

1 cup (½ of 15-ounce can) CONTADINA® Pizza Sauce

½ cup (2 ounces) shredded mozzarella cheese

1. Wash and dry mushrooms; remove stems.

2. Chop ¼ cup stems. In small bowl, combine chopped stems, bell pepper, meat and pizza sauce.

3. Spoon mixture into mushroom caps; top with cheese.

4. Broil 6 to 8 inches from heat for 2 to 3 minutes or until cheese is melted and mushrooms are heated through.

Makes 12 large or 24 medium appetizers

Prep Time: 15 minutes
Cook Time: 3 minutes

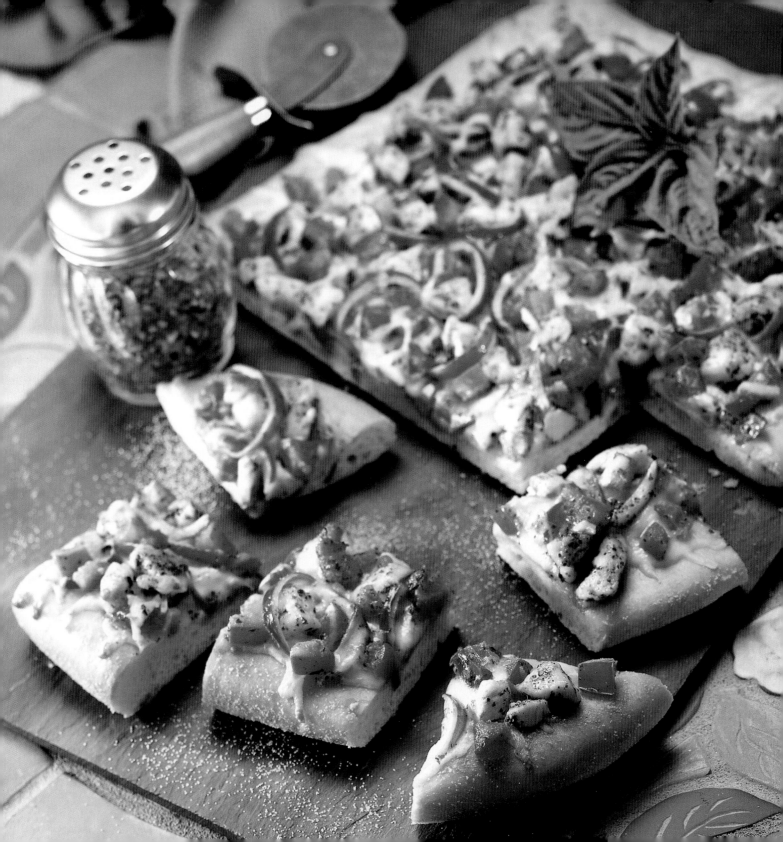

Bruschetta

1 can (14½ ounces)
   DEL MONTE® Diced
   Tomatoes, drained

2 tablespoons chopped fresh
   basil *or* ½ teaspoon dried
   basil

1 small clove garlic, finely
   minced

½ French bread baguette, cut
   into ⅜-inch-thick slices

2 tablespoons olive oil

1. Combine tomatoes, basil and garlic in 1-quart bowl; cover and refrigerate at least ½ hour.

2. Preheat broiler. Place bread slices on baking sheet; lightly brush both sides of bread with oil. Broil until lightly toasted, turning to toast both sides. Cool on wire rack.

3. Bring tomato mixture to room temperature. Spoon tomato mixture over bread and serve immediately. Sprinkle with additional fresh basil leaves, if desired.   *Makes 8 appetizer servings*

Note: For a fat-free version, omit olive oil. For a lower-fat variation, spray the bread with olive oil cooking spray.

Prep Time: 15 minutes
Cook Time: 30 minutes

BelGioioso® Fontina Melt

1 loaf Italian or French bread

2 fresh tomatoes, cubed

   Basil leaves, julienned

   BELGIOIOSO® Fontina
   Cheese, sliced

Cut bread lengthwise into halves. Top each half with tomatoes and sprinkle with basil. Top with BelGioioso Fontina Cheese. Place in oven at 350°F for 10 to 12 minutes or until cheese is golden brown.   *Makes 6 to 8 servings*

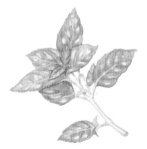

Bruschetta

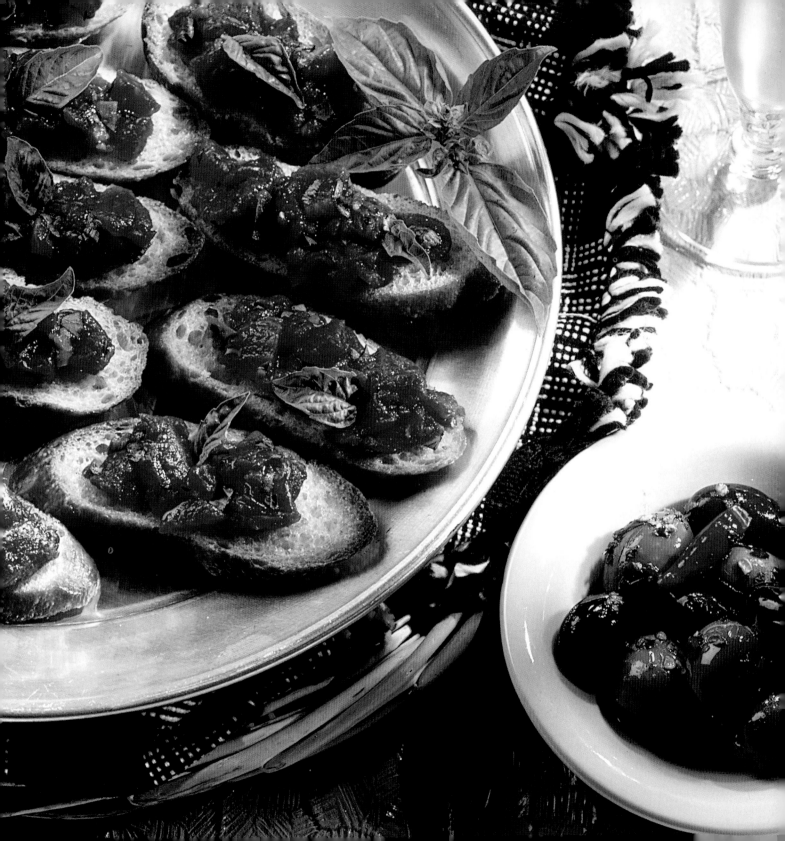

Pizzette with Basil

1 can (6 ounces) CONTADINA® Italian Paste with Italian Seasonings

2 tablespoons softened cream cheese

2 tablespoons chopped fresh basil *or* 2 teaspoons dried basil leaves

1 loaf (1 pound) Italian bread, sliced ¼ inch thick

8 ounces mozzarella cheese, thinly sliced

Whole basil leaves (optional)

Freshly ground black pepper (optional)

1. Combine tomato paste, cream cheese and chopped basil in small bowl.

2. Toast bread slices on *ungreased* baking sheet under broiler, 6 to 8 inches from heat, turning after 1 minute, until lightly browned on both sides; remove from broiler.

3. Spread 2 teaspoons tomato mixture onto each toasted bread slice; top with 1 slice (about ¼ ounce) mozzarella cheese.

4. Broil 6 to 8 inches from heat for 1 to 2 minutes or until cheese begins to melt. Top with whole basil leaves and pepper, if desired.

Makes about 30 pizzettes

Prep Time: 7 minutes
Cook Time: 10 minutes

Fast Pesto Focaccia

1 can (10 ounces) pizza crust dough

2 tablespoons prepared pesto

4 sun-dried tomatoes packed in oil, drained

1. Preheat oven to 425°F. Lightly grease 8×8×2-inch pan. Unroll pizza dough; fold in half and pat into pan.

2. Spread pesto evenly over dough. Chop tomatoes or snip with kitchen scissors; sprinkle over pesto. Press tomatoes into dough. Make indentations in dough every 2 inches using wooden spoon handle.

3. Bake 10 to 12 minutes or until golden brown. Cut into squares and serve warm or at room temperature.

Makes 16 squares

Prep and Cook Time: 20 minutes

Pizzette with Basil

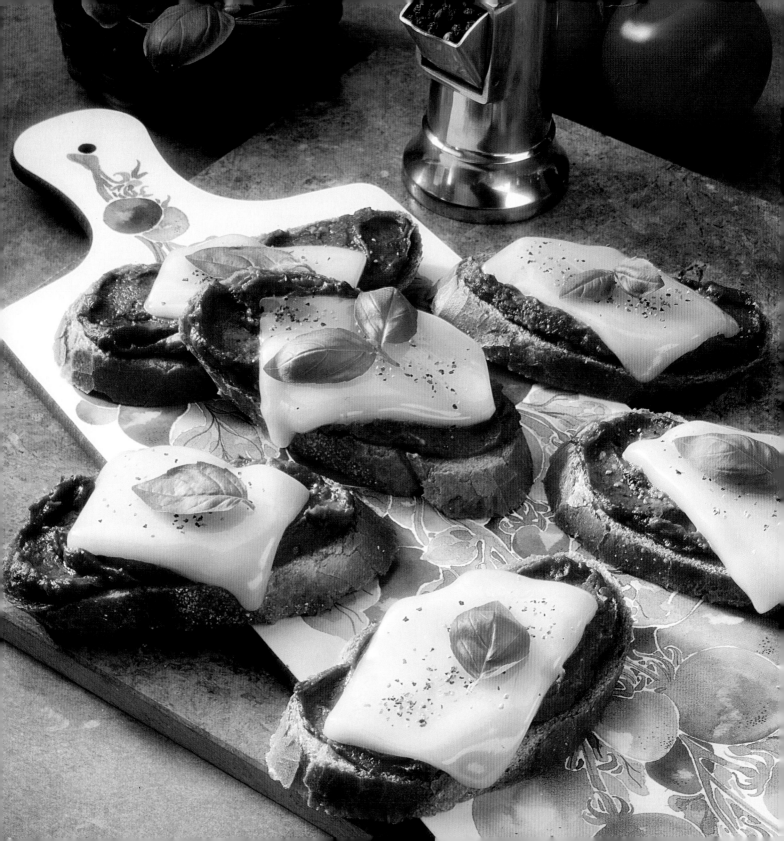

Artichoke Crostini

1 jar (6 ounces) marinated
   artichoke hearts, drained
   and chopped

3 green onions, chopped

5 tablespoons grated
   Parmesan cheese, divided

2 tablespoons mayonnaise

12 slices French bread (½ inch
   thick)

1. Preheat broiler. Combine artichokes, green onions, 3 tablespoons cheese and mayonnaise in small bowl; mix well.

2. Arrange bread slices on baking sheet. Broil 4 to 5 inches from heat source 2 to 3 minutes on each side or until lightly browned.

3. Remove baking sheet from broiler. Spoon about 1 tablespoon artichoke mixture on each bread slice and sprinkle with remaining 2 tablespoons cheese. Broil 1 to 2 minutes or until cheese is melted and lightly browned.

Makes 4 servings

Tip: Garnish crostini with red bell pepper, if desired.

Prep and Cook Time: 25 minutes

Italian Bread with Tomato Appetizers

3 medium tomatoes, seeded
   and finely chopped

2 tablespoons finely chopped
   red onion

1 tablespoon chopped fresh
   basil leaves

¼ teaspoon ground black
   pepper (optional)

8 tablespoons WISH-BONE®
   Italian Dressing*

1 loaf Italian or French bread
   (about 18 inches long)

*Also terrific with WISH-BONE® Robusto
Italian or Lite Italian Dressing.*

In small bowl, combine tomatoes, onion, basil, pepper and 2 tablespoons Italian dressing; set aside.

Slice bread diagonally into 18 slices. Brush one side of each slice with remaining 6 tablespoons dressing. Grill or broil bread until golden, turning once. Evenly top grilled slices with tomato mixture. *Makes 18 servings*

Note: Tomato mixture can be prepared ahead.

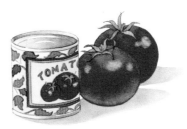

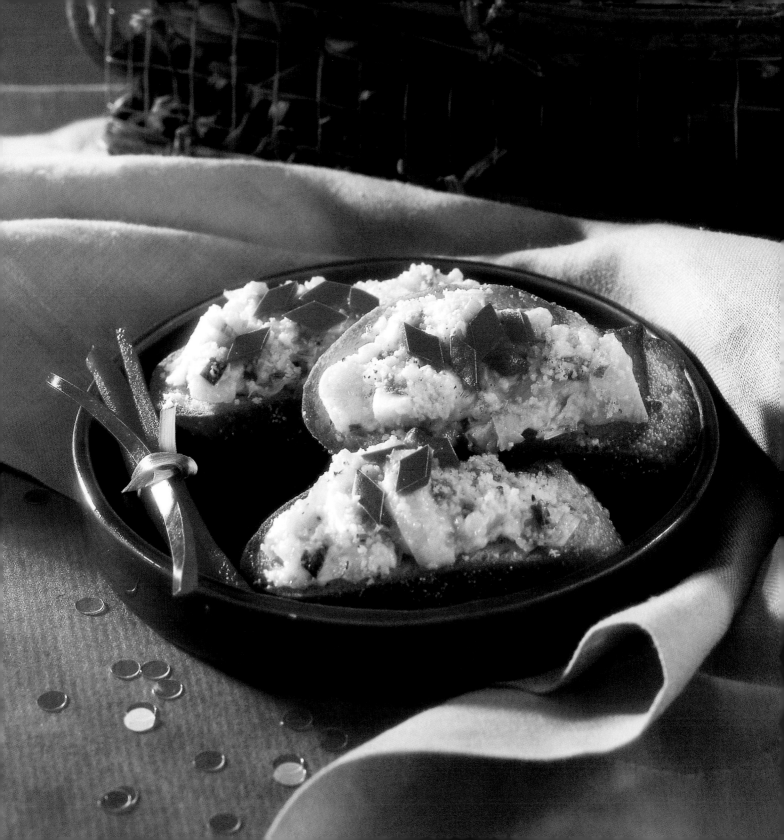

Tortellini Kabobs with Pesto Ranch Dip

½ bag (16 ounces) frozen
   tortellini

1¼ cups ranch salad dressing

½ cup grated Parmesan cheese

3 cloves garlic, minced

2 teaspoons dried basil leaves

1. Cook tortellini according to package directions. Rinse and drain under cold water. Thread tortellini onto bamboo skewers, 2 tortellini per skewer.

2. Combine salad dressing, cheese, garlic and basil in small bowl. Serve tortellini kabobs with dip.   *Makes 6 to 8 servings*

Serving suggestion: For an even quicker dip, combine purchased spaghetti sauce or salsa with some finely chopped black olives.

Prep and Cook Time: 30 minutes

Caponata

1 pound eggplant, cut into
   ½-inch cubes

3 large cloves garlic, minced

¼ cup olive oil

1 can (14½ ounces)
   DEL MONTE® Diced
   Tomatoes with Basil,
   Garlic & Oregano

1 medium green pepper, finely
   chopped

1 can (2¼ ounces) chopped
   ripe olives, drained

2 tablespoons lemon juice

1 teaspoon dried basil, crushed

1 baguette French bread,
   cut into ¼-inch slices

1. Cook eggplant and garlic in oil in large skillet over medium heat 5 minutes. Season with salt and pepper, if desired.

2. Stir in remaining ingredients except bread. Cook, uncovered, 10 minutes or until thickened.

3. Cover and chill. Serve with bread.   *Makes approximately 4½ cups*

Prep Time: 10 minutes
Cook Time: 15 minutes
Chill Time: 2 hours

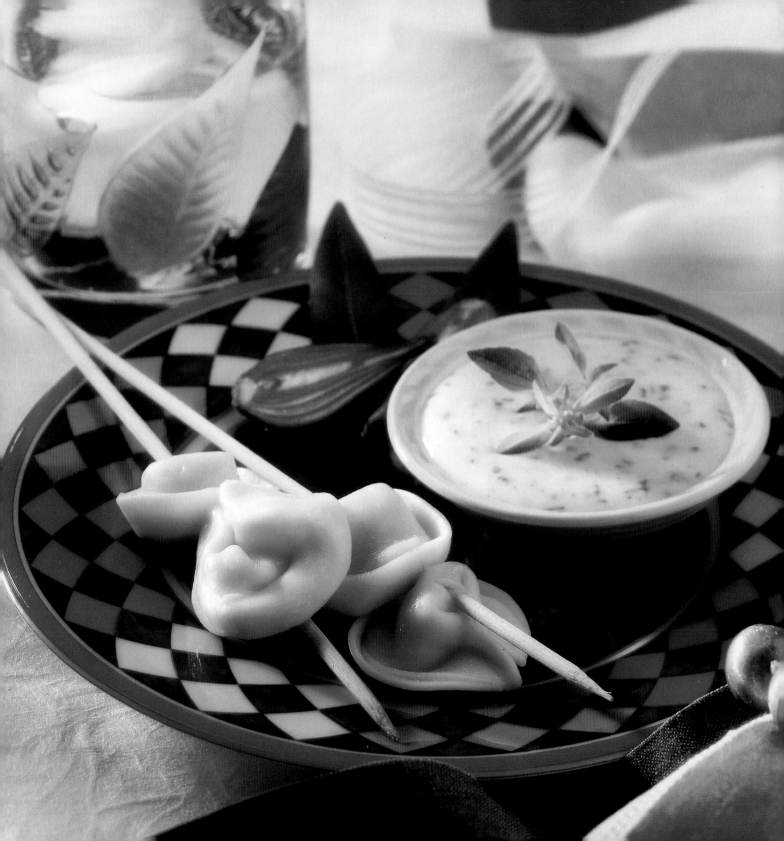

Soups & Salads

Italian Rustico Soup

1 cup BARILLA® Elbows

2 tablespoons olive or
 vegetable oil

1 pound fresh escarole or
 spinach, chopped

1 small onion, chopped

2 teaspoons minced garlic

4 cups water

2 cans (14½ ounces each)
 chicken broth

1 jar (26 ounces) BARILLA®
 Lasagna & Casserole
 Sauce or Marinara
 Pasta Sauce

1 can (15 ounces) white
 beans, drained

2 teaspoons balsamic or red
 wine vinegar

 Grated Parmesan cheese
 (optional)

1. Cook elbows according to package directions; drain.

2. Heat oil in 4-quart Dutch oven or large pot. Add escarole, onion and garlic; cook over medium heat, stirring occasionally, about 5 minutes or until onion is tender.

3. Stir in cooked elbows and remaining ingredients except cheese; heat to boiling. Reduce heat; cook, uncovered, 15 minutes, stirring occasionally. Serve with cheese, if desired. *Makes 12 servings*

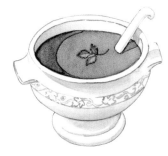

Italian Rustico Soup

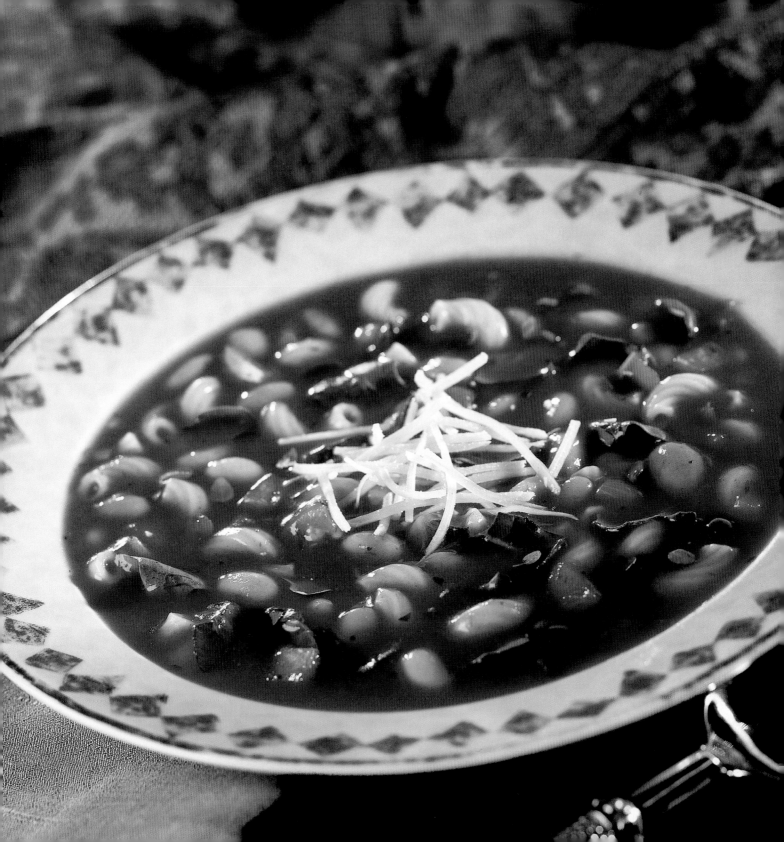

Sicilian-Style Pasta Salad

1 pound dry rotini pasta

2 cans (14.5 ounces each)
   CONTADINA® Recipe
   Ready Diced Tomatoes
   with Italian Herbs,
   undrained

1 cup sliced yellow bell pepper

1 cup sliced zucchini

8 ounces cooked bay shrimp

1 can (2.25 ounces) sliced
   pitted ripe olives, drained

2 tablespoons balsamic vinegar

1. Cook pasta according to package directions; drain.

2. Combine pasta, undrained tomatoes, bell pepper, zucchini, shrimp, olives and vinegar in large bowl; toss well.

3. Cover. Chill before serving.

Makes 10 servings

Italian Artichoke and Rotini Salad

4 ounces uncooked tri-colored
   rotini pasta

1 can (14 ounces) quartered
   artichoke hearts, drained

4 ounces (½ cup) sliced
   pimientos

1 can (2½ ounces) sliced black
   olives, drained

2 tablespoons finely chopped
   yellow onion

2 teaspoons dried basil leaves

½ clove garlic, minced

⅛ teaspoon black pepper

3 tablespoons cider vinegar

1 tablespoon extra-virgin olive
   oil

¼ teaspoon salt

1. Cook pasta according to package directions. Combine artichokes, pimientos, olives, onion, basil, garlic and pepper in medium bowl.

2. Drain pasta in colander; rinse under cold running water to cool completely. Drain well. Add to artichoke mixture and toss to blend. Just before serving, combine vinegar, oil and salt; whisk until well blended. Toss with pasta mixture to coat.

Makes 6 servings

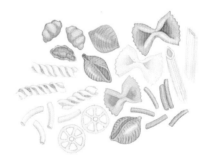

Sicilian-Style Pasta Salad

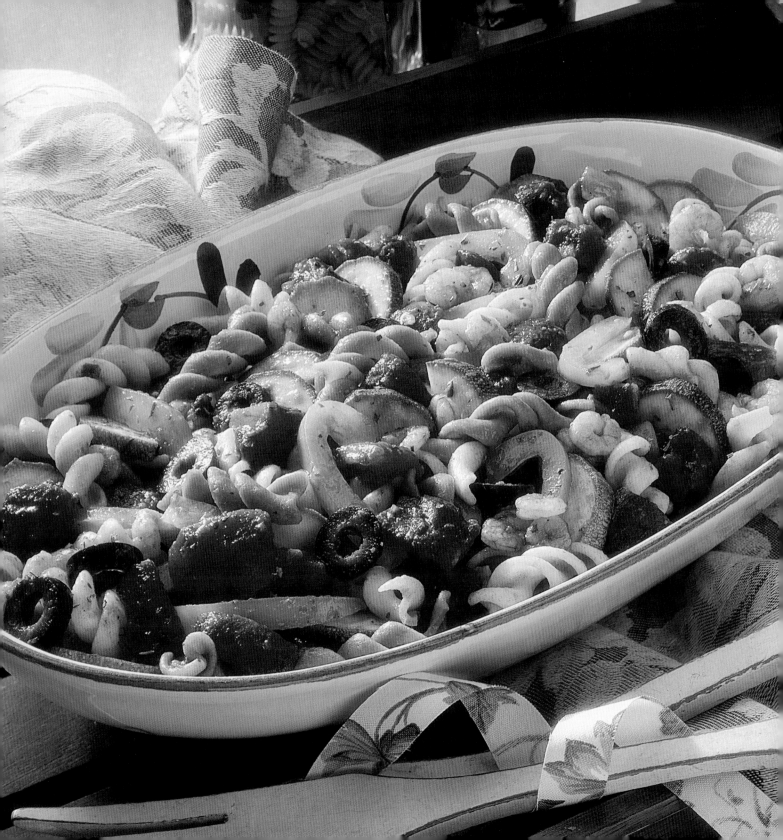

Quick Tuscan Bean, Tomato and Spinach Soup

2 cans (14½ ounces each) diced tomatoes with onions, undrained

1 can (14½ ounces) fat-free, reduced-sodium chicken broth

2 teaspoons sugar

2 teaspoons dried basil leaves

¾ teaspoon reduced-sodium Worcestershire sauce

1 can (15 ounces) small white beans, rinsed and drained

3 ounces fresh baby spinach leaves or chopped spinach leaves, stems removed

2 teaspoons extra-virgin olive oil

1. Combine tomatoes with juice, chicken broth, sugar, basil and Worcestershire sauce in Dutch oven or large saucepan; bring to a boil over high heat. Reduce heat and simmer, uncovered, 10 minutes.

2. Stir in beans and spinach; cook 5 minutes longer or until spinach is tender.

3. Remove from heat; stir in oil just before serving.

Makes 4 (1½-cup) servings

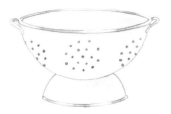

Green Bean Salad

1 pound fresh green beans, trimmed

3 tablespoons lemon juice

1 tablespoon FILIPPO BERIO® Extra Virgin Olive Oil

½ teaspoon dried oregano leaves

Salt

In medium saucepan, cook beans in boiling salted water 10 to 15 minutes or until tender. Drain well; cool slightly. In small bowl, whisk together lemon juice, olive oil and oregano. Pour over green beans; toss until lightly coated. Cover; refrigerate several hours or overnight before serving. Season to taste with salt.

Makes 6 servings

Note: Salad may also be served as an appetizer.

Quick Tuscan Bean, Tomato and Spinach Soup

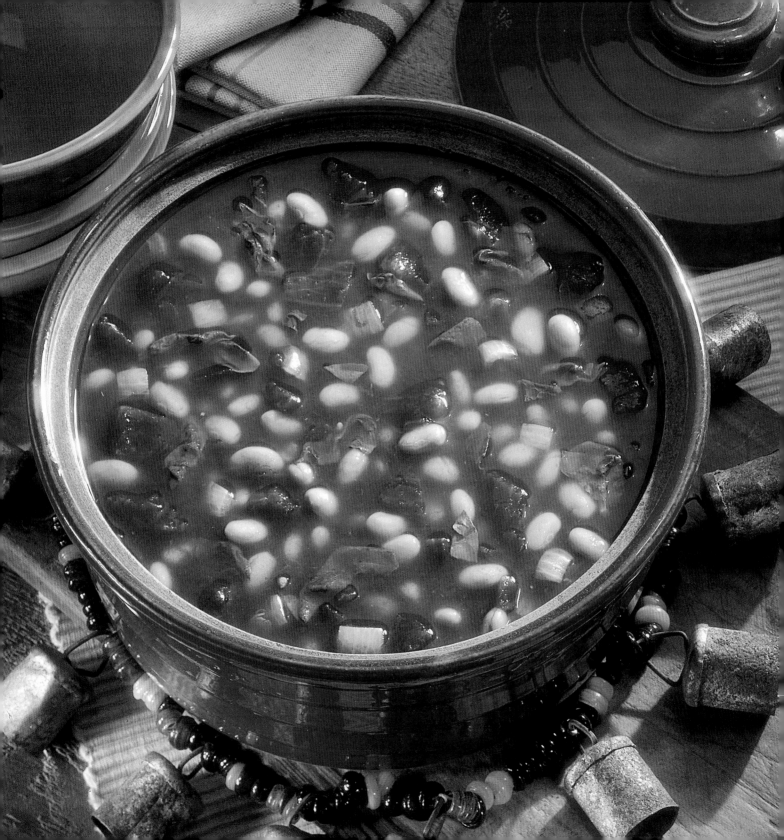

Isle of Capri Salad

8 ounces BARILLA® Farfalle

1 can (6 ounces) tuna packed in water, drained

6 plum tomatoes, seeded and chopped into large pieces

8 ounces fresh mozzarella cheese, diced

½ cup fresh basil leaves, coarsely chopped

2 cloves garlic, minced

¾ cup bottled Italian salad dressing

Salt and pepper

1. Cook farfalle according to package directions; drain.

2. Place tuna in large salad bowl with tomatoes, mozzarella, basil and garlic. Add salad dressing and cooked farfalle; toss to coat. Chill before serving.

3. Add salt and pepper to taste. Stir in additional salad dressing before serving, if necessary.

Makes 6 to 8 servings

Minute Minestrone Soup

½ pound turkey sausage, cut into small pieces

2 cloves garlic, crushed

3 cans (14½ ounces each) low-sodium chicken broth

2 cups frozen Italian blend vegetables

1 can (15 ounces) white kidney beans, rinsed and drained

1 can (14½ ounces) Italian stewed tomatoes, undrained

1 cup cooked ditalini or small shell pasta (½ cup uncooked)

3 tablespoons French's® Worcestershire Sauce

1. In medium saucepan, stir-fry sausage and garlic 5 minutes or until sausage is cooked; drain. Add broth, vegetables, beans and tomatoes. Heat to boiling. Simmer, uncovered, 5 minutes or until vegetables are crisp-tender.

2. Stir in pasta and Worcestershire. Cook until heated through. Serve with grated cheese and crusty bread, if desired.

Makes 6 servings

Prep Time: 10 minutes
Cook Time: about 10 minutes

Isle of Capri Salad

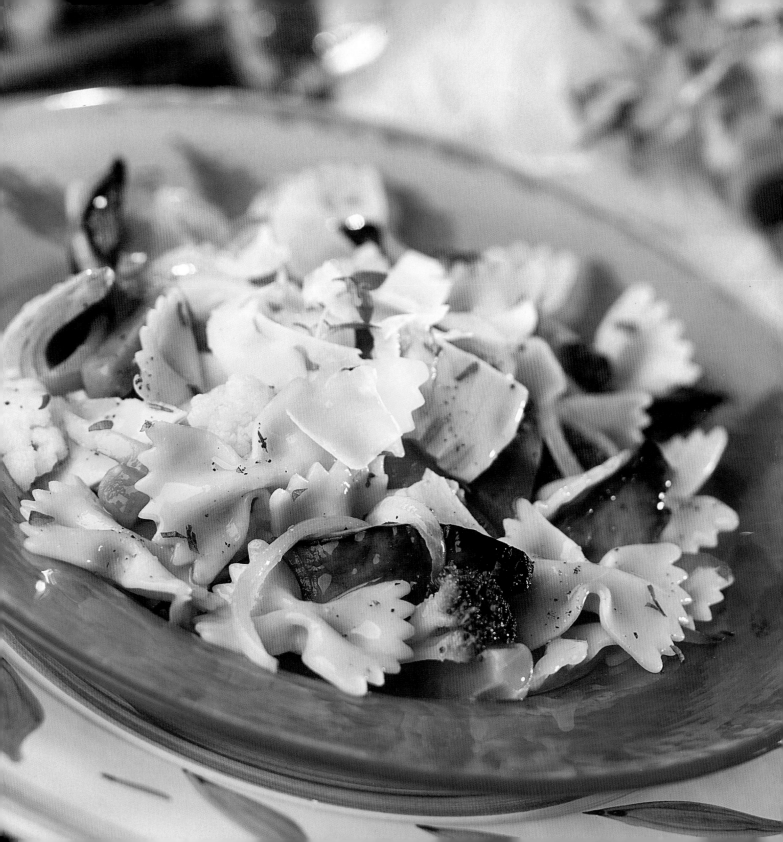

Veg•All® Italian Soup

2 tablespoons butter

1 cup diced onion

1 cup shredded cabbage

2 cups water

2 cans (14½ ounces each)
stewed tomatoes

1 can (15 ounces) VEG•ALL®
Original Mixed Vegetables,
drained

1 tablespoon chopped fresh
parsley

½ teaspoon dried basil

½ teaspoon dried oregano

½ teaspoon black pepper

In large saucepan, melt butter. Stir in onion and cabbage. Heat for 2 minutes. Add water; cover and simmer for 10 minutes. Stir in tomatoes, Veg•All and seasonings. Simmer for 10 minutes.

Makes 6 servings

Oven-Broiled Italian Style Salad

¼ cup FILIPPO BERIO® Olive Oil

1 clove garlic, crushed

2 medium red onions, thinly
sliced into rounds

3 large beefsteak tomatoes,
thinly sliced into rounds

1 (8-ounce) package thinly
sliced part-skim mozzarella
cheese

1 tablespoon balsamic vinegar

3 tablespoons shredded fresh
basil *or* 1 tablespoon dried
basil leaves

Salt and freshly ground black
pepper

In small bowl, combine olive oil and garlic. Brush 2 tablespoons olive oil mixture over onion slices. In large nonstick skillet, cook onions over medium heat 5 minutes or until beginning to brown, turning halfway through cooking time. In large, shallow, heatproof serving dish, arrange slightly overlapping slices of onion, tomato and mozzarella. Whisk vinegar into remaining 2 tablespoons olive oil mixture; drizzle over onion mixture. Broil, 4 to 5 inches from heat, 4 to 5 minutes or until cheese just begins to melt. Sprinkle with basil. Season to taste with salt and pepper.

Makes 4 servings

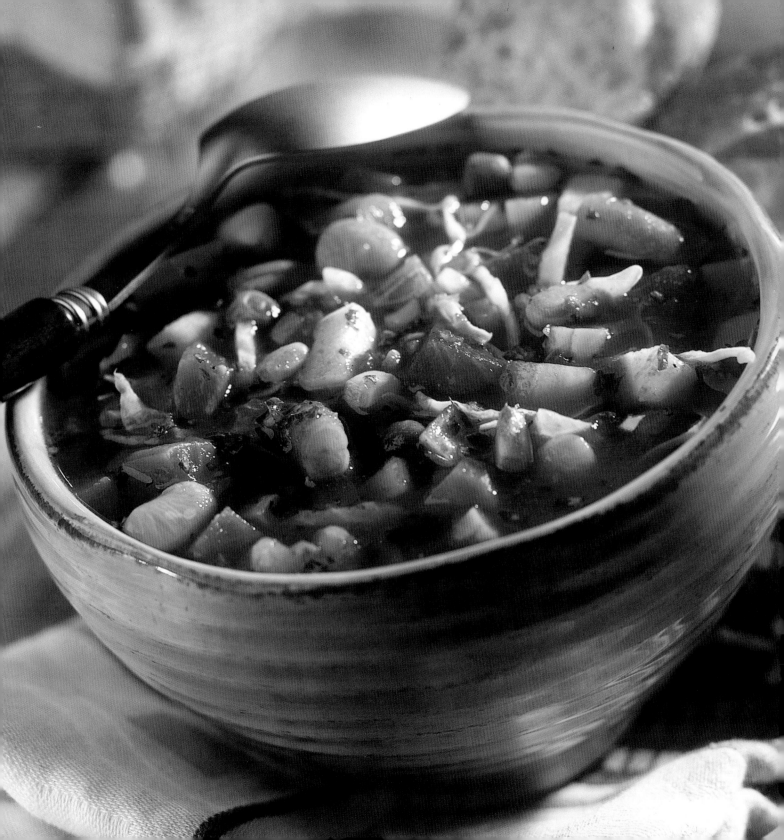

Pasta Fagioli

1 jar (1 pound 10 ounces)
  RAGÚ® Chunky Gardenstyle
  Pasta Sauce

1 can (19 ounces) white kidney
  beans, rinsed and drained

1 box (10 ounces) frozen
  chopped spinach, thawed

8 ounces ditalini pasta, cooked
  and drained (reserve
  2 cups pasta water)

1. In 6-quart saucepot, combine Ragú Pasta Sauce, beans, spinach, pasta and reserved pasta water; heat through.

2. Season, if desired, with salt, ground black pepper and grated Parmesan cheese.

Makes 4 servings

Prep Time: 10 minutes
Cook Time: 10 minutes

Italian Peasant Salad

1 (6.9-ounce) package
  RICE-A-RONI® Chicken
  Flavor

2 tablespoons vegetable oil

1 (16-ounce) can cannellini
  beans, Great Northern
  beans or navy beans,
  rinsed and drained

2 cups chopped cooked
  chicken

2 medium tomatoes, chopped

1 cup frozen or canned peas,
  drained

½ cup Italian dressing

1 teaspoon dried basil *or*
  ½ teaspoon dried rosemary
  leaves, crushed

1. In large skillet over medium heat, sauté rice-vermicelli mix with oil until vermicelli is golden brown.

2. Slowly stir in 2½ cups water and Special Seasonings; bring to a boil. Reduce heat to low. Cover; simmer 15 to 20 minutes or until rice is tender. Cool 10 minutes.

3. In large bowl, combine rice mixture, beans, chicken, tomatoes, peas, Italian dressing and basil. Cover; chill 1 hour before serving.

Makes 6 servings

Prep Time: 10 minutes
Cook Time: 25 minutes

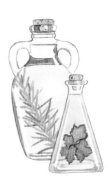

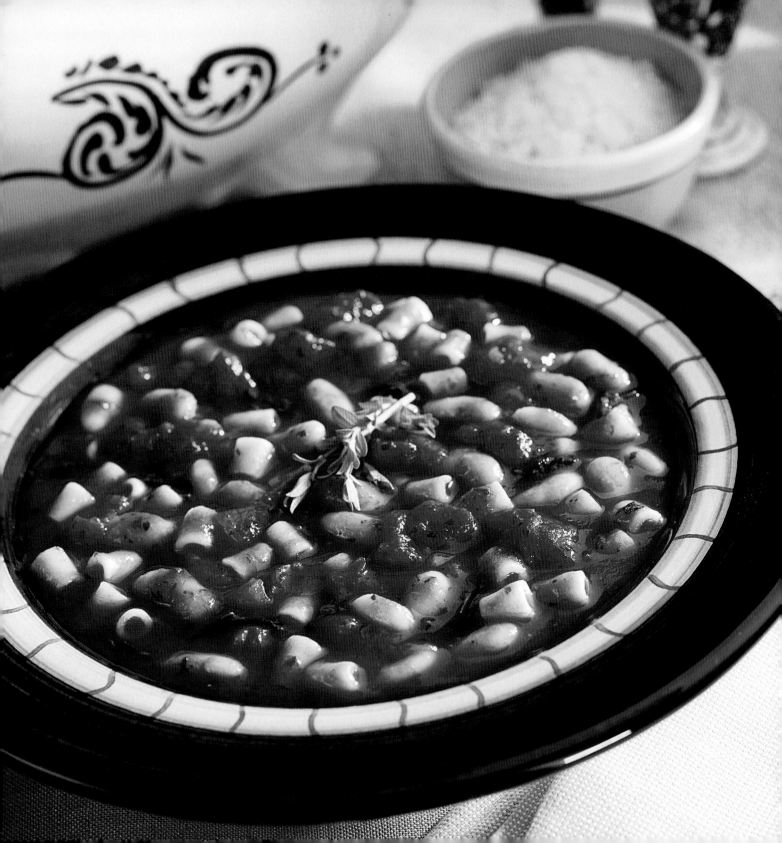

Primavera Tortellini en Brodo

2 cans (about 14 ounces each) reduced-sodium chicken broth

1 package (9 ounces) refrigerated fresh tortellini (cheese, chicken or sausage)

2 cups frozen mixed vegetables, such as broccoli, green beans, onions and red bell peppers

1 teaspoon dried basil leaves

Dash hot pepper sauce or to taste

2 teaspoons cornstarch

1 tablespoon water

¼ cup grated Romano or Parmesan cheese

1. Pour broth into large deep skillet. Cover and bring to a boil over high heat. Add tortellini; reduce heat to medium-high. Cook, uncovered, until pasta is tender, stirring occasionally. (Check package directions for approximate timing.)

2. Transfer tortellini to medium bowl with slotted spoon; keep warm.

3. Add vegetables, basil and hot pepper sauce to broth; bring to a boil. Reduce heat to medium; simmer about 3 minutes or until vegetables are crisp-tender.

4. Blend cornstarch and water in small cup until smooth. Stir into broth mixture. Cook about 2 minutes or until liquid thickens slightly, stirring frequently. Return tortellini to skillet; heat through. Ladle into shallow soup bowls; sprinkle with cheese.

Makes 2 servings

Serving Suggestion: Serve with salad and crusty Italian bread.

Prep and Cook Time: 20 minutes

Italian Vegetable Soup

1 package KNORR® Recipe Classics™ Tomato Basil Soup, Dip and Recipe Mix

4 cups water

2 cups sliced fennel or broccoli florets

1 large zucchini, diced (about 2 cups)

1 teaspoon dried oregano

Grated Parmesan cheese (optional)

• In 4-quart Dutch oven, combine recipe mix, water, fennel, zucchini and oregano. Stirring occasionally, bring to a boil over medium-high heat.

• Reduce heat, cover and simmer 15 minutes, stirring occasionally or until vegetables are tender.

• If desired, sprinkle lightly with Parmesan cheese.

Makes 6 (1-cup) servings

Prep Time: 20 minutes
Cook Time: 25 minutes

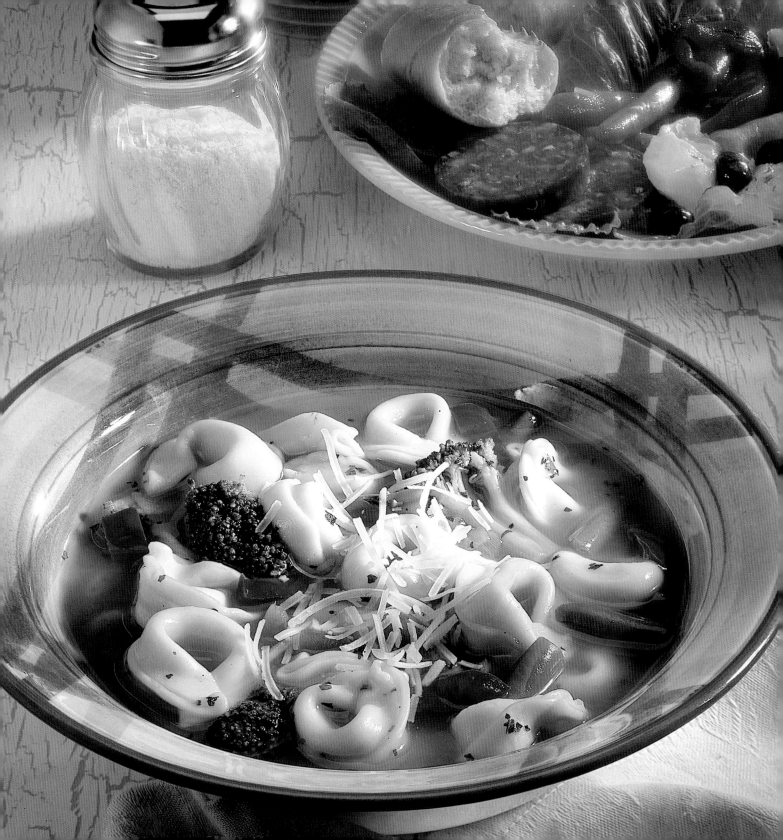

Easy Antipasto Salad

1 can (14.5 ounces)
  CONTADINA® Stewed
  Tomatoes, drained

½ cup thinly sliced cucumber

½ cup thinly sliced onion

2 jars (6 ounces each)
  marinated artichoke
  hearts, drained, cut in half

1 ounce thinly sliced salami
  (optional)

½ cup sliced pitted ripe olives,
  drained

½ cup thinly sliced green bell
  pepper

½ cup Italian dressing

  Lettuce leaves (optional)

1. Layer tomatoes, cucumber, onion, artichoke hearts, salami, olives and bell pepper in 1-quart casserole dish.

2. Pour dressing over salad; cover. Chill before serving. Serve over lettuce leaves, if desired.

Makes 6 servings

Prep Time: 10 minutes
Chill Time: 1 hour

Lentil Soup

1 tablespoon FILIPPO BERIO®
  Olive Oil

1 medium onion, diced

4 cups beef broth

1 cup dried lentils, rinsed and
  drained

¼ cup tomato sauce

1 teaspoon dried Italian herb
  seasoning

  Salt and freshly ground black
  pepper

In large saucepan, heat olive oil over medium heat until hot. Add onion; cook and stir 5 minutes or until softened. Add beef broth; bring mixture to a boil. Stir in lentils, tomato sauce and Italian seasoning. Cover; reduce heat to low and simmer 45 minutes or until lentils are tender. Season to taste with salt and pepper. Serve hot.

Makes 6 servings

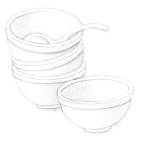

Noodle Soup Parmigiano

3 cups water

½ pound boneless skinless chicken breast halves, cut into ½-inch pieces

I cup chopped fresh tomatoes *or* I can (8 ounces) whole peeled tomatoes, undrained and chopped

I pouch LIPTON® Soup Secrets Noodle Soup Mix with Real Chicken Broth

½ teaspoon LAWRY'S® Garlic Powder with Parsley (optional)

½ cup shredded mozzarella cheese (about 2 ounces)

Grated Parmesan cheese (optional)

In medium saucepan, combine all ingredients except cheeses; bring to a boil. Reduce heat and simmer uncovered, stirring occasionally, 5 minutes or until chicken is thoroughly cooked. To serve, spoon into bowls; sprinkle with cheeses.

Makes about 5 (1-cup) servings

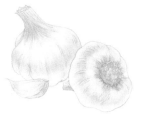

Pasta Pesto Salad

8 ounces BARILLA® Penne or Mostaccioli, cooked according to package directions and chilled

I container (about 7 ounces) prepared pesto sauce

4 plum tomatoes, cut into large chunks

I cup roasted red peppers, cut into strips*

I cup (4 ounces) crumbled feta cheese

Salt and pepper

1. Combine chilled penne and pesto sauce in large serving bowl.

2. Add tomatoes and red peppers; toss gently. Sprinkle with cheese. Add salt and pepper to taste.

Makes 6 to 8 servings

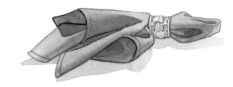

*Roasted red peppers are available in jars in Italian, deli or produce sections of supermarkets.

Antipasto Salad

1 package (12 ounces)
   HEBREW NATIONAL® Beef
   Polish Sausage

1 can (14½ ounces) quartered
   artichoke hearts, drained

12 small cherry tomatoes *or*
   1 large tomato, chopped

12 kalamata olives, drained

4 peperoncini peppers,
   drained, cut into rings

½ cup prepared Italian or light
   Italian salad dressing

¼ cup chopped fresh basil
   (optional)

6 cups prewashed torn salad
   greens or romaine lettuce

Cut sausage into ½-inch slices. Cut slices into quarters. Combine sausage, artichoke hearts, tomatoes, olives and pepper rings in medium bowl. Add dressing and basil; mix well. Add salad greens; toss.
Makes 4 servings

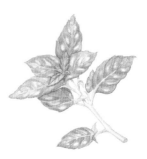

Hearty Minestrone Soup

2 cans (10¾ ounces each)
   condensed Italian tomato
   soup

3 cups water

3 cups cooked vegetables, such
   as zucchini, peas, corn or
   beans

2 cups cooked ditalini pasta

1⅓ cups *French's*® French Fried
   Onions

Combine soup and water in large saucepan. Add vegetables and pasta. Bring to a boil. Reduce heat. Cook until heated through, stirring often.

Place French Fried Onions in microwavable dish. Microwave on HIGH 1 minute or until onions are golden.

Ladle soup into individual bowls. Sprinkle with French Fried Onions.
Makes 6 servings

Prep Time: 10 minutes
Cook Time: 5 minutes

Antipasto Salad

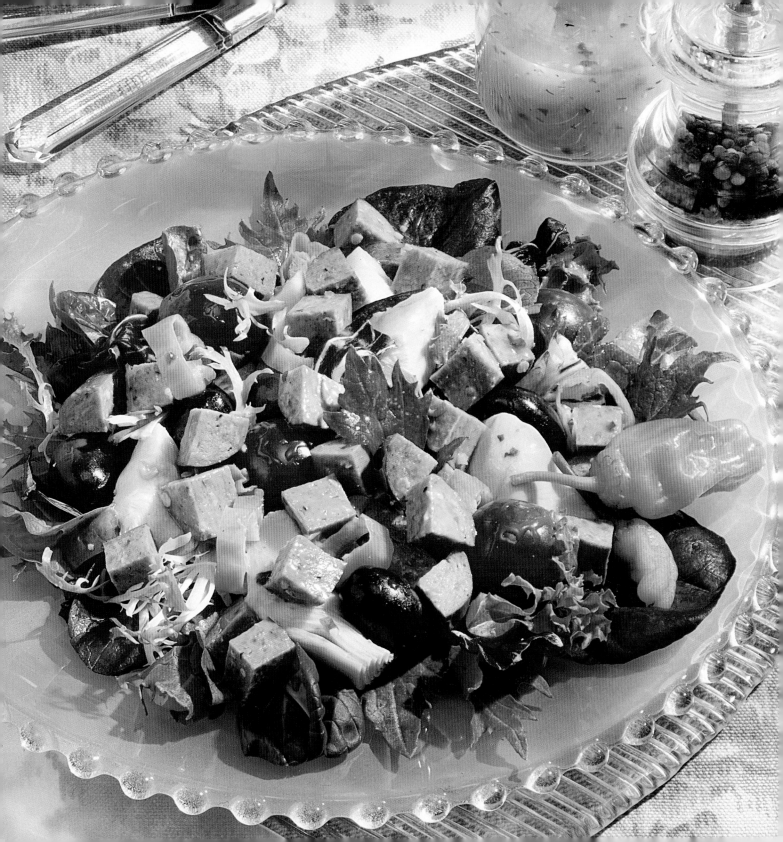

Ravioli Soup

1 package (9 ounces) fresh or frozen cheese ravioli or tortellini

¾ pound hot Italian sausage, crumbled

1 can (14½ ounces) DEL MONTE® Stewed Tomatoes - Italian Recipe

1 can (14½ ounces) beef broth

1 can (14½ ounces) DEL MONTE® Italian Beans, drained

2 green onions, sliced

1. Cook pasta according to package directions; drain.

2. Meanwhile, cook sausage in 5-quart pot over medium-high heat until no longer pink; drain. Add undrained tomatoes, broth and 1¾ cups water; bring to a boil.

3. Reduce heat to low; stir in pasta, green beans and green onions. Simmer until heated through. Season with pepper and sprinkle with grated Parmesan cheese, if desired. *Makes 4 servings*

Prep and Cook Time: 15 minutes

Italian Pasta & Vegetable Salad

8 ounces uncooked rotelle or spiral pasta

2½ cups assorted cut-up fresh vegetables (broccoli, carrots, tomatoes, bell peppers, cauliflower, onions and mushrooms)

½ cup cubed cheddar or mozzarella cheese

⅓ cup sliced pitted ripe olives (optional)

1 cup WISH-BONE® Italian Dressing*

Also terrific with WISH-BONE® Robusto Italian, Fat Free Italian, Ranch, Fat Free Ranch, Creamy Caesar and Red Wine Vinaigrette Dressing.

Cook pasta according to package directions; drain and rinse with cold water until completely cool.

In large bowl, combine all ingredients except Italian dressing. Add dressing; toss well. Serve chilled or at room temperature. *Makes 8 side-dish servings*

Note: If preparing a day ahead, refrigerate, then stir in ¼ cup additional Wish-Bone Dressing before serving.

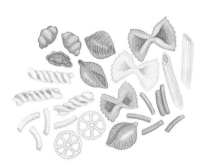

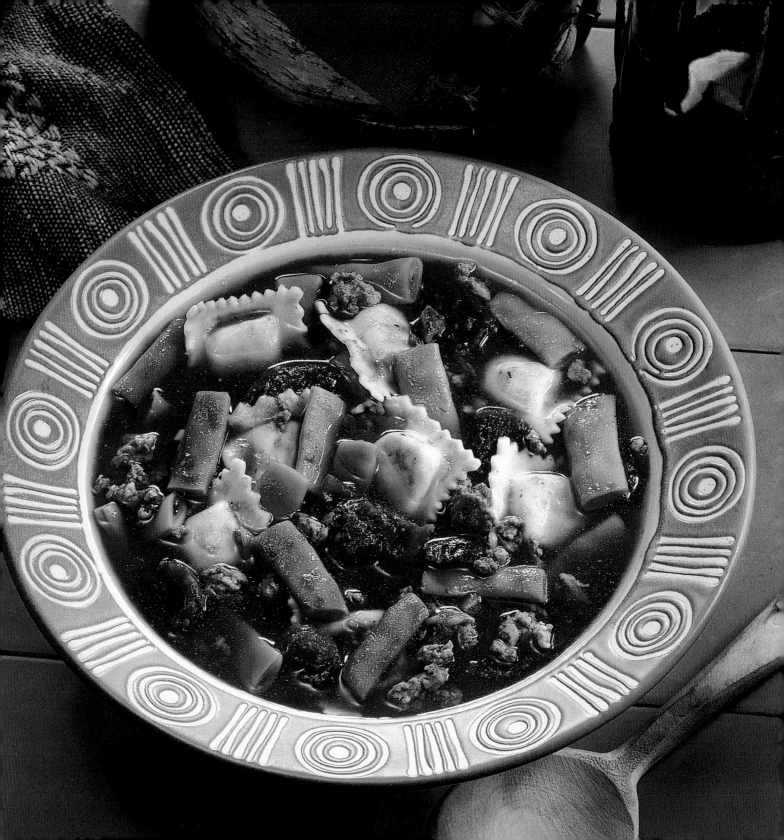

Tomato-Fresh Mozzarella Salad

**Vinaigrette Dressing
(recipe follows)**

1 pound fresh mozarella

1 pound ripe tomatoes

**Fresh whole large basil
leaves as needed**

Salt and ground pepper

Prepare Vinaigrette Dressing. Cut mozzarella into ¼-inch slices. Cut tomatoes into ¼-inch slices. Alternate mozzarella slices, tomato slices and basil leaves, overlapping on plate. Drizzle with dressing. Sprinkle with salt and pepper.

Makes 4 servings

Vinaigrette Dressing

**1 tablespoon balsamic or wine
vinegar**

¼ teaspoon Dijon-style mustard

Pinch salt, pepper and sugar

¼ cup olive oil

Whisk vinegar, mustard, salt, pepper and sugar in small bowl until smooth. Add oil in thin stream, whisking until mixture is smooth. Refrigerate until ready to serve. Whisk again before serving.

Quick & Easy Meatball Soup

**1 package (15 to 18 ounces)
frozen Italian sausage
meatballs without sauce**

**2 cans (about 14 ounces each)
Italian-style stewed
tomatoes**

**2 cans (about 14 ounces each)
beef broth**

**1 can (about 14 ounces) mixed
vegetables**

**½ cup uncooked rotini or small
macaroni**

**½ teaspoon dried oregano
leaves**

1. Thaw meatballs in microwave oven according to package directions.

2. Place remaining ingredients in large saucepan. Add meatballs. Bring to a boil. Reduce heat; cover and simmer 15 minutes or until pasta is tender.

Makes 4 to 6 servings

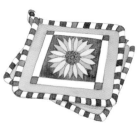

Tomato-Fresh Mozzarella Salad

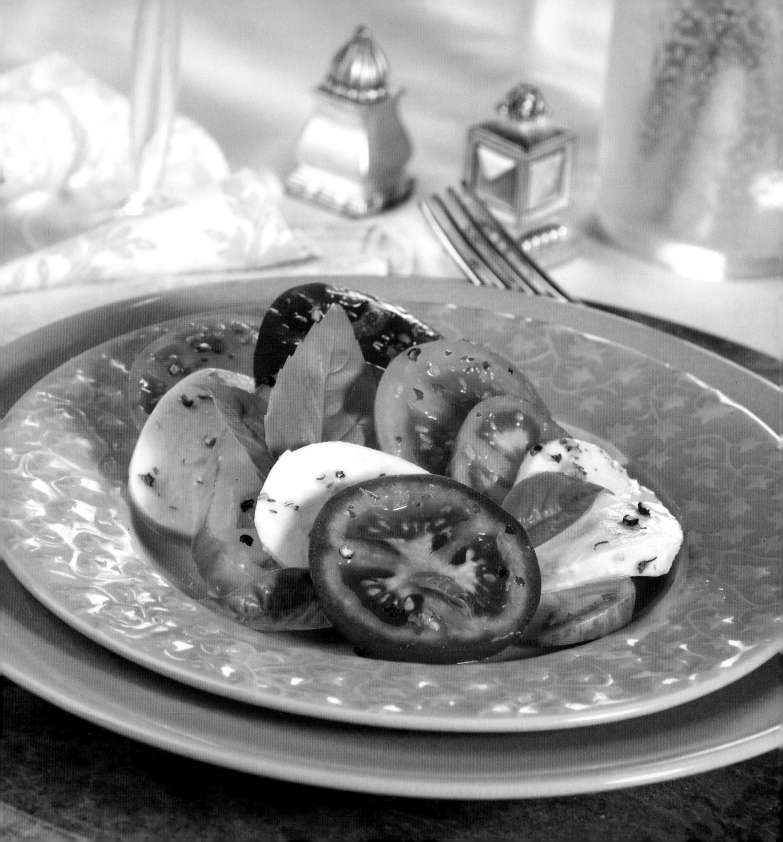

Cool Italian Tomato Soup

1 can (14.5 ounces)
   CONTADINA® Recipe
   Ready Diced Tomatoes,
   undrained

2 cups tomato juice

½ cup half-and-half

2 tablespoons lemon juice

1 large cucumber, peeled,
   diced (about 2 cups)

1 medium green bell pepper,
   diced (about ½ cup)

Chopped fresh basil
   (optional)

Croutons (optional)

1. Place tomatoes with juice, tomato juice, half-and-half and lemon juice in blender container; blend until smooth.

2. Pour into large bowl or soup tureen; stir in cucumber and bell pepper.

3. Sprinkle with basil and croutons just before serving, if desired.

Makes 6 cups

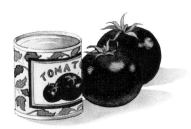

Italian Antipasto Salad

1 box (9 ounces) BIRDS EYE®
   frozen Deluxe Artichoke
   Heart Halves

1 box (9 ounces) BIRDS EYE®
   frozen Deluxe Whole
   Green Beans

12 lettuce leaves

1 pound salami, cut into ¾-inch
   cubes

¾ pound provolone cheese,
   cut into ¾-inch cubes

1 jar (7 ounces) roasted red
   peppers*

⅓ cup Italian salad dressing

Or, substitute pimientos, drained and cut into thin strips.

• In large saucepan, cook artichokes and green beans according to package directions; drain. Rinse under cold water to cool; drain again.

• Place lettuce on serving platter. Arrange cooked vegetables, salami, cheese and peppers in separate piles.

• Drizzle with dressing just before serving. *Makes 6 servings*

Serving Suggestion: Add pitted ripe olives and jarred pepperoncini, if desired.

Prep Time: 5 minutes
Cook Time: 10 minutes

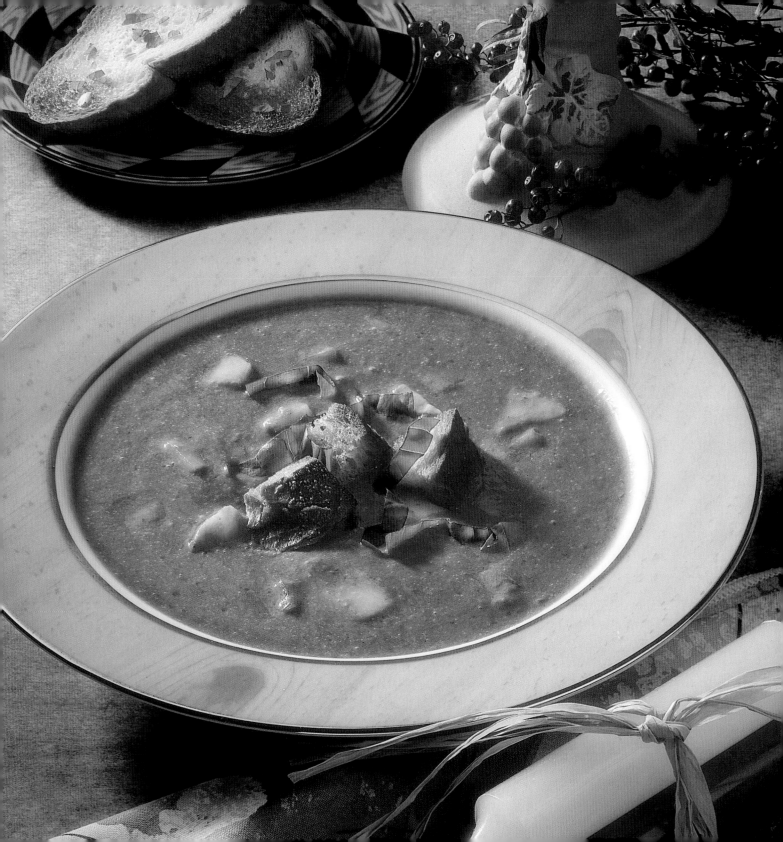

Pepperoni Pasta Salad

1 package (16 ounces)
   BARILLA® Castellane,
   cooked according to
   package directions

6 ounces sliced pepperoni,
   cut into quarters

4 ounces shredded Cheddar
   cheese

½ red onion, chopped

½ green pepper, chopped

1 small tomato, cubed

½ small can chopped black
   olives

¾ cup Italian salad dressing

1. Thoroughly rinse castellane in cold water; drain and place in large serving bowl. Add remaining ingredients except salad dressing.

2. About 1 hour before serving, add salad dressing and toss to coat. Toss again just before serving, adding additional salad dressing if necessary.

Makes 8 to 10 servings

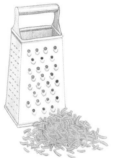

Italian Bow Tie Vegetable Soup

3 cans (14½ ounces each)
   chicken broth

1 can (14½ ounces) Italian-style
   or regular stewed tomatoes

½ teaspoon Italian seasoning

1½ cups (4 ounces) uncooked
   bow tie pasta (farfalle)

1 package (about 1 pound)
   small frozen precooked
   meatballs

1 medium zucchini, cut into
   ¼-inch slices

½ cup diced red or green bell
   pepper

1½ cups *French's®* French Fried
   Onions

1. Combine broth, tomatoes and Italian seasoning in large saucepan. Bring to a boil.

2. Stir in pasta, meatballs, zucchini and bell pepper. Simmer for 12 minutes or until pasta is cooked al dente and meatballs are heated through, stirring occasionally. Spoon soup into serving bowls; top with French Fried Onions.

Makes 6 servings

Prep Time: 5 minutes
Cook Time: 12 minutes

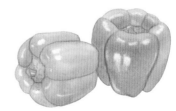

Pepperoni Pasta Salad

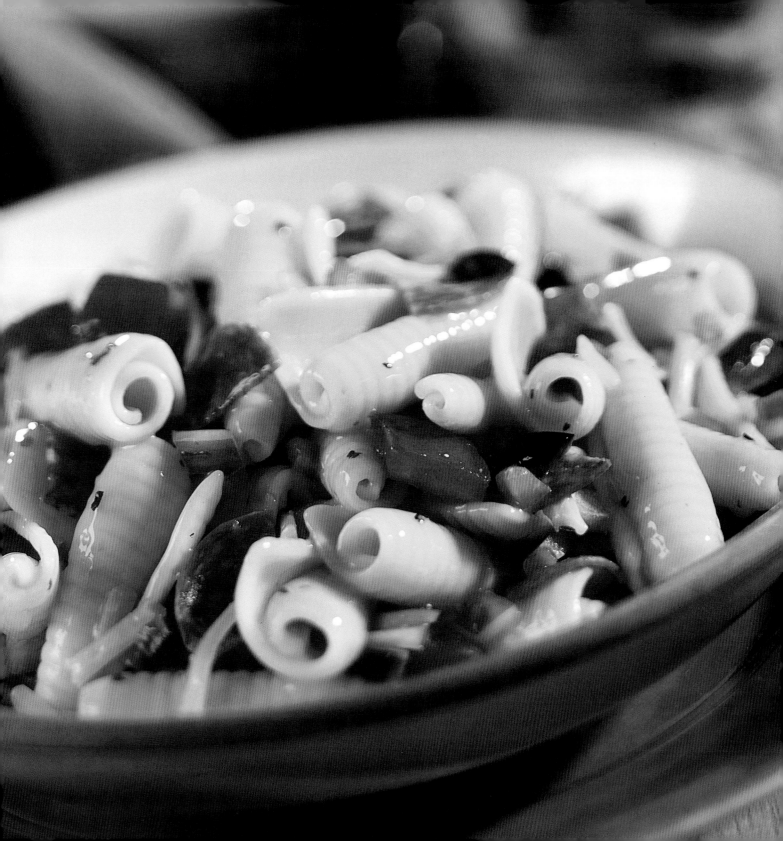

Italian Bread Salad

1 loaf (about 12 ounces) hearty peasant-style bread (such as sourdough, rosemary-olive oil or roasted garlic)

1 cup sliced red onion

1 teaspoon minced garlic

⅓ cup bottled balsamic and olive oil vinaigrette

1½ cups grape tomatoes or cherry tomatoes, halved

⅓ cup pitted oil- or salt-cured black and green olives

1 package European salad mix or 1 package pre-washed baby spinach

Grated Parmesan cheese

Freshly ground black pepper to taste

1. Preheat oven to 250°F. Tear bread into large cubes, about the size of marshmallows. Place on baking sheet. Bake 10 to 15 minutes or until slightly dry but not browned. Set aside to cool.

2. Place onion slices and garlic in large salad bowl. Add vinaigrette and stir to coat. Set aside a few minutes to allow flavors to mellow.

3. Add tomatoes and olives; stir gently to coat with dressing. Add greens, bread cubes and Parmesan; toss gently. Add more vinaigrette if needed and season with black pepper.   *Makes 4 servings*

Tip: You can use day-old bread that has started to dry out for this recipe. Bread that is a little too hard or stale can be softened by sprinkling it with water. Gently squeeze the bread in your hands to remove excess moisture.

Mixed Spring Vegetable Salad

8 ounces fresh green beans, trimmed and cut into thirds

1 medium zucchini (about ½ pound), sliced

1 large tomato *or* 3 plum tomatoes, sliced

3 tablespoons FILIPPO BERIO® Extra Virgin Olive Oil

3 tablespoons lemon juice

Salt and freshly ground black pepper

Cook or steam green beans and zucchini separately until tender-crisp. Cover; refrigerate until chilled. Stir in tomato. Just before serving, drizzle olive oil and lemon juice over vegetables. Season to taste with salt and pepper.   *Makes 6 servings*

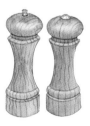

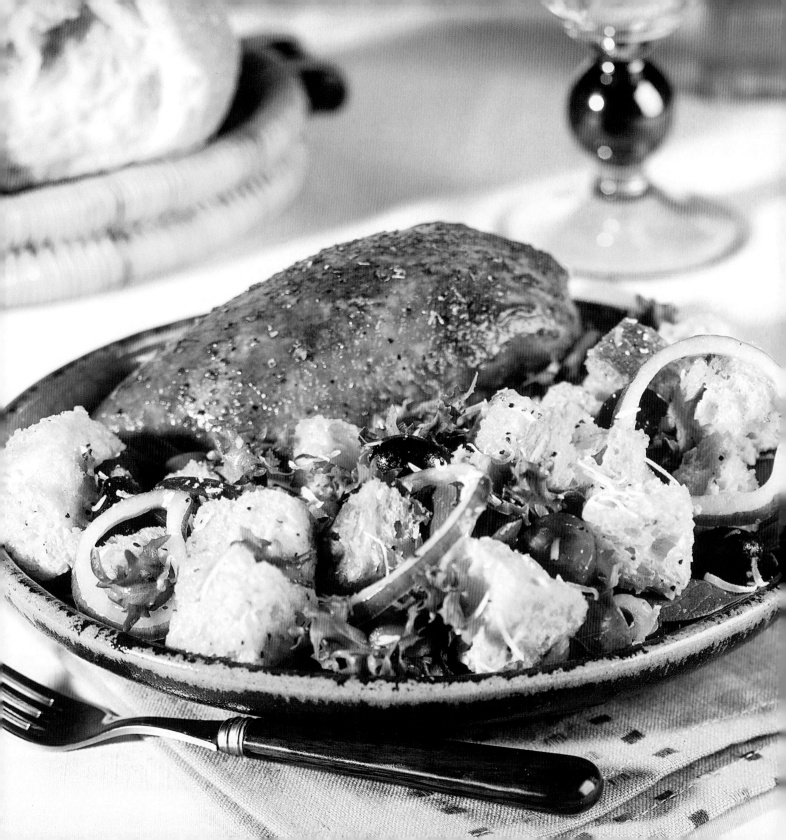

Pasta

Zesty Artichoke Pesto Sauce

1 jar (6 ounces) marinated
    artichoke hearts,
    chopped, marinade
    reserved

1 cup sliced onion

1 can (14.5 ounces)
    CONTADINA® Recipe
    Ready Diced Tomatoes,
    undrained

1 can (6 ounces) CONTADINA
    Italian Paste with Tomato
    Pesto

1 cup water

½ teaspoon salt

    Hot cooked pasta

1. Heat reserved artichoke marinade in large saucepan over medium-high heat until warm.

2. Add onion; cook for 3 to 4 minutes or until tender. Add artichoke hearts, tomatoes and juice, tomato paste, water and salt.

3. Bring to a boil; reduce heat to low. Cook, stirring occasionally, for 10 to 15 minutes or until flavors are blended. Serve over pasta.   *Makes 6 to 8 servings*

Savory Caper and Olive Sauce: Eliminate artichoke hearts. Heat 2 tablespoons olive oil in large saucepan over medium-high heat. Add onion; cook for 3 to 4 minutes or until tender. Add tomatoes and juice, tomato paste, water, salt, ¾ cup sliced and quartered zucchini, ½ cup (2¼-ounce can) drained sliced ripe olives and 2 tablespoons capers. Proceed as above.

Prep time: 5 minutes
Cook Time: 19 minutes

Zesty Artichoke Pesto Sauce

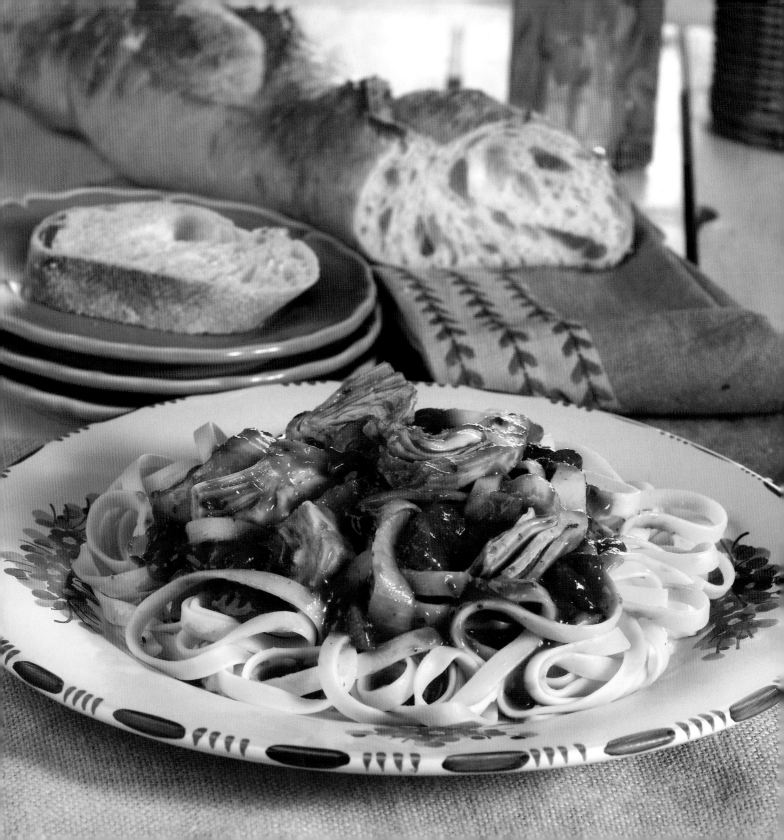

Tuscan Chicken and Pasta

8 ounces BARILLA® Rotini

¼ cup chopped dry-pack sun-dried tomatoes

2 medium zucchini, cut into matchstick strips

1 tablespoon olive or vegetable oil

1 jar (26 ounces) BARILLA® Tomato and Basil Pasta Sauce

1 cup (about 5 ounces) cooked chicken strips (purchased ready-to-eat, frozen or homemade)

¼ cup (1 ounce) grated Parmesan cheese

1. Begin cooking rotini according to package directions. Add sun-dried tomatoes to pasta during last 5 minutes of cooking; drain rotini and tomatoes.

2. Meanwhile, combine zucchini and oil in large (6-cup or more) microwave-safe bowl; cover with plastic wrap. Microwave on HIGH 4 minutes, stirring twice.

3. Stir in pasta sauce and chicken. Cover with plastic wrap; microwave on HIGH 4 minutes, stirring twice. Combine sauce mixture, hot drained rotini with sun-dried tomatoes and cheese; toss to coat.   *Makes 6 to 8 servings*

Tip: Firm cheeses such as Parmesan should be wrapped airtight in a plastic bag or foil and stored in your refrigerator's cheese compartment (or its warmest location) for up to several weeks.

Pasta Alfredo

½ pound thin vegetable-flavored noodles, cooked and drained

½ cup grated Parmesan cheese

½ cup prepared HIDDEN VALLEY® The Original Ranch® Dressing

2 tablespoons chopped parsley

Additional Parmesan cheese and freshly ground black pepper, to taste

In large pot, toss noodles, cheese, salad dressing and parsley. Warm over medium heat until cheese melts. Sprinkle individual servings with additional cheese and black pepper.   *Makes 4 servings*

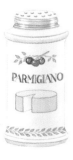

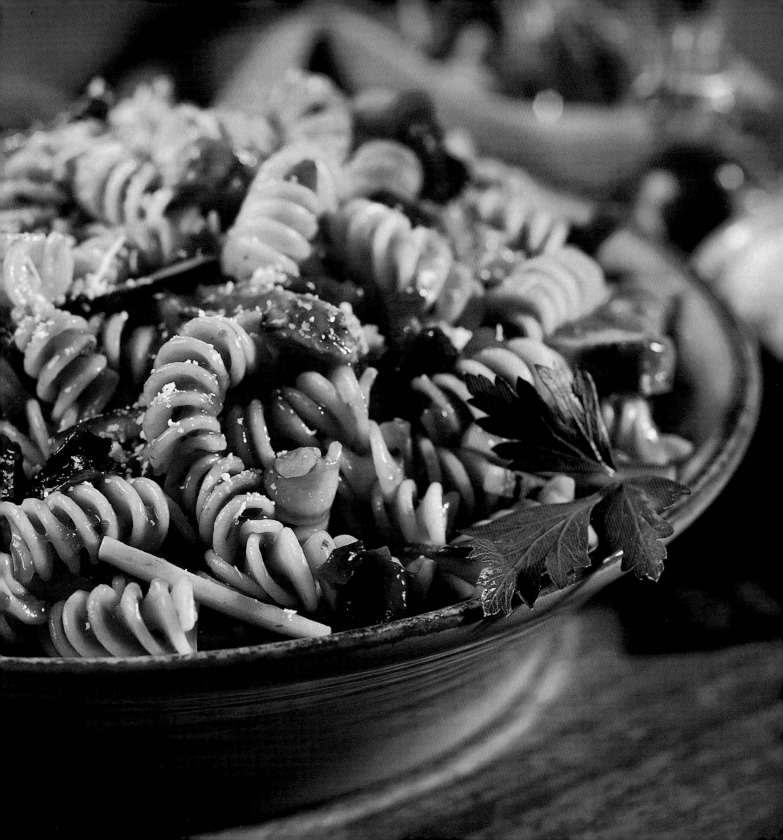

Angel Hair Al Fresco

¾ cup skim milk

1 tablespoon margarine or butter

1 package (4.8 ounces) PASTA RONI® Angel Hair Pasta with Herbs

1 can (6⅛ ounces) white tuna in water, drained, flaked *or* 1½ cups chopped cooked chicken

2 medium tomatoes, chopped

⅓ cup sliced green onions

¼ cup dry white wine or water

¼ cup slivered almonds, toasted (optional)

1 tablespoon chopped fresh basil *or* 1 teaspoon dried basil

1. In 3-quart saucepan, combine 1⅓ cups water, skim milk and margarine. Bring just to a boil.

2. Stir in pasta, Special Seasonings, tuna, tomatoes, onions, wine, almonds and basil. Return to a boil; reduce heat to medium.

3. Boil, uncovered, stirring frequently, 6 to 8 minutes. Sauce will be thin, but will thicken upon standing.

4. Let stand 3 minutes or until desired consistency. Stir before serving.

Makes 4 servings

Linguine with White Clam Sauce

2 tablespoons CRISCO® Oil*

2 cloves garlic, minced

2 cans (6½ ounces *each*) chopped clams, undrained

½ cup chopped fresh parsley

¼ cup dry white wine or clam juice

1 teaspoon dried basil leaves

1 pound linguine, cooked (without salt or fat) and well drained

*Use your favorite Crisco Oil product.

1. Heat oil and garlic in medium skillet on medium heat.

2. Drain clams, reserving liquid. Add reserved liquid and parsley to skillet. Reduce heat to low. Simmer 3 minutes, stirring occasionally.

3. Add clams, wine and basil. Simmer 5 minutes, stirring occasionally. Add to hot linguine. Toss lightly to coat.

Makes 8 servings

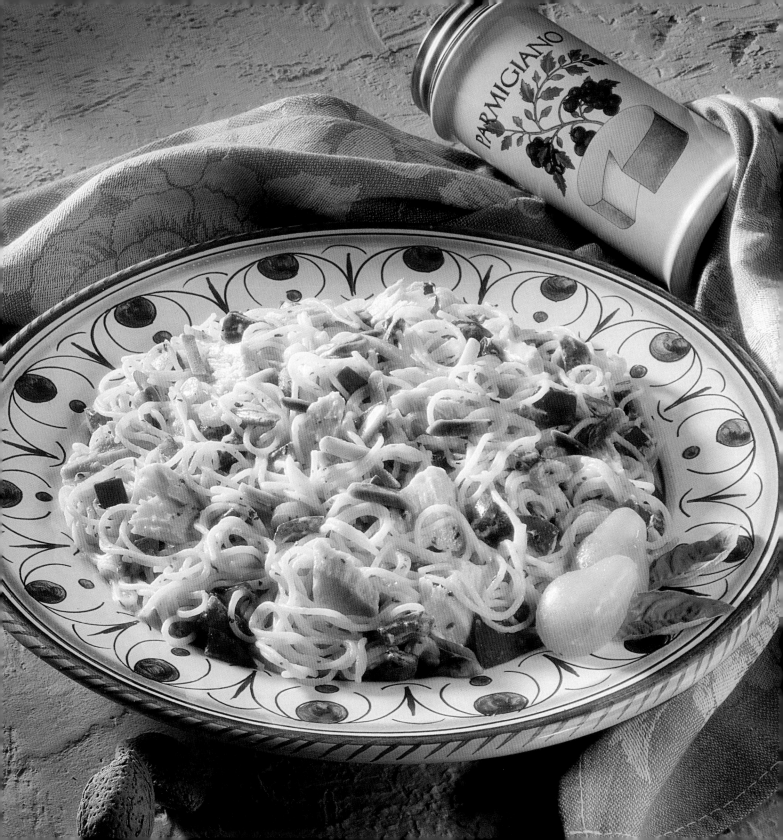

Giardiniera Sauce

1 pound dry pasta

1 tablespoon olive or vegetable oil

2 cups sliced fresh mushrooms

1 cup chopped onion

½ cup sliced green bell pepper

2 cloves garlic, minced

1 can (14.5 ounces) CONTADINA® Stewed Tomatoes, undrained

½ cup chicken broth

1 can (6 ounces) CONTADINA® Tomato Paste

2 teaspoons Italian herb seasoning

½ teaspoon salt (optional)

1. Cook pasta according to package directions; drain and keep warm.

2. Meanwhile, heat oil in large skillet. Add mushrooms, onion, bell pepper and garlic; sauté 3 to 4 minutes or until vegetables are tender.

3. Stir in undrained tomatoes, chicken broth, tomato paste, Italian seasoning and salt, if desired. Bring to a boil.

4. Reduce heat to low; simmer, uncovered, 10 minutes, stirring occasionally. Serve over pasta.

Makes 8 servings

Prep Time: 8 minutes
Cook Time: 15 minutes

Pasta Primavera with Lemon Pepper Sauce

1 package (8 ounces) linguine

1 bag (16 ounces) BIRDS EYE® frozen Farm Fresh Mixtures Broccoli, Cauliflower & Carrots

1 packet (1.8 ounces) white sauce mix

¼ cup grated Parmesan cheese

2 teaspoons grated lemon peel

¼ teaspoon pepper

• In large saucepan, cook pasta according to package directions. Add vegetables during last 8 minutes; drain and set aside.

• In same saucepan, prepare sauce according to package directions; stir in cheese, lemon peel and pepper. Stir in vegetables and pasta; cook over medium heat until heated through.

Makes 4 servings

Variation: Add 2 cans (6 ounces each) drained and flaked tuna when you add pasta and vegetables to sauce.

Prep Time: 5 minutes
Cook Time: 20 minutes

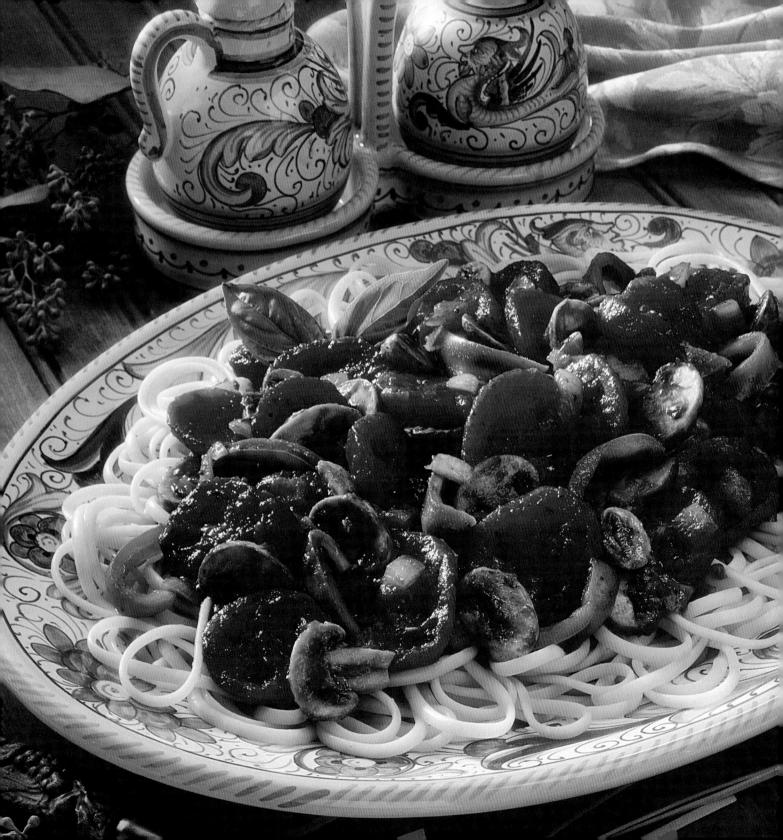

Tortellini Carbonara

1 package (15 ounces) cheese
  tortellini

1 box (10 ounces) frozen
  broccoli florets, thawed

1 jar (1 pound) RAGÚ® Cheese
  Creations!® Roasted Garlic
  Parmesan Sauce

½ cup diced drained roasted
  red peppers

4 ounces bacon, crisp-cooked
  and crumbled

In 3-quart saucepan, cook tortellini according to package directions, adding broccoli during last 2 minutes of cooking; drain. Return pasta mixture to saucepan. Stir in Ragú Cheese Creations! Sauce and peppers. Spoon onto platter and top with bacon. Garnish, if desired, with Parmesan cheese.

Makes 4 servings

Fusilli with Fresh Red & Yellow Tomato Sauce

½ cup (1 stick) I CAN'T
  BELIEVE IT'S NOT
  BUTTER!® Spread

1 medium onion, chopped

2 cloves garlic, finely chopped
  (optional)

1½ pounds red and/or yellow
  cherry tomatoes, halved

⅓ cup chopped fresh basil
  leaves

1 box (16 ounces) fusilli (long
  curly pasta) or linguine,
  cooked and drained

Grated Parmesan cheese

In 12-inch nonstick skillet, melt I Can't Believe It's Not Butter! Spread over medium heat and cook onion, stirring occasionally, 2 minutes or until softened. Stir in garlic and tomatoes and cook, stirring occasionally, 5 minutes or until tomatoes soften but do not lose their shape and sauce thickens slightly. Stir in basil and season, if desired, with salt and ground black pepper.

In large serving bowl, toss sauce with hot fusilli and sprinkle with cheese.

Makes 4 servings

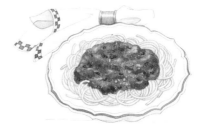

Tortellini Carbonara

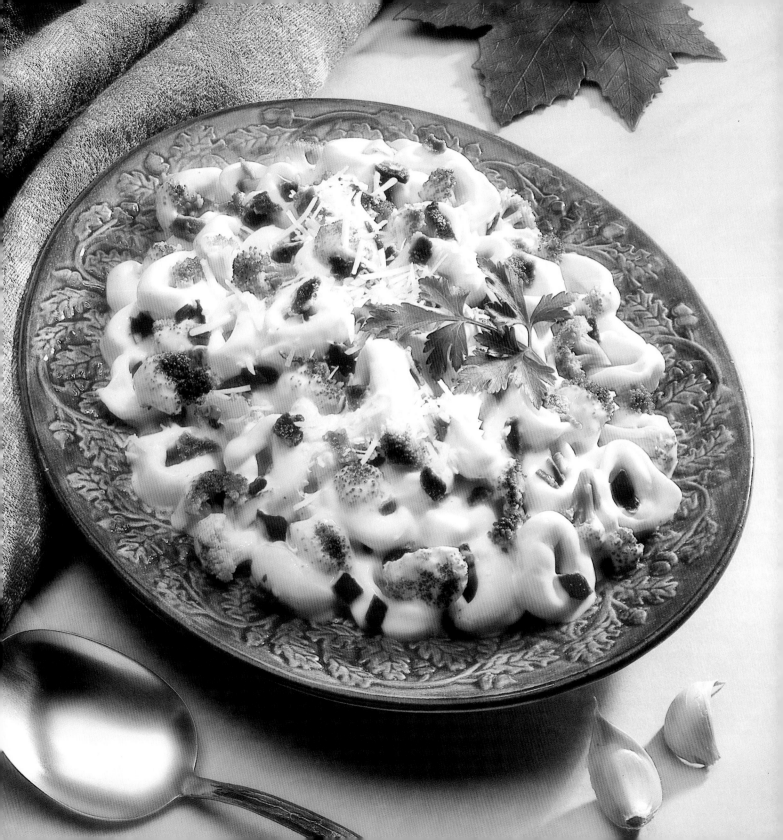

Ravioli Stew

1 tablespoon BERTOLLI®
Olive Oil

3 medium carrots, chopped

2 medium ribs celery, chopped

1 medium onion, chopped

1 jar (1 pound 10 ounces)
RAGÚ® Robusto!™ Pasta
Sauce

1 can (14½ ounces) chicken
broth

1 cup water

1 package (12 to 16 ounces)
fresh or frozen mini ravioli,
cooked and drained

1. In 6-quart saucepot, heat oil over medium-high heat and cook carrots, celery and onion, stirring occasionally, 8 minutes or until golden.

2. Stir in Ragú Robusto! Pasta Sauce, broth and water. Bring to a boil over high heat. Reduce heat to low and simmer covered 15 minutes.

3. Just before serving, stir in hot ravioli and season, if desired, with salt and ground black pepper. Garnish, if desired, with fresh basil.

Makes 6 servings

Prep Time: 10 minutes
Cook Time: 30 minutes

Saucepot Spinach Lasagne

1 package KNORR® Recipe
Classics™ Leek Soup, Dip
and Recipe Mix

3 cups water

8 ounces uncooked wide egg
noodles (about 6 cups)

1 cup milk

1 package (10 ounces) frozen
leaf spinach, thawed

2 cups shredded mozzarella
cheese, divided (about
8 ounces)

⅓ cup grated Parmesan cheese

• In 4-quart saucepot, combine recipe mix and water. Add noodles and milk. Stirring frequently, heat to boiling. Reduce heat; stirring occasionally, simmer 5 minutes.

• Add spinach; heat to simmering. Stir in 1 cup mozzarella and Parmesan cheese. Spoon into shallow serving bowl and sprinkle with remaining mozzarella cheese.

Makes 4 servings

Prep Time: 20 minutes

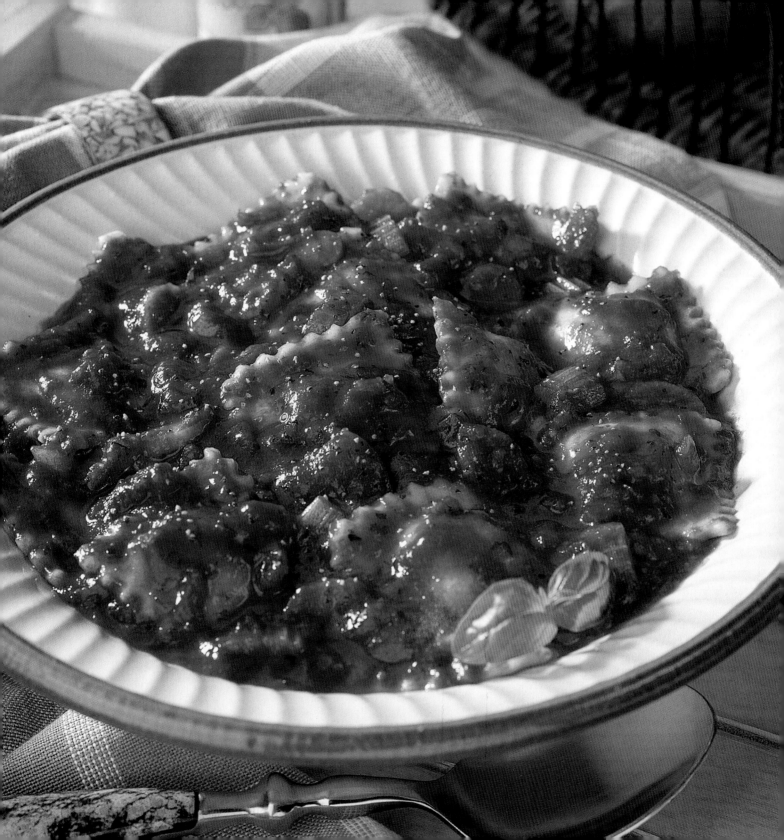

Penne with Creamy Tomato Sauce

1 tablespoon olive or vegetable oil

½ cup diced onion

2 tablespoons dry vermouth, white wine or chicken broth

1 can (14.5 ounces) CONTADINA® Recipe Ready Diced Tomatoes with Italian Herbs, undrained

½ cup heavy whipping cream

8 ounces dry penne or rigatoni, cooked, drained, kept warm

1 cup pitted ripe olives, drained, sliced

½ cup (2 ounces) grated Parmesan cheese

¼ cup sliced green onions

1. Heat oil in large skillet. Add diced onion; sauté 2 to 3 minutes or until onion is tender.

2. Add vermouth; cook 1 minute.

3. Stir in undrained tomatoes, cream, pasta, olives and Parmesan cheese; heat thoroughly, stirring occasionally. Sprinkle with green onions.

Makes 4 servings

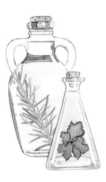

Spaghetti with Garlic

12 ounces uncooked spaghetti

4½ teaspoons FILIPPO BERIO® Olive Oil

1 clove garlic, sliced

Salt and freshly ground black pepper

Grated Parmesan cheese

Cook pasta according to package directions until al dente (tender but still firm). Drain; transfer to large bowl. In small skillet, heat olive oil over medium heat until hot. Add garlic; cook and stir 2 to 3 minutes or until golden. Discard garlic. Pour oil over hot pasta; toss until lightly coated. Season to taste with salt and pepper. Top with cheese.

Makes 4 servings

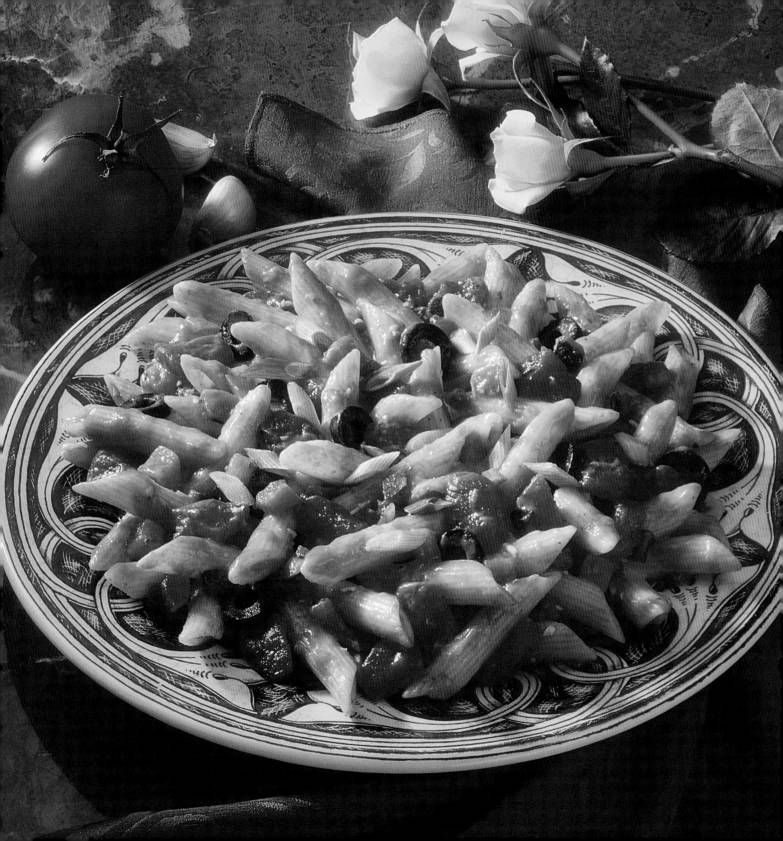

Greens and Gemelli

8 ounces BARILLA® Gemelli

1 tablespoon olive oil

1 bag (10 ounces) spinach, washed and trimmed

1 jar (26 ounces) BARILLA® Green & Black Olive Pasta Sauce

8 ounces Italian sausage, cooked and crumbled

¼ cup crumbled feta cheese

1. Cook gemelli according to package directions; drain.

2. Meanwhile, add olive oil to large skillet. Add spinach; cook and stir 1 minute over medium-high heat.

3. Reduce heat; stir in pasta sauce and cooked sausage. Cook 5 minutes.

4. Pour sauce over hot drained gemelli; sprinkle with cheese.

Makes 4 to 6 servings

Fast-Track Fettuccine

1 cup SONOMA® Dried Tomato Halves, snipped into strips

1 tablespoon olive oil

4 cloves garlic, chopped

1 can (2¼ ounces) sliced ripe olives, drained

3 tablespoons chopped fresh basil *or* 1 tablespoon dried basil leaves

12 ounces dry fettuccine, cooked and drained

2 cups (8 ounces) grated mozzarella or crumbled feta cheese

In small bowl, cover tomatoes with boiling water; set aside 10 minutes. Meanwhile, heat oil in large skillet. Add garlic and sauté 2 minutes. Drain tomatoes. Add tomatoes, olives and basil to skillet; cook and toss 2 minutes. Add hot fettuccine and cheese. Toss just until heated through and thoroughly blended. Serve immediately. *Makes 4 to 6 servings*

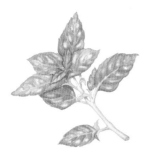

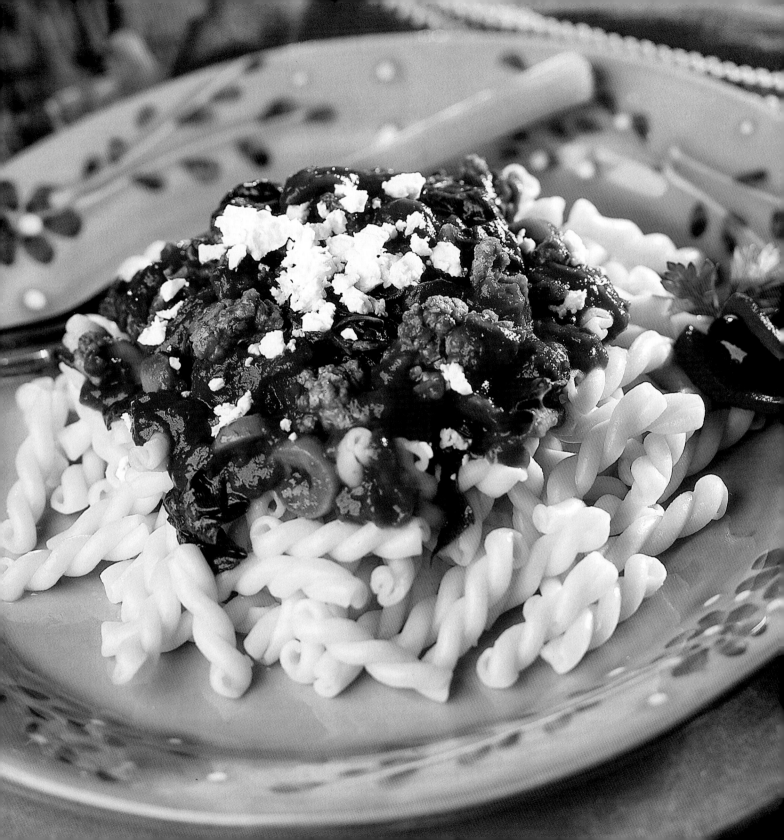

Mama's Best Ever Spaghetti & Meatballs

1 pound lean ground beef

½ cup Italian seasoned dry bread crumbs

1 egg

1 jar (1 pound 10 ounces) RAGÚ® Old World Style® Pasta Sauce

8 ounces spaghetti, cooked and drained

1. In medium bowl, combine ground beef, bread crumbs and egg; shape into 12 meatballs.

2. In 3-quart saucepan, bring Ragú Pasta Sauce to a boil over medium-high heat. Gently stir in meatballs.

3. Reduce heat to low and simmer covered, stirring occasionally, 20 minutes or until meatballs are no longer pink in center. Serve over hot spaghetti; sprinkle with shredded Parmesan cheese if desired. *Makes 4 servings*

Prep Time: 10 minutes
Cook Time: 20 minutes

Pizza Casserole

2 cups uncooked rotini or other spiral pasta

1½ to 2 pounds ground beef

1 medium onion, chopped

Salt and pepper

1 can (about 15 ounces) pizza sauce

1 can (8 ounces) tomato sauce

1 can (6 ounces) tomato paste

½ teaspoon sugar

½ teaspoon garlic salt

½ teaspoon dried oregano leaves

2 cups (8 ounces) shredded mozzarella cheese

12 to 15 slices pepperoni

1. Preheat oven to 350°F. Cook rotini according to package directions. Set aside.

2. Meanwhile, cook and stir ground beef and onion in large skillet over medium-high heat until meat is no longer pink. Season with salt and pepper. Set aside.

3. Combine rotini, pizza sauce, tomato sauce, tomato paste, sugar, garlic salt and oregano in large bowl. Add beef mixture and combine.

4. Place half of mixture in 3-quart casserole and top with 1 cup cheese. Repeat layers. Arrange pepperoni slices on top. Bake 25 to 30 minutes or until heated through and cheese melts. *Makes 6 servings*

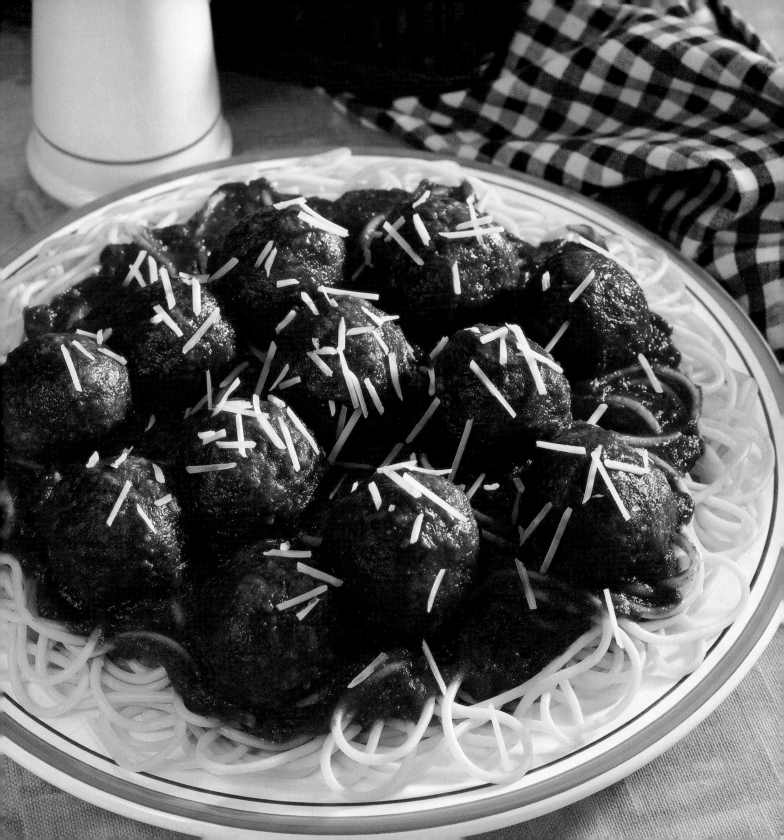

Ravioli with Tomatoes and Zucchini

2 packages (9 ounces each) fresh or frozen cheese ravioli or tortellini

¾ pound hot Italian sausage, crumbled

2 cans (14½ ounces each) DEL MONTE® Diced Tomatoes

1 medium zucchini, thinly sliced and quartered

1 teaspoon dried basil leaves

½ cup ricotta cheese *or* 2 tablespoons grated Parmesan cheese

1. Cook pasta according to package directions; drain.

2. Brown sausage in large skillet or saucepan over medium-high heat until no longer pink; drain, reserving sausage in skillet.

3. Add undrained tomatoes, zucchini and basil to skillet. Cook about 8 minutes or until zucchini is just tender-crisp, stirring occasionally. Season with pepper, if desired.

4. Spoon sauce over hot pasta. Top with ricotta cheese. Garnish, if desired.

Makes 4 servings

Prep and Cook Time: 20 minutes

Turkey Sausage & Pasta Toss

8 ounces uncooked penne or gemelli pasta

1 can (14½ ounces) stewed tomatoes, undrained

6 ounces turkey kielbasa or smoked turkey sausage

2 cups fresh asparagus pieces (1 inch) or broccoli florets

2 tablespoons prepared pesto sauce

2 tablespoons grated Parmesan cheese

1. Cook pasta according to package directions.

2. Meanwhile, heat tomatoes in medium saucepan. Cut sausage crosswise into ¼-inch slices; add to tomatoes. Stir in asparagus and pesto; cover and simmer about 6 minutes or until asparagus is crisp-tender.

3. Drain pasta; toss with tomato mixture and sprinkle with cheese.

Makes 4 servings

Prep and Cook Time: 25 minutes

Pasta with Tuna Sauce

3 cups bow tie pasta, uncooked

1 box (9 ounces) BIRDS EYE® frozen Italian Green Beans

1 jar (15 ounces) prepared spaghetti sauce

1 can (6⅛ ounces) tuna packed in water, drained

Chopped Italian parsley (optional)

- Cook pasta according to package directions; drain.

- Cook beans according to package directions; drain.

- Combine pasta, beans, spaghetti sauce, tuna and parsley. Cook and stir over medium-high heat 5 minutes or until heated through.

Makes about 2 servings

Prep Time: 5 minutes
Cook Time: 20 minutes

Mushroom-Laced Fettuccine

3 tablespoons margarine or butter

½ pound assorted fresh mushrooms*

1 envelope LIPTON® RECIPE SECRETS® Savory Herb with Garlic Soup Mix**

1½ cups milk

8 ounces fettuccine or linguine, cooked and drained

*Use any of the following, sliced: portobello, crimini, shiitake, white, morels, porcini or enoki mushrooms.

**Also terrific with LIPTON® Recipe Secrets® Golden Onion Soup Mix.

In 10-inch skillet, melt margarine over medium heat and cook mushrooms, stirring occasionally, 4 minutes or until tender. Add savory herb with garlic soup mix blended with milk. Bring to a boil over high heat. Reduce heat to low and simmer 3 minutes, stirring frequently. Toss with hot fettuccine. Serve immediately.

Makes about 2 main-dish servings

Tuscan Baked Rigatoni

1 pound Italian sausage, casings removed

1 pound rigatoni pasta, cooked, drained and kept warm

2 cups (8 ounces) shredded fontina cheese

2 tablespoons olive oil

2 fennel bulbs, thinly sliced

4 cloves garlic, minced

1 can (28 ounces) crushed tomatoes

1 cup heavy cream

1 teaspoon salt

1 teaspoon pepper

8 cups coarsely chopped spinach

1 can (15 ounces) cannellini beans, rinsed and drained

2 tablespoons pine nuts

½ cup grated Parmesan cheese

1. Preheat oven to 350°F. Spray 4-quart casserole with nonstick cooking spray. Crumble sausage in large skillet over medium-high heat. Cook and stir until no longer pink; drain. Transfer sausage to large bowl. Add cooked pasta and fontina cheese; mix well.

2. Combine oil, fennel and garlic in same skillet. Cook and stir over medium heat 3 minutes or until fennel is tender. Add tomatoes, cream, salt and pepper; cook and stir until slightly thickened. Stir in spinach, beans and pine nuts; cook until heated through.

3. Pour sauce over pasta and sausage; toss to coat. Transfer to prepared casserole; sprinkle evenly with Parmesan cheese. Bake 30 minutes or until hot and bubbly. *Makes 6 to 8 servings*

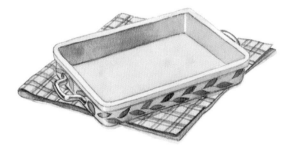

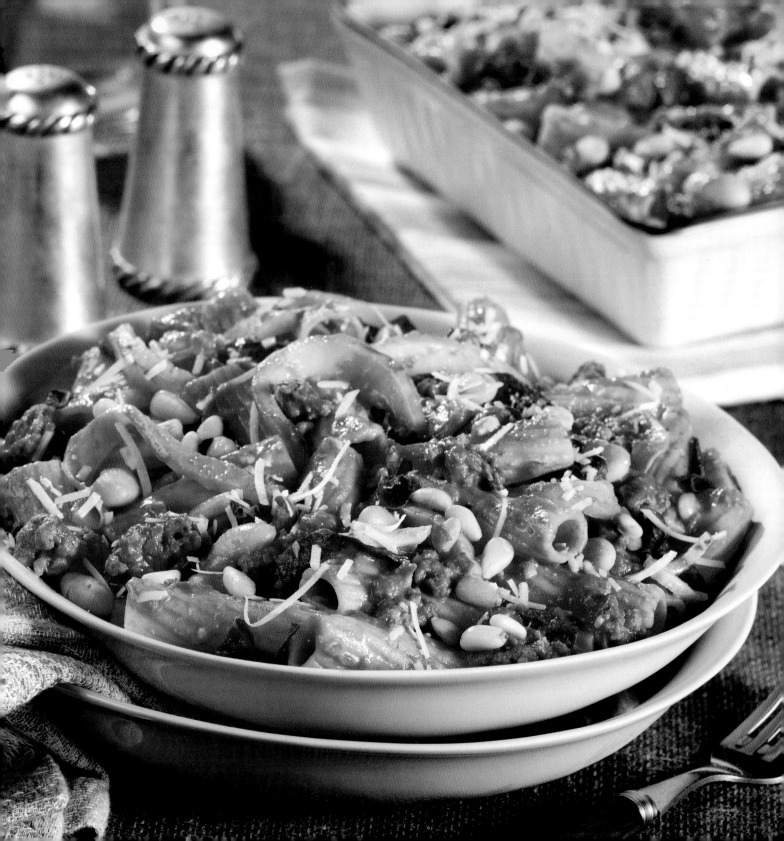

Roma Artichoke and Tomato Ragu

1 can (14.5 ounces)
CONTADINA® Recipe
Ready Diced Tomatoes,
drained

1 jar (6 ounces) marinated
artichoke hearts, sliced,
undrained

¼ cup sliced ripe olives,
drained

2 tablespoons chopped fresh
parsley *or* 2 teaspoons
dried parsley flakes

2 tablespoons chopped fresh
basil *or* 2 teaspoons dried
basil leaves, crushed

1 clove garlic, minced

¼ teaspoon salt

⅛ teaspoon black pepper

1. Combine tomatoes, artichoke hearts and juice, olives, parsley, basil, garlic, salt and pepper in large bowl.

2. Cover; chill for several hours to blend flavors.

3. Toss with pasta or serve at room temperature on toasted Italian bread slices or pizza.

Makes 4 servings

Prep Time: 6 minutes
Chill Time: several hours

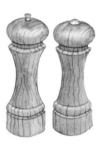

Simply Delicious Pasta Primavera

¼ cup margarine or butter

1 envelope LIPTON® RECIPE
SECRETS® Vegetable
Soup Mix

1½ cups milk

8 ounces linguine or spaghetti,
cooked and drained

¼ cup grated Parmesan cheese
(about 1 ounce)

1. In medium saucepan, melt margarine over medium heat and stir in soup mix and milk. Bring just to a boil over high heat.

2. Reduce heat to low and simmer uncovered, stirring occasionally, 10 minutes or until vegetables are tender. Toss hot linguine with sauce and Parmesan cheese.

Makes 4 servings

Prep Time: 5 minutes
Cook Time: 12 minutes

Roma Artichoke and Tomato Ragu

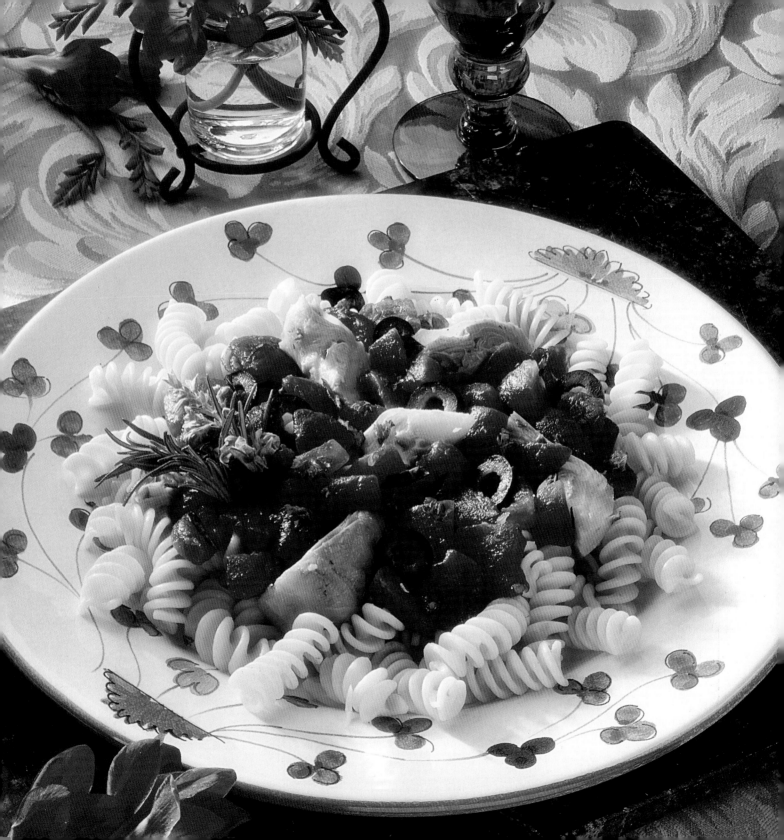

Penne with Arrabiatta Sauce

½ pound uncooked penne or other tube-shaped pasta

2 tablespoons olive oil or oil from sun-dried tomatoes

8 cloves garlic

1 can (28 ounces) crushed tomatoes in purée

¼ cup chopped sun-dried tomatoes packed in oil

3 tablespoons *Frank's® RedHot®* Cayenne Pepper Sauce

8 kalamata olives, pitted and chopped*

6 fresh basil leaves *or* 1½ teaspoons dried basil leaves

1 tablespoon capers

To pit olives, place olives on cutting board. Press with side of knife until olives split. Remove pits.

1. Cook pasta according to package directions; drain.

2. Heat oil in large nonstick skillet over medium heat. Add garlic; cook until golden, stirring frequently. Add remaining ingredients. Bring to a boil. Simmer, partially covered, 10 minutes. Stir occasionally.

3. Toss pasta with half of the sauce mixture. Spoon into serving bowl. Pour remaining sauce mixture over pasta. Garnish with fresh basil or parsley, if desired. *Makes 4 servings (3 cups sauce)*

Prep Time: 15 minutes
Cook Time: 20 minutes

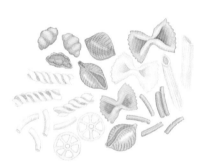

Spicy Sausage and Roasted Garlic Sauce for Spaghetti

1 package (16 ounces) BARILLA® Thin Spaghetti

1 tablespoon olive or vegetable oil

1 pound bulk hot Italian sausage

2 jars (26 ounces each) BARILLA® Roasted Garlic and Onion Pasta Sauce

1. Cook spaghetti according to package directions; drain.

2. Meanwhile, heat oil in large nonstick skillet over medium heat. Add sausage; cook 5 to 6 minutes or until brown, stirring to break up sausage. Drain off excess fat from skillet.

3. Add pasta sauce to skillet. Reduce heat; cook and stir 10 minutes. Combine hot drained spaghetti with sauce mixture. *Makes 8 servings*

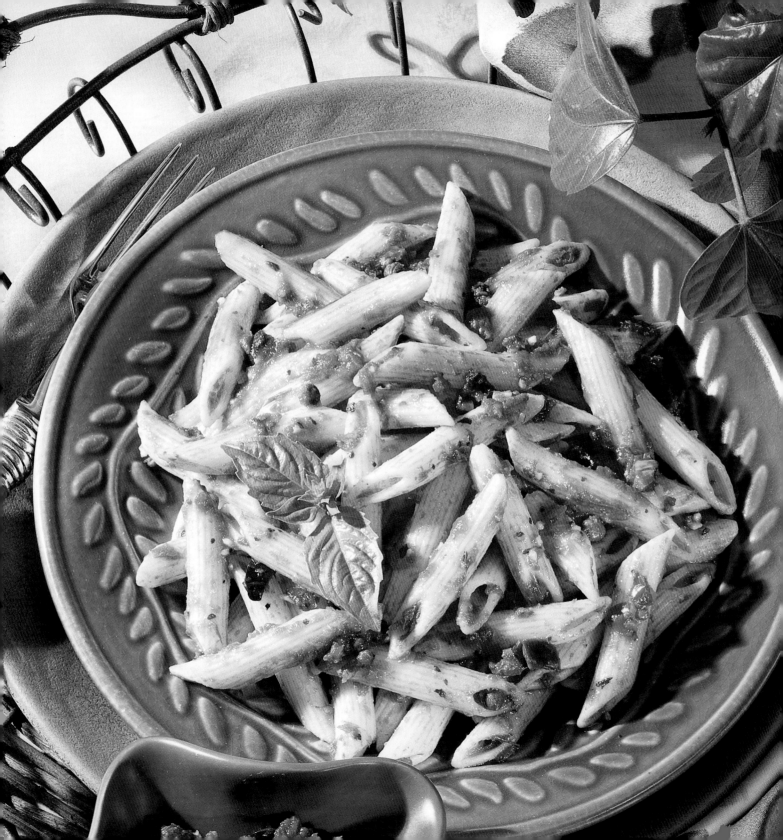

Chicken and Linguine in Creamy Tomato Sauce

1 tablespoon BERTOLLI®
Olive Oil

1 pound boneless, skinless
chicken breasts, cut into
½-inch strips

1 jar (1 pound 10 ounces)
RAGÚ® Old World Style®
Pasta Sauce

2 cups water

8 ounces linguine or spaghetti

½ cup whipping or heavy cream

1 tablespoon fresh basil leaves,
chopped or ½ teaspoon
dried basil leaves, crushed

1. In 12-inch skillet, heat oil over medium heat and brown chicken. Remove chicken and set aside.

2. In same skillet, stir in Ragú Pasta Sauce and water. Bring to a boil over high heat. Stir in uncooked linguine and return to a boil. Reduce heat to low and simmer covered, stirring occasionally, 15 minutes or until linguine is tender.

3. Stir in cream and basil. Return chicken to skillet and cook 5 minutes or until chicken is thoroughly cooked.   *Makes 4 servings*

Prep Time: 10 minutes
Cook Time: 30 minutes

Penne with Sausage and Kalamata Olives

8 ounces penne pasta

1 pound sweet Italian sausage

½ cup ricotta cheese

1 large tomato, quartered

2 teaspoons TABASCO® brand
Pepper Sauce

1 teaspoon salt

¼ cup sliced kalamata olives

2 tablespoons chopped fresh
parsley

Heat 4 quarts salted water to boiling in large saucepan. Add penne; cook until tender. Drain.

Meanwhile, remove casing from sausage. Cook sausage in 10-inch skillet over medium-high heat until well browned, stirring to crumble. Remove sausage to paper towels with slotted spoon.

Combine ricotta cheese, tomato, TABASCO® Sauce and salt in food processor or blender; process until smooth. Toss penne with sausage, ricotta mixture, olives and chopped parsley in large bowl; mix well.   *Makes 4 servings*

*Chicken and Linguine in
Creamy Tomato Sauce*

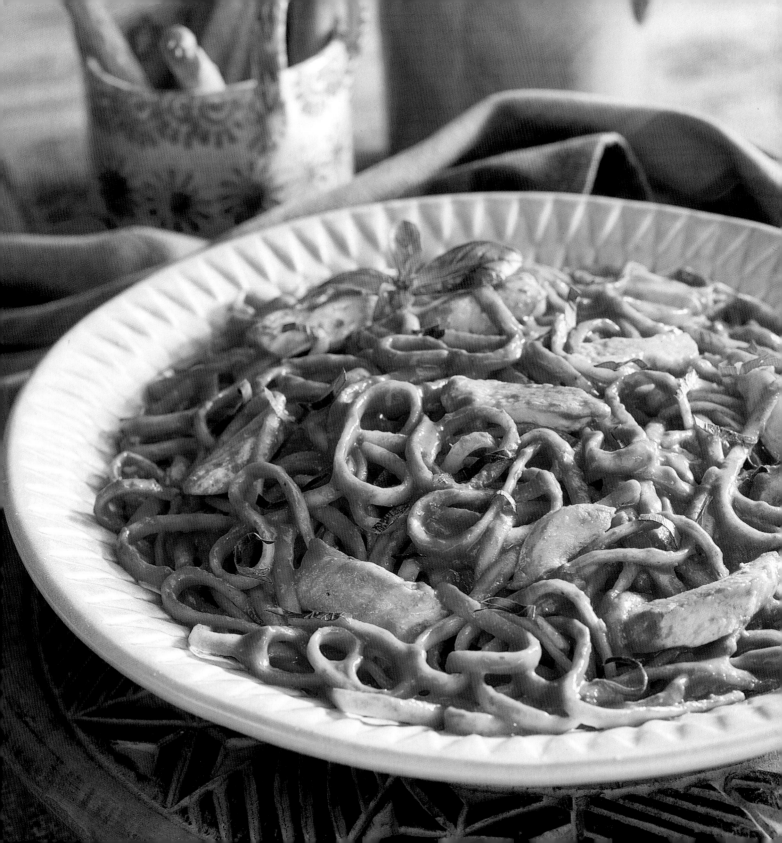

Portofino Primavera

1 pound dry pasta

2 tablespoons olive oil

1 small onion, chopped

1 large clove garlic, minced

1 can (14.5 ounces) CONTADINA® Recipe Ready Diced Tomatoes, undrained

1 can (6 ounces) CONTADINA® Tomato Paste

1 cup chicken broth or water

1 cup quartered sliced zucchini

½ cup sliced pitted ripe olives, drained

2 tablespoons capers

½ teaspoon salt

1. Cook pasta according to package directions; drain and keep warm.

2. Heat oil in medium saucepan. Add onion and garlic; sauté for 1 minute.

3. Add undrained tomatoes, tomato paste, broth, zucchini, olives, capers and salt.

4. Bring to a boil. Reduce heat to low; simmer, uncovered, for 15 to 20 minutes or until heated through. Serve over pasta.   *Makes 8 servings*

Prep Time: 6 minutes
Cook Time: 22 minutes

Pasta with BelGioioso® Gorgonzola Sauce

1½ cups whipping cream

1½ cups (12 ounces) creamy BELGIOIOSO® Gorgonzola Cheese

1 pound fettuccine, cooked and drained

Fresh grated BELGIOIOSO® Parmesan Cheese

Fresh cracked black pepper

Chopped fresh basil

In medium saucepan, bring cream to a boil over medium heat. Simmer about 5 minutes. Reduce heat to low and stir in BelGioioso Gorgonzola Cheese until melted.

Place cooked pasta into large warm bowl; pour sauce over and toss. Sprinkle with BelGioioso Parmesan Cheese, pepper and basil.   *Makes 6 servings*

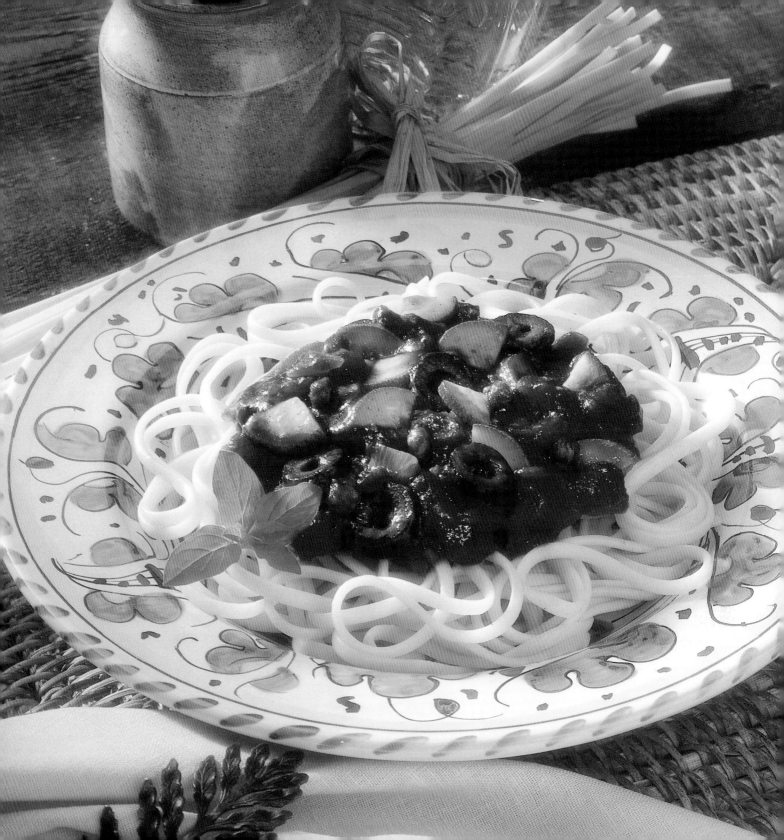

Quick Pasta Puttanesca

1 package (16 ounces)
    spaghetti or linguine,
    uncooked

3 tablespoons plus 1 teaspoon
    olive oil, divided

¼ to 1 teaspoon red pepper
    flakes*

2 cans (6 ounces each) chunk
    light tuna packed in water,
    drained

1 tablespoon dried minced
    onion

1 teaspoon minced garlic

1 can (28 ounces) diced
    tomatoes, undrained

1 can (8 ounces) tomato sauce

24 pitted Kalamata or ripe
    olives

2 tablespoons capers, drained

*For a mildly spicy dish, use ¼ teaspoon red
pepper. For a very spicy dish, use 1 teaspoon
red pepper.

1. Cook spaghetti according to package directions.

2. While pasta is cooking, heat remaining 3 tablespoons oil in large skillet over medium-high heat. Add red pepper flakes; cook and stir 1 to 2 minutes or until they sizzle. Add tuna; cook and stir 2 to 3 minutes. Add onion and garlic; cook and stir 1 minute. Add tomatoes with juice, tomato sauce, olives and capers. Cook over medium-high heat, stirring frequently, until sauce is heated through.

3. Drain pasta; do not rinse. Return pasta to pan; add 1 teaspoon oil and toss to coat.

4. Add sauce to pasta; mix well. Divide pasta among individual bowls or plates. *Makes 6 to 8 servings*

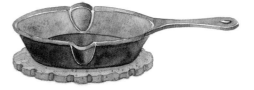

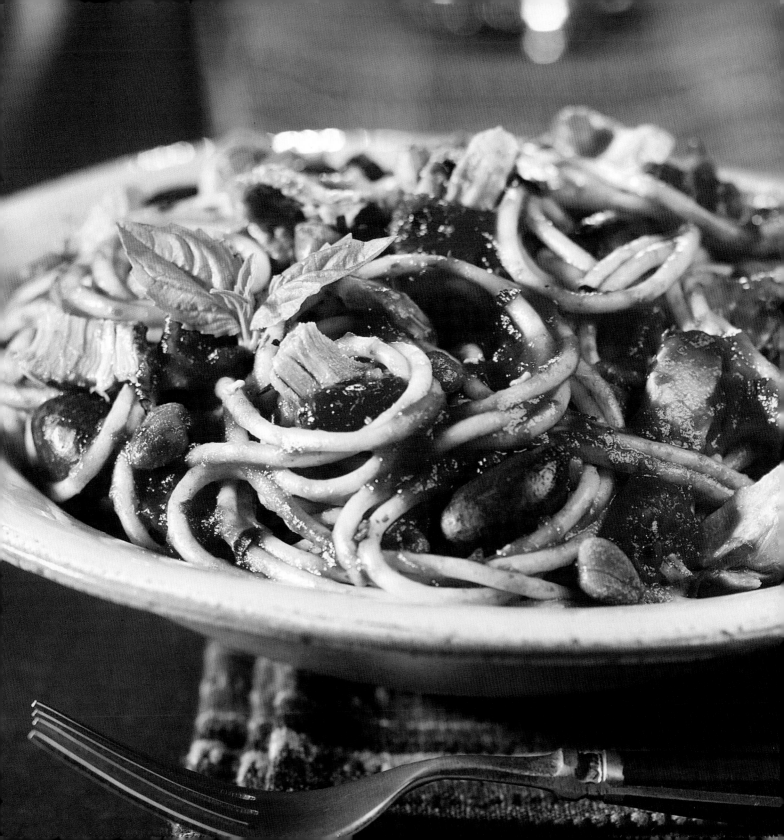

Entreés

Polenta with Pasta Sauce & Vegetables

1 can (about 14 ounces) reduced-sodium chicken broth

1½ cups water

1 cup yellow cornmeal

2 teaspoons olive oil

12 ounces assorted cut vegetables, such as broccoli florets, bell peppers, red onions, zucchini squash and julienned carrots

2 teaspoons minced garlic

2 cups prepared tomato-basil pasta sauce

½ cup grated Asiago cheese

¼ cup chopped fresh basil (optional)

1. To prepare polenta, whisk together chicken broth, water and cornmeal in large microwavable bowl. Cover with waxed paper; microwave at HIGH 5 minutes. Whisk well and microwave at HIGH 4 to 5 minutes more or until polenta is very thick. Whisk again; cover and keep warm.

2. Meanwhile, heat oil in large deep nonstick skillet over medium heat. Add vegetables and garlic; cook and stir 5 minutes. Add pasta sauce; reduce heat, cover and simmer 5 to 8 minutes or until vegetables are tender.

3. Spoon polenta onto serving plates; top with pasta sauce mixture. Sprinkle with cheese and basil, if desired.

Makes 4 servings

Prep Time: 5 minutes
Cook Time: 15 minutes

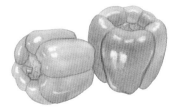

Polenta with Pasta Sauce & Vegetables

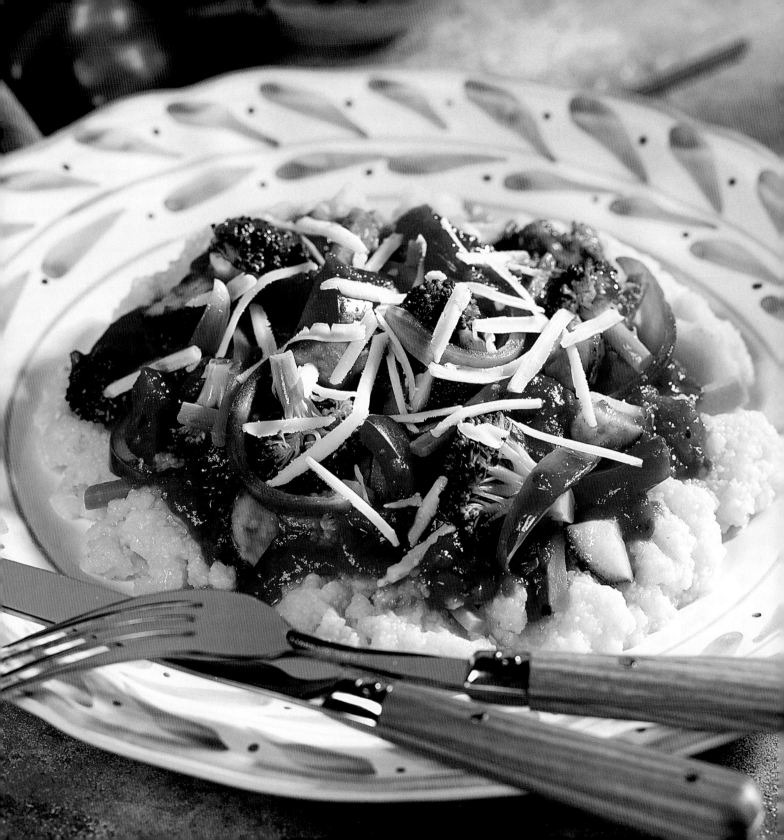

Chicken Cacciatore

8 ounces uncooked noodles

1 can (15 ounces) chunky Italian-style tomato sauce

1 cup chopped green bell pepper

1 cup sliced onion

1 cup sliced mushrooms

4 boneless skinless chicken breast halves (1 pound)

1. Cook noodles according to package directions; drain.

2. While noodles are cooking, combine tomato sauce, bell pepper, onion and mushrooms in microwavable dish. Cover loosely with plastic wrap or waxed paper; microwave at HIGH 6 to 8 minutes, stirring halfway through cooking time.

3. While sauce mixture is cooking, coat large skillet with nonstick cooking spray and heat over medium-high heat. Cook chicken breasts 3 to 4 minutes per side or until lightly browned.

4. Add sauce mixture to skillet with salt and pepper to taste. Reduce heat to medium and simmer 12 to 15 minutes. Serve over noodles.

Makes 4 servings

Veal Piccata

1 pound veal cutlets (or chicken)

2 garlic cloves, crushed

Flour

2 tablespoons oil

4 tablespoons butter, divided

½ cup HOLLAND HOUSE® Vermouth Cooking Wine

2 tablespoons lemon juice

1 tablespoon chopped fresh parsley

Freshly ground pepper

1. Rub veal or chicken with garlic; coat with flour. Heat oil and 2 tablespoons butter in large skillet over medium heat. Add veal or chicken; brown on both sides until cooked through. Transfer to serving platter; keep warm.

2. In small saucepan, combine cooking wine, remaining 2 tablespoons butter, lemon juice, parsley and pepper. Bring to boil, stirring constantly. Cook 1 minute over high heat. Pour sauce over veal or chicken.

Makes 4 servings

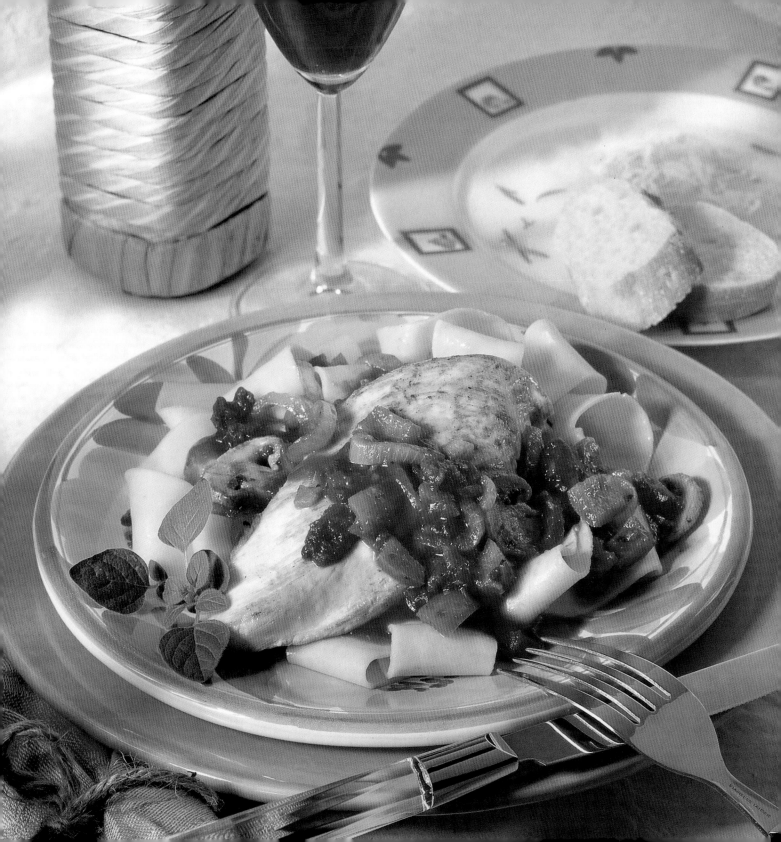

Chicken Puttanesca-Style

2 tablespoons BERTOLLI®
  Olive Oil

1 (2½- to 3-pound) chicken,
  cut into pieces

1 medium onion, sliced

¼ cup balsamic vinegar

1 jar (1 pound 10 ounces)
  RAGÚ® Old World Style®
  Pasta Sauce

1 cup pitted ripe olives

1 tablespoon drained capers

In 12-inch skillet, heat oil over medium-high heat and brown chicken. Remove chicken and set aside; drain.

In same skillet, add onion and vinegar and cook over medium heat, stirring occasionally, 3 minutes. Stir in Ragú Pasta Sauce. Return chicken to skillet and simmer covered 25 minutes or until chicken is thoroughly cooked. Stir in olives and capers; heat through. Serve, if desired, over hot cooked rice and garnish with chopped fresh parsley.

Makes 4 servings

Recipe Tip: Be sure to use the best quality balsamic vinegar you can afford. In general, the longer it's been aged, the deeper and tastier the flavor.

Ragú® Steak Pizzaiola

4 eye-round steaks
  (1½ pounds)

2 tablespoons finely chopped
  garlic

4 tablespoons grated
  Parmesan cheese

½ teaspoon salt

½ teaspoon ground black
  pepper

2 cups frozen French-cut green
  beans, thawed

1 jar (1 pound 10 ounces)
  RAGÚ® Robusto!
  Pasta Sauce

Preheat oven to 400°F. In bottom of 13×9-inch baking pan, arrange steaks; sprinkle with garlic, 2 tablespoons of the Parmesan cheese, salt and pepper. Add green beans and Ragú Robusto! Pasta Sauce. Bake 20 minutes or until desired doneness. Sprinkle with remaining cheese. Serve, if desired, over hot cooked noodles.

Makes 4 servings

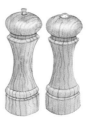

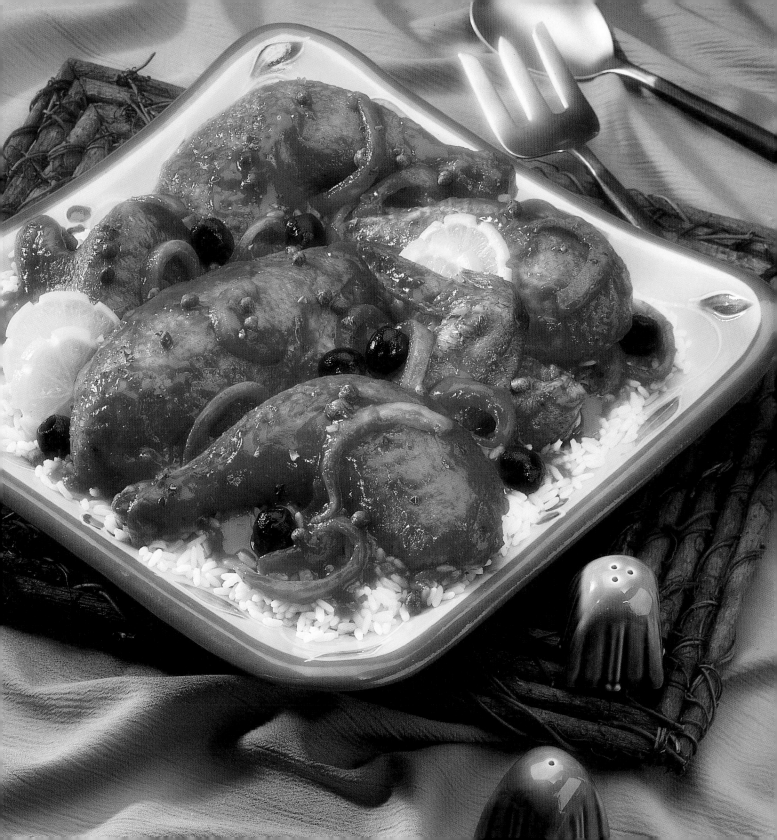

Shrimp Scampi

2 tablespoons olive or
  vegetable oil

½ cup diced onion

1 large clove garlic, minced

1 small green bell pepper,
  cut into strips

1 small yellow bell pepper,
  cut into strips

8 ounces medium shrimp,
  peeled, deveined

1 can (14.5 ounces)
  CONTADINA® Recipe
  Ready Diced Tomatoes
  with Italian Herbs,
  undrained

2 tablespoons chopped fresh
  parsley *or* 2 teaspoons
  dried parsley flakes

1 tablespoon lemon juice

½ teaspoon salt

  Hot cooked orzo pasta

1. Heat oil in large skillet over medium-high heat. Add onion and garlic; sauté 1 minute.

2. Add bell peppers; sauté 2 minutes. Add shrimp; cook 2 minutes or until shrimp turn pink.

3. Add undrained tomatoes, parsley, lemon juice and salt; cook 2 to 3 minutes or until heated through. Serve over hot cooked orzo pasta, if desired.

Makes 4 servings

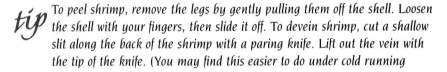

tip *To peel shrimp, remove the legs by gently pulling them off the shell. Loosen the shell with your fingers, then slide it off. To devein shrimp, cut a shallow slit along the back of the shrimp with a paring knife. Lift out the vein with the tip of the knife. (You may find this easier to do under cold running water.)*

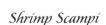

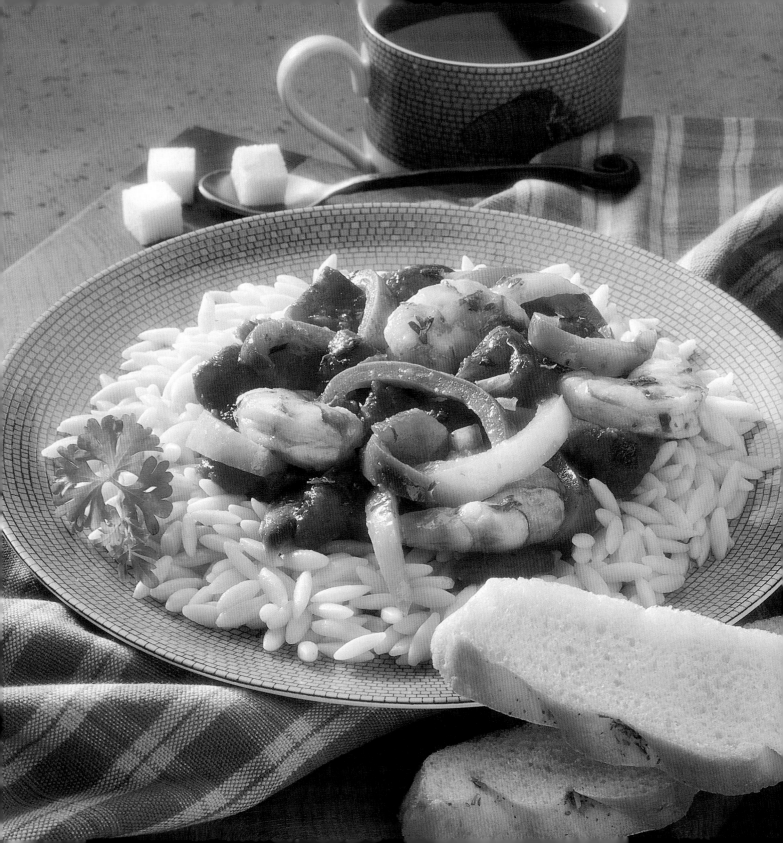

Wish-Bone® Marinade Italiano

¾ **cup WISH-BONE® Italian Dressing***

2½ **to 3 pounds chicken pieces****

Also terrific with Wish-Bone® Robusto Italian or Just 2 Good Italian Dressing.

**Variations: Use 1 (2- to 2½-pound) T-bone, boneless sirloin or top loin steak or 6 boneless, skinless chicken breast halves (about 1½ pounds) or 2½ pounds center cut pork chops (about 1 inch thick).*

In large, shallow nonaluminum baking dish or plastic bag, pour ½ cup Italian dressing over chicken. Cover, or close bag, and marinate in refrigerator, turning occasionally, 3 to 24 hours.

Remove chicken from marinade; discard marinade. Grill or broil chicken, turning once and brushing frequently with remaining ¼ cup dressing, until chicken is thoroughly cooked and juices run clear.   *Makes about 4 servings*

Creamy Parmesan Rice with Chicken

1 tablespoon oil

4 boneless, skinless chicken breasts (about 1 pound)

3 cloves garlic, minced

1½ cups UNCLE BEN'S® ORIGINAL CONVERTED® Brand Rice

2 cans (14½ ounces each) low-sodium chicken broth

1 cup grated Parmesan cheese

1 cup frozen peas, thawed

1. Heat oil in medium skillet. Add chicken, cook over medium-high heat 5 to 7 minutes or until lightly browned on both sides. Season with salt and pepper, if desired.

2. Add garlic; cook briefly. Stir in rice and chicken broth. Bring to boil. Cover; reduce heat and simmer 20 minutes or until chicken is no longer pink in center.

3. Remove from heat; stir in Parmesan cheese and peas. Cover and let stand 5 minutes.   *Makes 4 servings*

Cook's Tip: For extra creaminess, stir in 2 tablespoons butter and/or 2 tablespoons cream with the Parmesan cheese; proceed with recipe as directed.

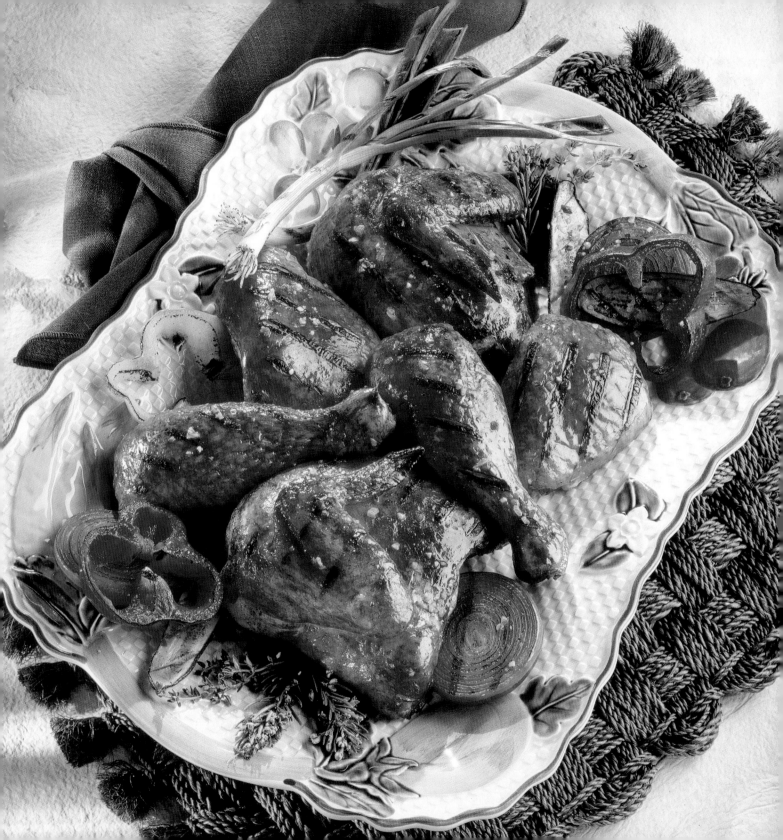

Italian Vegetable Stew

1 teaspoon BERTOLLI®
   Olive Oil

2 medium zucchini, halved
   lengthwise and thinly sliced

1 medium eggplant, chopped

1 large onion, thinly sliced

⅛ teaspoon ground black
   pepper

1 jar (1 pound 10 ounces)
   RAGÚ® Light Pasta Sauce

3 tablespoons grated
   Parmesan cheese

1 box (10 ounces) couscous

1. In 12-inch nonstick skillet, heat oil over medium heat and cook zucchini, eggplant, onion and pepper, stirring occasionally, 15 minutes or until vegetables are golden.

2. Stir in Ragú Pasta Sauce and cheese. Bring to a boil over high heat. Reduce heat to low and simmer covered 10 minutes.

3. Meanwhile, prepare couscous according to package directions. Serve vegetable mixture over hot couscous. *Makes 4 servings*

Prep Time: 10 minutes
Cook Time: 25 minutes

Tuscan Pork with Peppers

1 pound boneless pork chops,
   cut into 1-inch cubes

1 medium onion, peeled and
   chopped

2 cloves garlic, minced

1 teaspoon olive oil

1 (14½-ounce) can Italian-style
   tomatoes, undrained

½ cup dry white wine

1 sweet red bell pepper,
   seeded and sliced

1 green bell pepper, seeded
   and sliced

In large nonstick skillet over medium-high heat, sauté pork cubes, onion and garlic in olive oil until pork starts to brown, about 4 to 5 minutes. Add remaining ingredients; lower heat to a simmer. Cover and cook gently for 12 to 15 minutes. Taste for seasoning, adding salt and black pepper if desired. Serve with hot cooked rigatoni or penne, if desired. *Makes 4 servings*

Prep Time: 30 minutes

Favorite recipe from **National Pork Board**

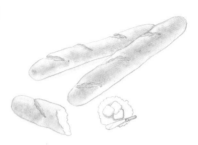

Italian Vegetable Stew

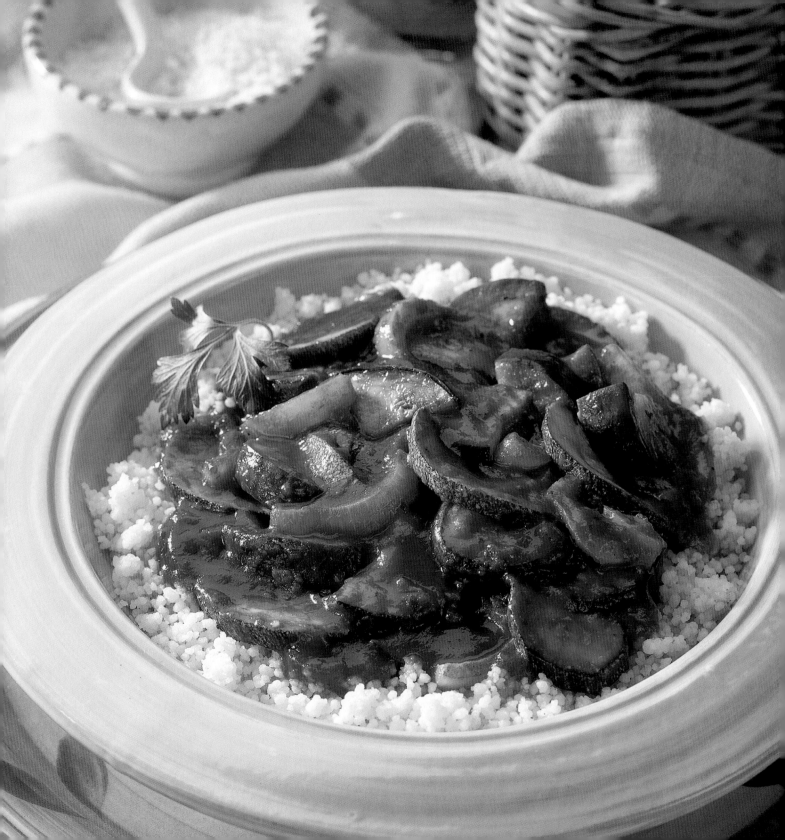

Oven-Baked Chicken Parmesan

4 boneless, skinless chicken breast halves (about 1¼ pounds)

1 egg, lightly beaten

¾ cup Italian seasoned dry bread crumbs

1 jar (1 pound 10 ounces) RAGÚ® Old World Style® Pasta Sauce

1 cup shredded mozzarella cheese (about 4 ounces)

1. Preheat oven to 400°F. Dip chicken in egg, then bread crumbs, coating well.

2. In 13×9-inch glass baking dish, arrange chicken. Bake uncovered 20 minutes.

3. Pour Ragú Pasta Sauce over chicken, then top with cheese. Bake an additional 10 minutes or until chicken is thoroughly cooked. Serve, if desired, with hot cooked pasta.

Makes 4 servings

Prep Time: 10 minutes
Cook Time: 30 minutes

Easy Italian Skillet Supper

1 pound Italian sausage, casing removed and crumbled, or ground beef

1 medium onion, cut into wedges

1 medium green bell pepper, cut into strips

2 cloves garlic, minced

1 (6.8-ounce) package RICE-A-RONI® Spanish Rice

2 tablespoons margarine or butter

1 (14½-ounce) can diced tomatoes, undrained

½ cup sliced pimiento-stuffed olives

1 teaspoon dried oregano

1. In large skillet, sauté sausage, onion, bell pepper and garlic until sausage is well cooked. Remove with slotted spoon; set aside.

2. In same skillet over medium heat, sauté rice-vermicelli mix with margarine until vermicelli is golden brown.

3. Slowly stir in 2 cups water, tomatoes, olives, oregano and Special Seasonings; bring to a boil. Reduce heat to low. Cover; simmer 15 to 20 minutes or until rice is tender. Stir in sausage mixture; serve.

Makes 4 servings

Tip: Only have canned whole tomatoes on hand? Simply snip them directly in the can using kitchen shears.

Prep Time: 10 minutes
Cook Time: 30 minutes

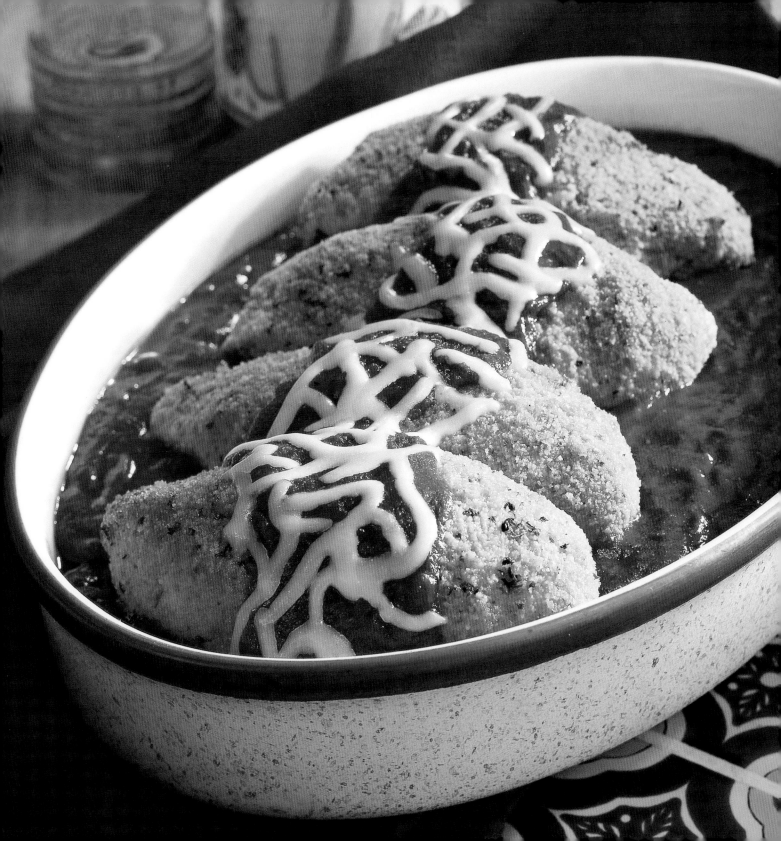

Swordfish Messina Style

2 tablespoons olive or
vegetable oil

½ cup chopped fresh parsley

2 tablespoons chopped fresh
basil *or* 2 teaspoons dried
basil leaves, crushed

2 cloves garlic, minced

1 can (8 ounces) CONTADINA®
Tomato Sauce

¾ cup sliced fresh mushrooms

1 tablespoon capers

1 tablespoon lemon juice

⅛ teaspoon ground black
pepper

3 pounds swordfish or halibut
steaks

1. Heat oil in small saucepan. Add parsley, basil and garlic; sauté for 1 minute. Reduce heat to low. Add tomato sauce, mushrooms and capers; simmer, uncovered, for 5 minutes.

2. Stir in lemon juice and pepper. Place swordfish in single layer in greased 13×9-inch baking dish; cover with sauce.

3. Bake in preheated 400°F oven for 20 minutes or until fish flakes easily when tested with fork.

Makes 8 servings

Prep Time: 5 minutes
Cook Time: 26 minutes

 tip *Firm fish such as swordfish or halibut can be prepared in almost any manner—baking, broiling, grilling, pan-frying or poaching.*

Cutlets Milanese

1 package (about 1 pound)
PERDUE® FIT 'N EASY®
Thin-Sliced Turkey Breast
Cutlets or Chicken Breast

Salt and ground pepper
to taste

½ cup Italian seasoned bread
crumbs

½ cup grated Parmesan cheese

1 large egg beaten with
1 teaspoon water

2 to 3 tablespoons olive oil

Season cutlets with salt and pepper. On wax paper, combine bread crumbs and Parmesan cheese. Dip cutlets in egg mixture and roll in bread crumb mixture. In large nonstick skillet over medium-high heat, heat oil. Add cutlets and sauté 3 minutes per side, until golden brown and cooked through.

Makes 4 servings

Prep Time: 6 to 8 minutes
Cook Time: 6 minutes

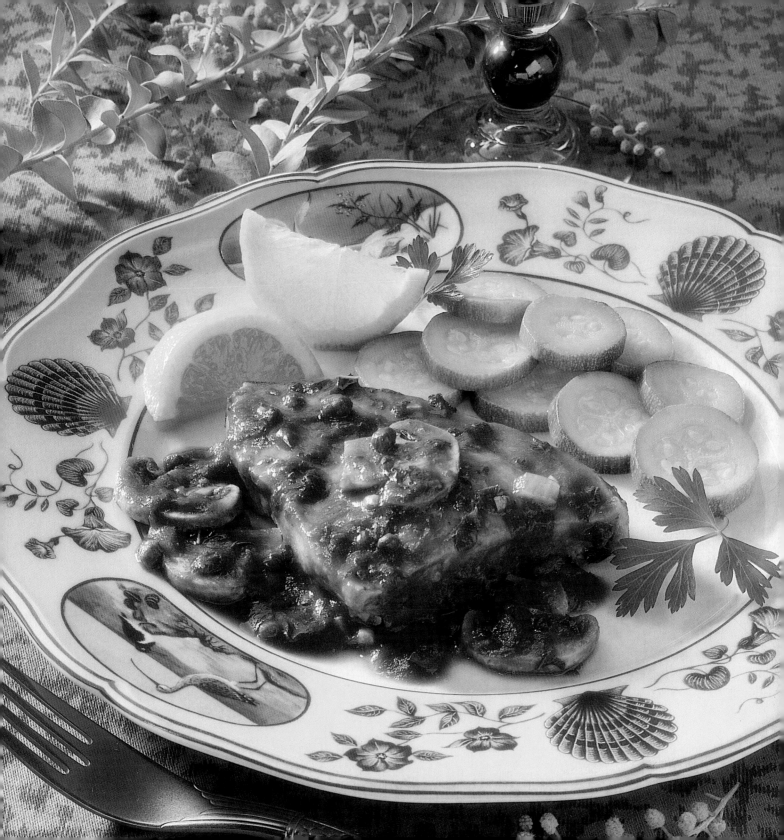

Italian Sausage and Vegetable Stew

1 pound hot or mild Italian sausage links, cut into 1-inch pieces

1 package (16 ounces) frozen mixed vegetables, such as onions and green, red and yellow bell peppers

2 medium zucchini, sliced

1 can (14½ ounces) diced Italian-style tomatoes, undrained

1 jar (4½ ounces) sliced mushrooms, drained

4 cloves garlic, minced

1. Cook sausage in large saucepan, covered, over medium to medium-high heat 5 minutes or until browned; pour off drippings.

2. Add frozen vegetables, zucchini, tomatoes with juice, mushrooms and garlic; bring to a boil. Reduce heat and simmer, covered, 10 minutes. Cook uncovered 5 to 10 minutes or until juices have thickened slightly.

Makes 6 (1-cup) servings

Serving Suggestion: Serve with garlic bread.

Prep and Cook Time: 30 minutes

Shrimp Classico

⅔ cup milk

2 tablespoons margarine or butter

1 package (4.8 ounces) PASTA RONI® Angel Hair Pasta with Herbs

1 clove garlic, minced

1 package (10 ounces) frozen chopped spinach, thawed and well drained

1 package (10 ounces) frozen precooked shrimp, thawed and well drained

1 jar (2 ounces) chopped pimentos, drained

Microwave Directions:

1. In 3-quart round microwavable glass casserole, combine 1⅔ cups water, milk and margarine. Microwave, uncovered, at HIGH 4 to 5 minutes or until boiling.

2. Gradually add pasta while stirring. Separate pasta with a fork, if needed. Stir in Special Seasonings and garlic.

3. Microwave, uncovered, at HIGH 4 minutes, stirring gently after 2 minutes. Separate pasta with a fork, if needed. Stir in spinach, shrimp and pimentos. Microwave at HIGH 1 to 2 minutes. Sauce will be very thin, but will thicken upon standing.

4. Let stand, uncovered, 2 minutes or until desired consistency. Stir before serving.

Makes 4 servings

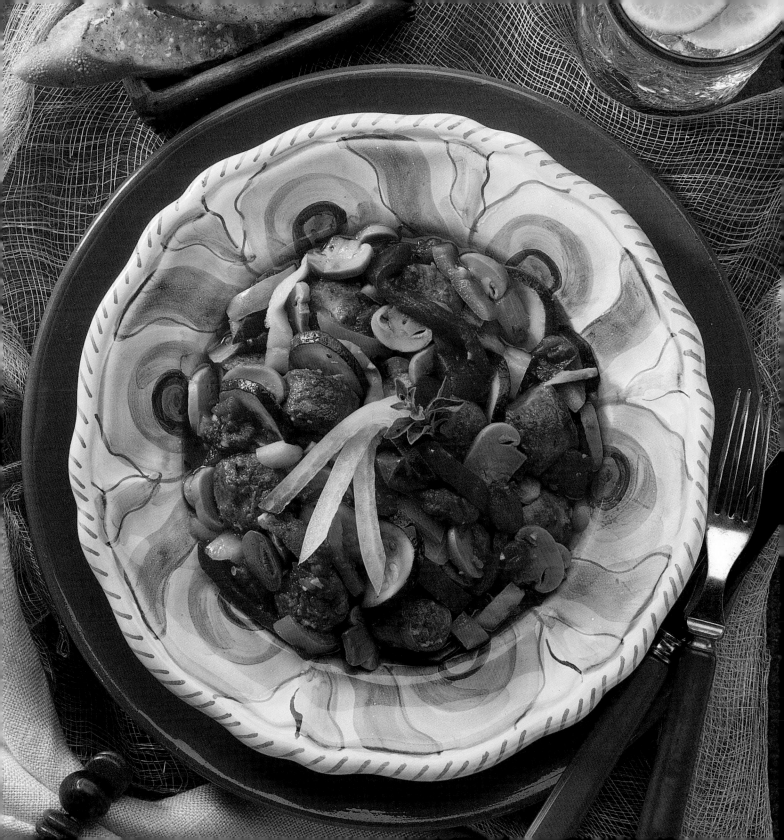

Red Snapper Scampi

¼ cup butter or margarine, softened

1 tablespoon white wine

1½ teaspoons minced garlic

½ teaspoon grated lemon peel

⅛ teaspoon black pepper

1½ pounds red snapper, orange roughy or grouper fillets (about 4 to 5 ounces each)

1. Preheat oven to 450°F. Combine butter, wine, garlic, lemon peel and pepper in small bowl; stir to blend.

2. Place fish on foil-lined shallow baking pan. Top with seasoned butter. Bake 10 to 12 minutes or until fish begins to flake easily when tested with fork.

Makes 4 servings

Tip: Serve fish over mixed salad greens, if desired. Or, add sliced carrots, zucchini and bell pepper cut into matchstick-size strips to the fish in the baking pan for an easy vegetable side dish.

Simmered Tuscan Chicken

2 tablespoons BERTOLLI® Olive Oil

1 pound boneless, skinless chicken breasts, cut into 1-inch cubes

2 cloves garlic, finely chopped

4 medium potatoes, cut into ½-inch cubes (about 4 cups)

1 medium red bell pepper, cut into large pieces

1 jar (1 pound 10 ounces) RAGÚ® Old World Style® Pasta Sauce

1 pound fresh or frozen cut green beans

1 teaspoon dried basil leaves, crushed

Salt and ground black pepper to taste

In 12-inch skillet, heat oil over medium-high heat and cook chicken with garlic until chicken is thoroughly cooked. Remove chicken and set aside.

In same skillet, add potatoes and bell pepper. Cook over medium heat, stirring occasionally, 5 minutes. Stir in remaining ingredients. Bring to a boil over high heat. Reduce heat to low and simmer covered, stirring occasionally, 35 minutes or until potatoes are tender. Return chicken to skillet and heat through.

Makes 6 servings

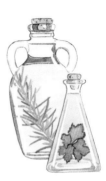

Red Snapper Scampi

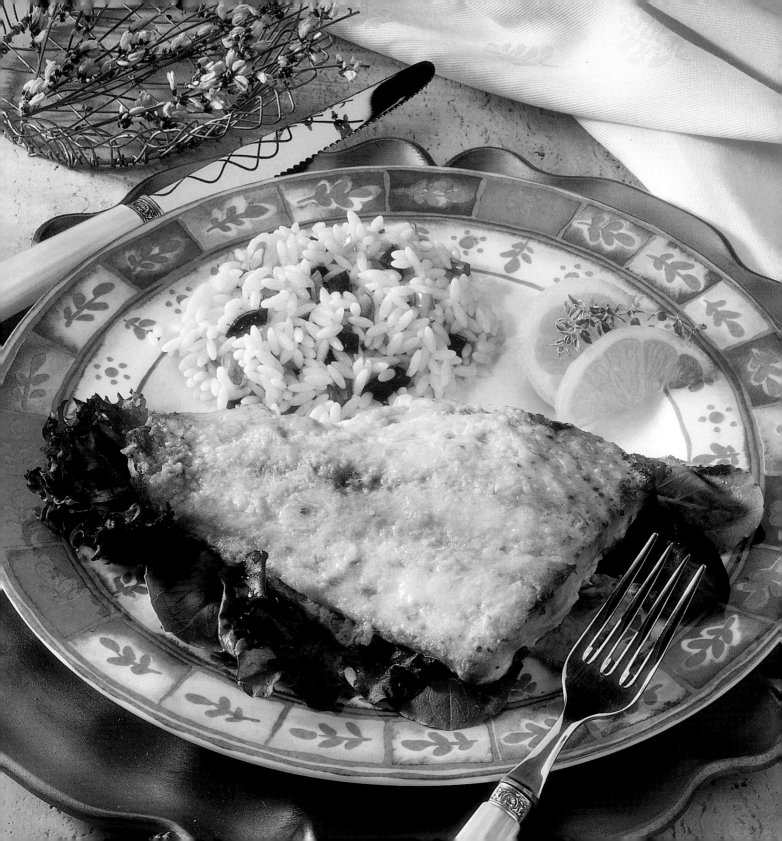

Chicken Milano

2 cloves garlic, minced

4 boneless, skinless chicken breast halves (about 1¼ pounds)

½ teaspoon dried basil leaves, crushed

⅛ teaspoon crushed red pepper flakes (optional)

Salt and black pepper

1 tablespoon olive oil

1 can (14½ ounces) DEL MONTE® Diced Tomatoes with Basil, Garlic & Oregano

1 can (14½ ounces) DEL MONTE Cut Green Italian Beans, drained

¼ cup whipping cream

1. Rub garlic over chicken. Sprinkle with basil and red pepper. Season with salt and black pepper.

2. Brown chicken in oil in skillet over medium-high heat. Stir in undrained tomatoes.

3. Cover; simmer 5 minutes. Uncover; reduce heat to medium and cook 8 to 10 minutes or until liquid is slightly thickened and chicken is tender.

4. Stir in green beans and cream; heat through. Do not boil.

Makes 4 servings

Prep and Cook Time: 25 minutes

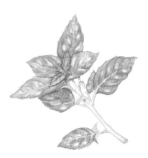

Grilled Italian Steak

¾ cup WISH-BONE® Italian Dressing*

2 tablespoons grated Parmesan cheese

2 teaspoons dried basil leaves, crushed

¼ teaspoon cracked black pepper

2 to 3-pound boneless sirloin or top round steak

*Also terrific with WISH-BONE® Robusto Italian or Just 2 Good Italian Dressing.

In large, shallow nonaluminum baking dish or plastic bag, combine all ingredients except steak. Add steak; turn to coat. Cover or close bag and marinate in refrigerator, turning occasionally, 3 to 24 hours.

Remove steak from marinade, reserving marinade. Grill or broil steak, turning once, until steak is done.

Meanwhile, in small saucepan, bring reserved marinade to a boil and continue boiling 1 minute. Pour over steak.

Makes 8 servings

Chicken Milano

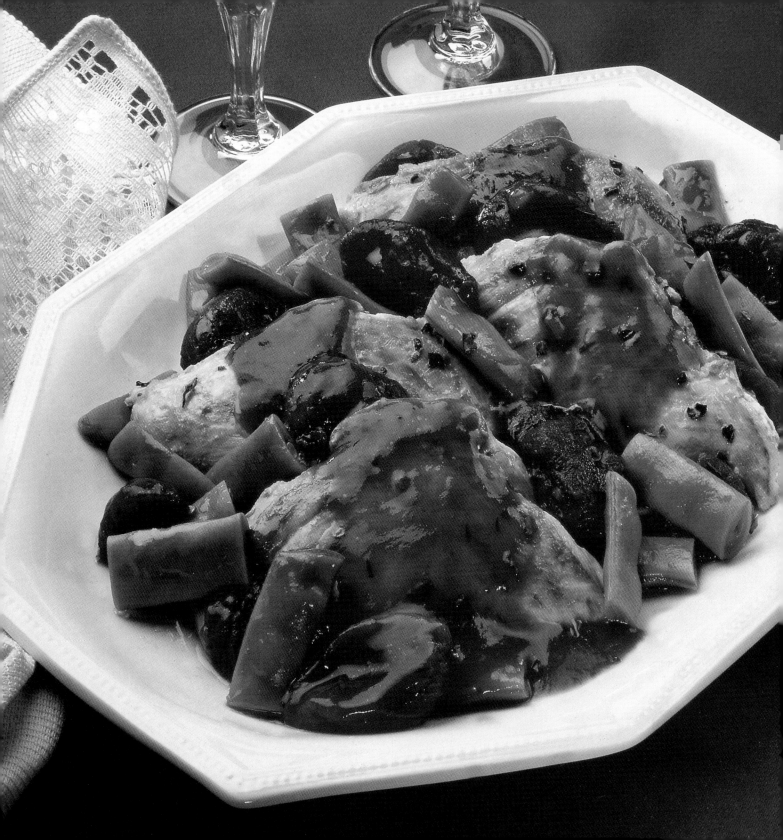

Poached Seafood Italiano

1 tablespoon olive or vegetable oil

1 large clove garlic, minced

¼ cup dry white wine or chicken broth

4 (6-ounce) salmon steaks or fillets

1 can (14.5 ounces) CONTADINA® Recipe Ready Diced Tomatoes with Italian Herbs, undrained

⅓ cup sliced olives (black, green or a combination)

2 tablespoons chopped fresh basil (optional)

1. Heat oil in large skillet. Add garlic; sauté 30 seconds. Add wine. Bring to boil.

2. Add salmon; cover. Reduce heat to medium; simmer 6 minutes.

3. Add undrained tomatoes and olives; simmer 2 minutes or until salmon flakes easily when tested with fork. Sprinkle with basil just before serving, if desired.

Makes 4 servings

Italian Marinated Chicken

1 bottle (8 ounces) LAWRY'S® Herb & Garlic Marinade with Lemon Juice

2 tablespoons finely chopped onion

2 tablespoons lemon juice

¾ teaspoon LAWRY'S® Seasoned Pepper

6 boneless, skinless chicken breast halves (about 1½ pounds)

In large resealable plastic food storage bag, combine all ingredients except chicken; mix well. Add chicken to marinade; seal bag. Marinate in refrigerate at least 1 hour, turning occasionally. Remove chicken; discard used marinade. Grill or broil chicken 10 to 15 minutes or until no longer pink in center and juices run clear when cut.

Makes 6 to 8 servings

Serving Suggestion: Perfect served with any pasta or crisp green salad.

Hint: Chill leftover chicken and slice for use in salads or sandwiches.

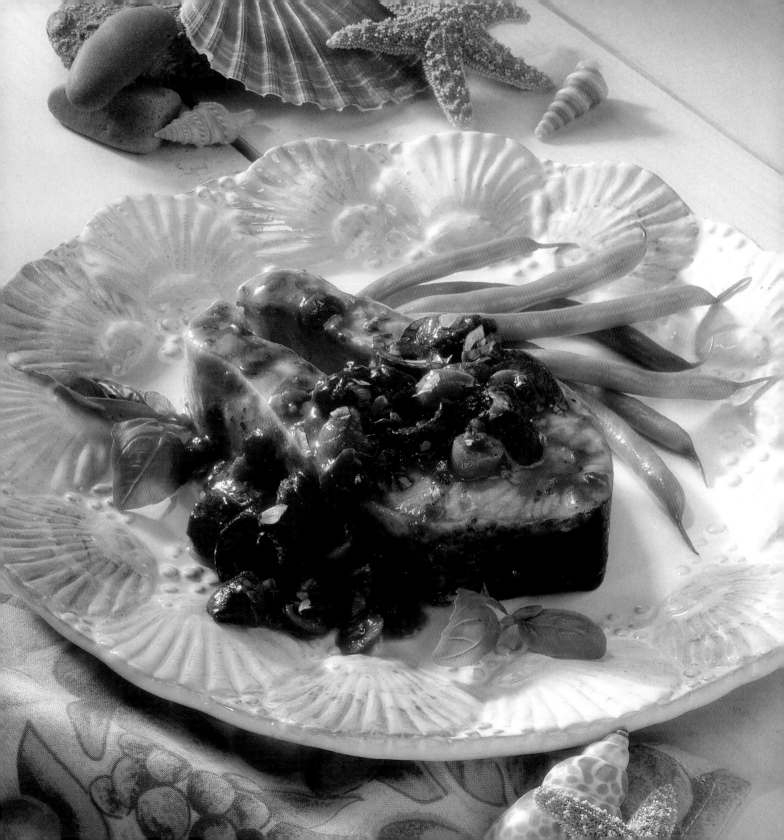

Italian-Glazed Pork Chops

1 tablespoon BERTOLLI®
   Olive Oil

8 bone-in pork chops

1 medium zucchini, thinly
   sliced

1 medium red bell pepper,
   chopped

1 medium onion, thinly sliced

3 cloves garlic, finely chopped

¼ cup dry red wine or beef
   broth

1 jar (1 pound 10 ounces)
   RAGÚ® Chunky Gardenstyle
   Pasta Sauce

1. In 12-inch skillet, heat oil over medium-high heat and brown chops. Remove chops and set aside.

2. In same skillet, cook zucchini, red bell pepper, onion and garlic, stirring occasionally, 4 minutes. Stir in wine and Ragú Pasta Sauce.

3. Return chops to skillet, turning to coat with sauce. Simmer covered 15 minutes or until chops are tender and barely pink in the center. Serve, if desired, over hot cooked couscous or rice.   *Makes 8 servings*

Prep Time: 10 minutes
Cook Time: 25 minutes

Hearty Italian Medley

1 pound hot Italian sausage,
   cut into bite-size pieces

1 onion, chopped

3 zucchini, chunked

1 eggplant, chunked

1 DOLE® Green Bell Pepper,
   seeded, chunked

¼ cup water

2 cups prepared marinara
   sauce

3 cups DOLE® Fresh Pineapple,
   cut into chunks

1 tomato, chunked

4 cups hot cooked noodles

• Brown sausage and onion in large skillet or Dutch oven. Add zucchini, eggplant, bell pepper and water. Cover, simmer 10 minutes until tender.

• Stir in marinara sauce, pineapple chunks and tomato. Simmer 5 minutes. Serve over hot cooked noodles.   *Makes 8 Servings*

Prep Time: 10 minutes
Cook Time: 17 minutes

Italian-Glazed Pork Chop

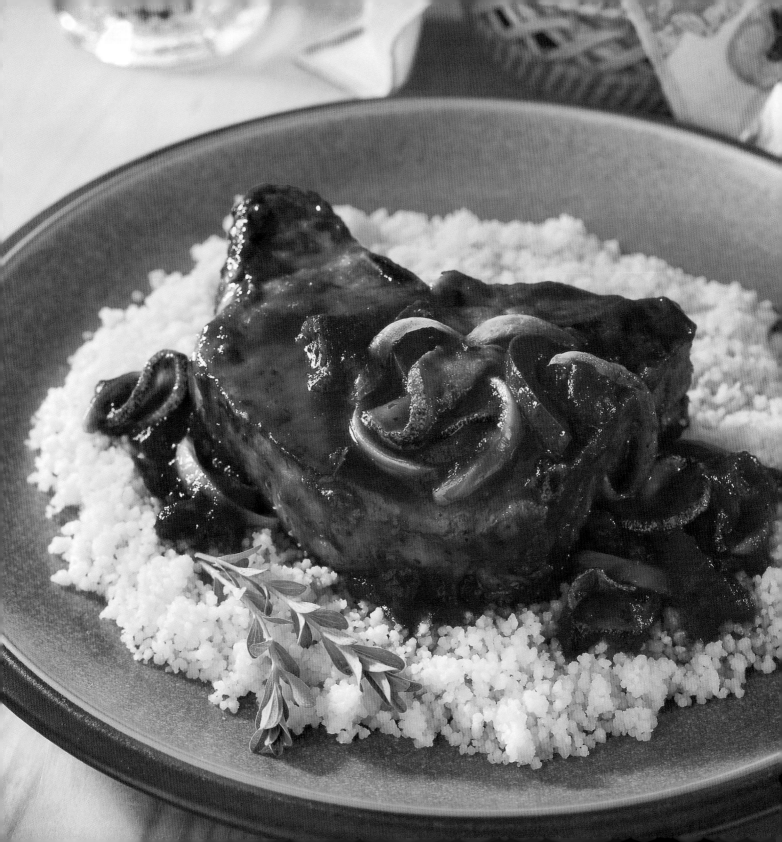

Chicken Rustigo

4 boneless skinless chicken breast halves

1 package (10 ounces) fresh mushrooms, sliced

¾ cup chicken broth

¼ cup dry red wine or water

3 tablespoons French's® Bold n' Spicy Brown Mustard

2 plum tomatoes, coarsely chopped

1 can (14 ounces) artichoke hearts, drained and quartered

2 teaspoons cornstarch

1. Season chicken with salt and pepper. Heat 1 *tablespoon oil* in large nonstick skillet over medium-high heat. Cook chicken 5 minutes or until browned on both sides. Remove and set aside.

2. Heat 1 *tablespoon oil* in same skillet over medium-high heat until hot. Add mushrooms. Cook and stir 5 minutes or until mushrooms are tender. Stir in broth, wine and mustard. Return chicken to skillet. Add tomatoes and artichoke hearts. Heat to boiling. Reduce heat to medium-low. Cook, covered, 10 minutes or until chicken is no longer pink in center.

3. Combine cornstarch and 1 *tablespoon cold water* in small bowl. Stir into skillet. Heat to boiling. Cook, stirring, over high heat about 1 minute or until sauce thickens. Serve with hot cooked orzo pasta, if desired.   *Makes 4 servings*

Prep Time: 10 minutes
Cook Time: 21 minutes

Chicken di Napolitano

1 tablespoon olive oil

2 boneless, skinless chicken breasts (about 8 ounces)

1 can (14½ ounces) diced tomatoes, undrained

1¼ cups water

1 box UNCLE BEN'S® COUNTRY INN® Rice Pilaf

¼ cup chopped fresh basil *or* 1½ teaspoons dried basil leaves

1. Heat oil in large skillet. Add chicken; cook over medium-high heat 8 to 10 minutes or until lightly browned on both sides.

2. Add tomatoes, water, rice and contents of seasoning packet. Bring to a boil. Cover; reduce heat and simmer 15 to 18 minutes or until chicken is no longer pink in center and liquid is absorbed.

3. Stir in basil. Slice chicken and serve over rice.   *Makes 2 servings*

Cook's Tip: For more flavor, substitute diced tomatoes with Italian herbs or roasted garlic for diced tomatoes.

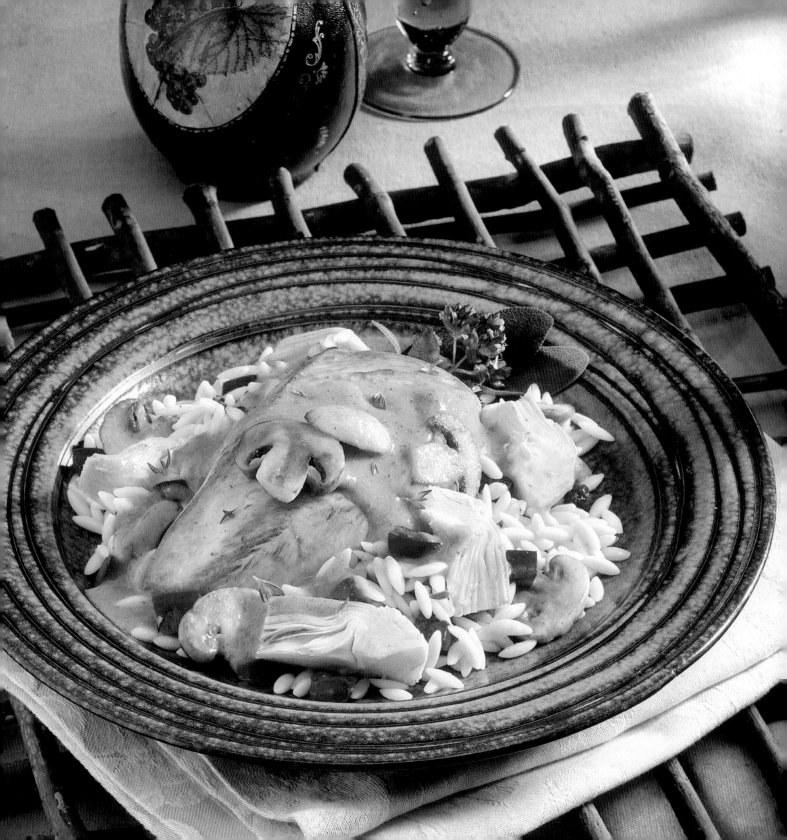

Chicken Marsala

1 tablespoon butter

2 boneless skinless chicken breasts, halved

1 cup sliced carrots

1 cup sliced fresh mushrooms

⅓ cup chicken broth

⅓ cup HOLLAND HOUSE® Marsala Cooking Wine

Melt butter in skillet over medium-high heat. Add chicken; cook 5 minutes. Turn chicken over, add remaining ingredients. Bring to a boil; simmer 15 to 20 minutes until juices run clear. Serve over cooked fettuccine, if desired.

Makes 4 servings

Savory Veal Ragú®

1 tablespoon BERTOLLI® Olive Oil

2 pounds veal shoulder, cubed

2 medium green or red bell peppers, sliced

1 small onion, chopped

2 ribs celery, chopped

2 carrots, chopped

2 cloves garlic, finely chopped

1 jar (1 pound 10 ounces) RAGÚ® Old World Style® Pasta Sauce

½ cup water

¼ cup Burgundy wine

½ teaspoon salt

Preheat oven to 350°F. In 6-quart Dutch oven, heat oil and brown veal in two batches. Return veal to Dutch oven. Stir in bell peppers, onion, celery, carrots and garlic and cook 5 minutes. Stir in remaining ingredients. Cover and bake 1 hour. Remove cover and stir. Continue baking uncovered 30 minutes or until veal and vegetables are tender.

Makes 4 servings

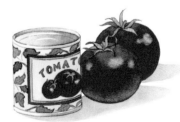

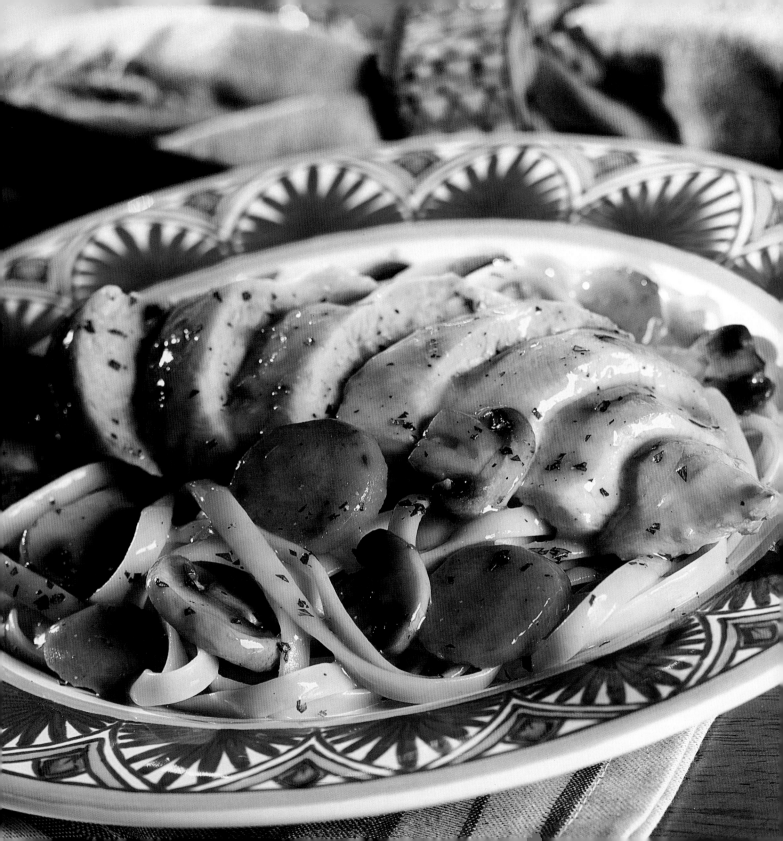

Skillet Chicken Cacciatore

2 tablespoons olive or vegetable oil

1 cup sliced red onion

1 medium green bell pepper, cut into strips (about 1 cup)

2 cloves garlic, minced

1 pound (about 4) boneless, skinless chicken breast halves

1 can (14.5 ounces) CONTADINA® Recipe Ready Diced Tomatoes with Italian Herbs, undrained

¼ cup dry white wine or chicken broth

½ teaspoon salt

¼ teaspoon ground black pepper

1 tablespoon chopped fresh basil *or* 1 teaspoon dried basil leaves, crushed

1. Heat oil in large skillet over medium-high heat. Add onion, bell pepper and garlic; sauté 1 minute.

2. Add chicken; cook 6 to 8 minutes or until chicken is no longer pink in center.

3. Add undrained tomatoes, wine, salt and black pepper. Simmer, uncovered, 5 minutes. Serve over hot cooked rice or pasta, if desired. Sprinkle with basil.

Makes 6 servings

 tip Cacciatore, Italian for "hunter," refers to dishes prepared "hunter's style." The most popular dish is Chicken Cacciatore, which usually includes chicken pieces, tomatoes or tomato sauce, mushrooms, onions, garlic, various herbs and spices and sometimes wine.

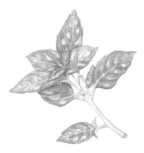

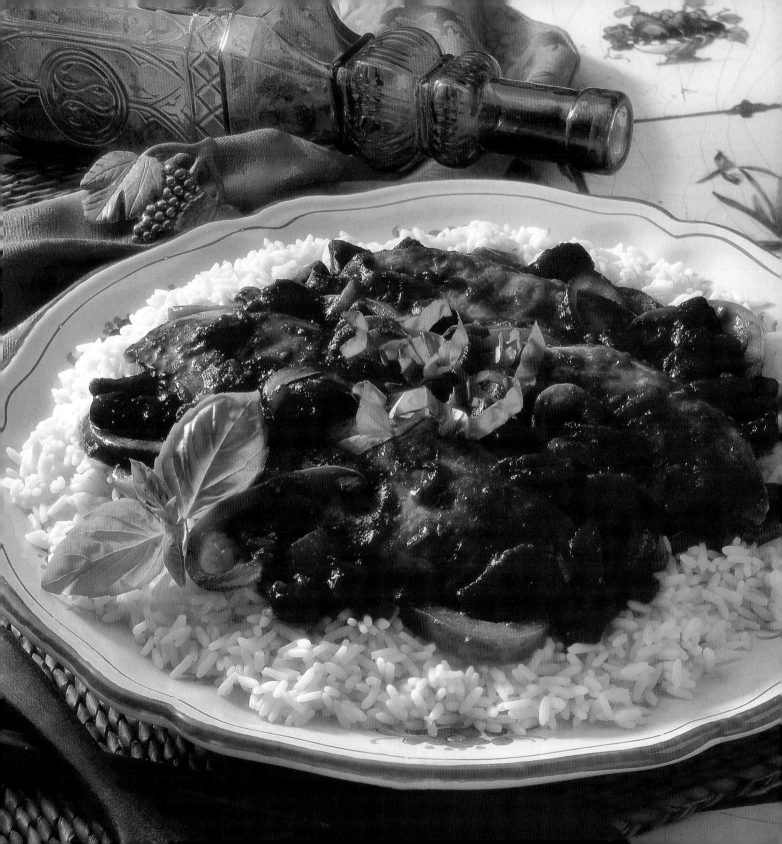

Light Meals

Chicken Cacciatore Melt

4 TYSON® Fresh Boneless, Skinless Chicken Thigh Cutlets

2 tablespoons garlic oil (see note)

1 jar (28 ounces) spaghetti sauce

1 cup shredded mozzarella cheese

4 large slices crusty Italian bread, lightly toasted

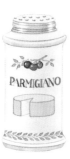

COOK: CLEAN: Wash hands. In large skillet, heat oil. Add chicken and cook 3 minutes per side or until browned. Stir in spaghetti sauce. Cover and cook over medium heat 20 minutes or until internal juices of chicken run clear. (Or insert instant-read meat thermometer in thickest part of chicken. Temperature should read 180°F.) Divide cheese evenly over chicken. Cover and cook over medium heat 1 minute or until cheese is melted slightly. Top each slice of toast with chicken thigh.   *Makes 4 servings*

CHILL: Refrigerate leftovers immediately.

Note: Use mixture of 1 clove garlic, minced, and 2 tablespoons olive oil if garlic oil is not available. Fresh sliced mushrooms may be added to spaghetti sauce before heating, if desired.

Tip: Serve with three bean salad, if desired

Prep Time: none
Cook Time: 30 minutes

Chicken Cacciatore Melt

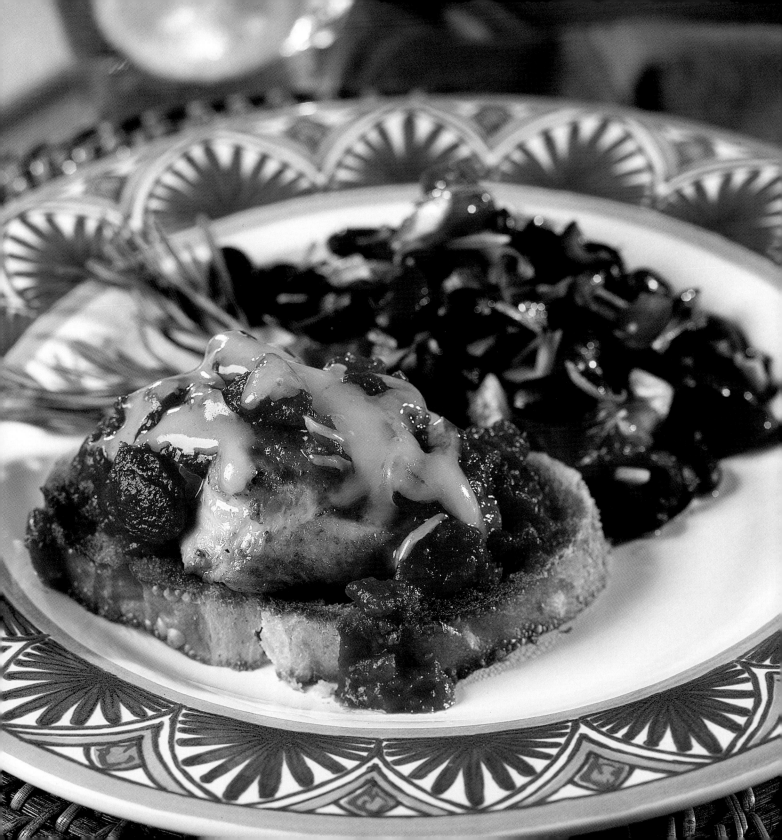

Pizza Primavera

¾ cup RAGÚ® Pizza Quick® Sauce

1 (10-inch) prebaked pizza crust

1 medium red bell pepper, thinly sliced

1 cup sliced zucchini

½ cup chopped red onion

1 cup shredded mozzarella cheese (about 4 ounces)

Preheat oven to 450°F. Evenly spread Ragú Pizza Quick Sauce on pizza crust, then top with remaining ingredients. Bake 12 minutes or until cheese is melted.

Makes 4 servings

Tuscan-Style Sausage Sandwiches

1 pound hot or sweet Italian sausage links, sliced

1 box (10 ounces) frozen chopped spinach, thawed and squeezed dry

1 small onion, sliced

½ cup fresh or drained canned sliced mushrooms

1 jar (1 pound 10 ounces) RAGÚ® Robusto! Pasta Sauce

1 loaf Italian or French bread (about 16 inches long), cut into 4 rolls

In 12-inch skillet, brown sausage over medium-high heat. Stir in spinach, onion and mushrooms. Cook, stirring occasionally, 5 minutes or until sausage is done. Stir in Ragú Robusto! Pasta Sauce; heat through.

For each sandwich, split open each roll and evenly spoon in sausage mixture. Sprinkle, if desired, with crushed red pepper flakes.

Makes 4 servings

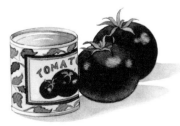

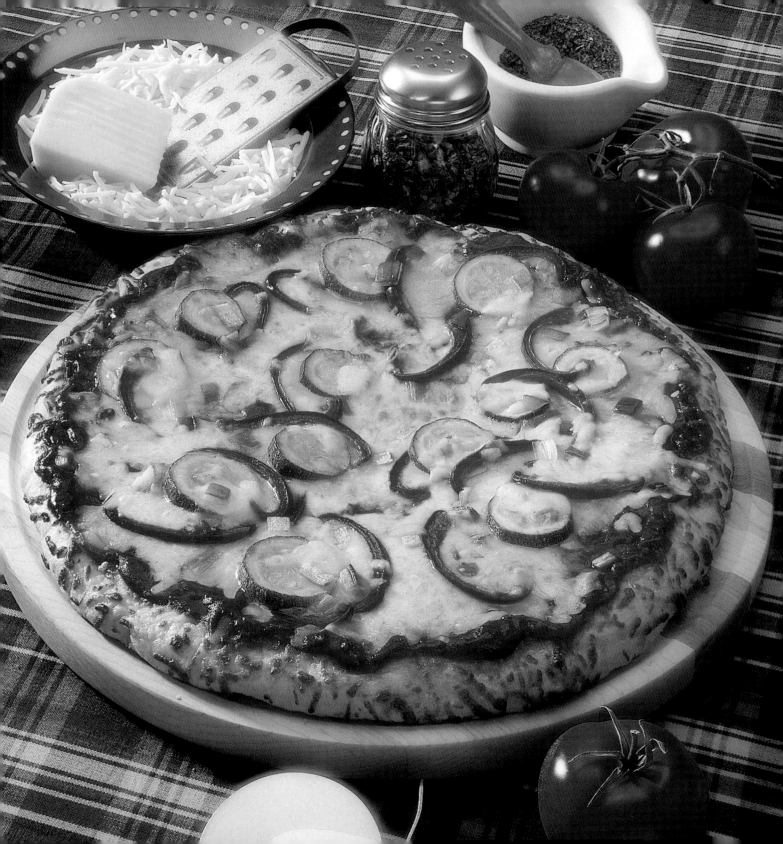

Vegetable Frittata

2 tablespoons butter or
  margarine
1 bag (16 ounces) BIRDS EYE®
  frozen Farm Fresh Mixtures
  Broccoli, Corn and Red
  Peppers
8 eggs
½ cup water
1 tablespoon TABASCO®*
  Pepper Sauce
¾ teaspoon salt

*Tabasco® is a registered trademark of
McIlhenny Company.

Melt butter in 12-inch nonstick skillet over medium heat. Add vegetables;
cook and stir 3 minutes.

Lightly beat eggs, water, Tabasco sauce and salt.

Pour egg mixture over vegetables in skillet. Cover and cook 10 to 15 minutes
or until eggs are set.

To serve, cut into wedges.   *Makes about 4 servings*

Serving Suggestion: Serve with warm crusty bread and a green salad.

Prep Time: 5 minutes
Cook Time: 20 minutes

Italian Grilled Sandwich

1 medium eggplant, cut into
  ½-inch-thick slices
  (about 1 pound)
1 medium zucchini,
  cut diagonally into
  ¼-inch-thick slices
  (about ¾ pound)
½ cup WISH-BONE® Italian or
  Classic House Italian
  Dressing
1 loaf Italian bread,
  cut lengthwise in half
  (about 14 inches)
1 jar (12 ounces) roasted
  red peppers, drained
  and rinsed
1 package (8 ounces) fresh
  mozzarella cheese, sliced

In large, shallow nonaluminum baking dish or plastic bag, combine eggplant,
zucchini and Italian dressing. Cover, or close bag, and marinate in refrigerator,
turning occasionally, 3 to 24 hours.

Remove vegetables, reserving marinade. Grill or broil vegetables, turning
once, until tender. Remove; set aside. Brush reserved marinade on bread.
Grill or broil until bread is toasted. Arrange roasted red peppers, vegetables
and cheese on bottom half of bread. Top with remaining bread and slice into
4 sandwiches.   *Makes about 4 generous servings*

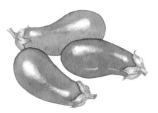

Vegetable Frittata

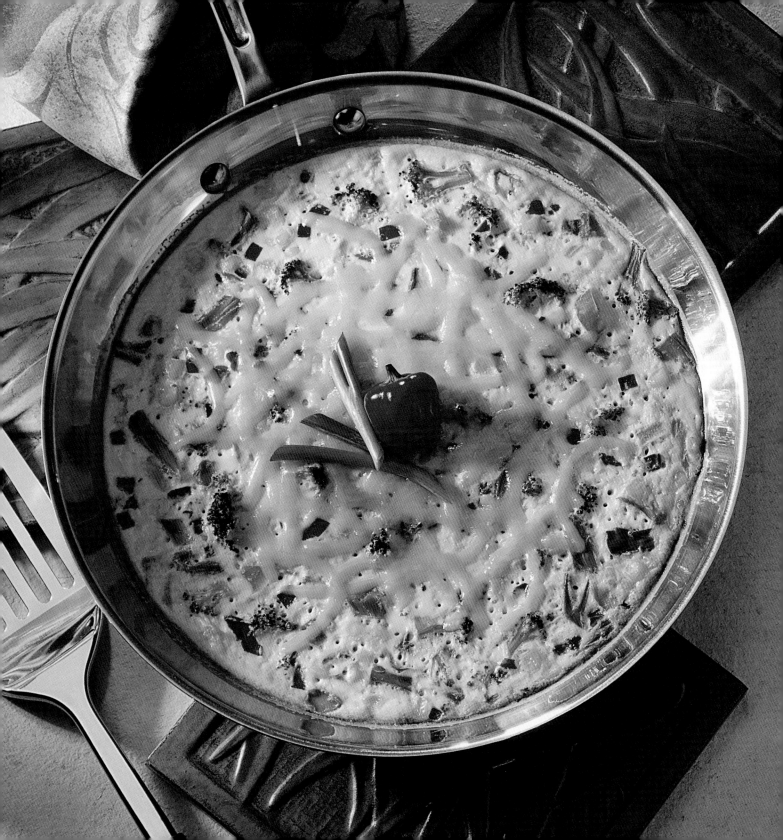

Chicken Parmesan Stromboli

1 pound boneless, skinless chicken breast halves

½ teaspoon salt

¼ teaspoon ground black pepper

2 teaspoons BERTOLLI® Olive Oil

2 cups shredded mozzarella cheese (about 8 ounces)

1 jar (1 pound 10 ounces) RAGÚ® Chunky Gardenstyle Pasta Sauce, divided

2 tablespoons grated Parmesan cheese

1 tablespoon finely chopped fresh parsley

1 pound fresh or thawed frozen bread dough

1. Preheat oven to 400°F. Season chicken with salt and pepper. In 12-inch skillet, heat oil over medium-high heat and brown chicken. Remove chicken from skillet and let cool; pull into large shreds.

2. In medium bowl, combine chicken, mozzarella cheese, ½ cup Ragú Chunky Gardenstyle Pasta Sauce, Parmesan cheese and parsley; set aside.

3. On greased jelly-roll pan, press dough to form 12×10-inch rectangle. Arrange chicken mixture down center of dough. Cover filling bringing one long side into center, then overlap with the other long side; pinch seam to seal. Fold in ends and pinch to seal. Arrange on pan, seam-side down. Gently press in sides to form 12×4-inch loaf. Bake 35 minutes or until dough is cooked and golden. Cut stromboli into slices. Heat remaining pasta sauce and serve with stromboli.

Makes 6 servings

Vegetable Pizza

2 to 3 cups BIRDS EYE® frozen Farm Fresh Mixtures Broccoli, Red Peppers, Onions and Mushrooms

1 Italian bread shell or pizza crust, about 12 inches

1 to 1½ cups shredded mozzarella cheese

Dried oregano, basil or Italian seasoning

• Preheat oven according to directions on pizza crust package.

• Rinse vegetables in colander under warm water. Drain well; pat with paper towel to remove excess moisture.

• Spread crust with half the cheese and all the vegetables. Sprinkle with herbs; top with remaining cheese.

• Follow baking directions on pizza crust package; bake until hot and bubbly.

Makes 3 to 4 servings

Prep Time: 5 minutes
Cook Time: 15 minutes

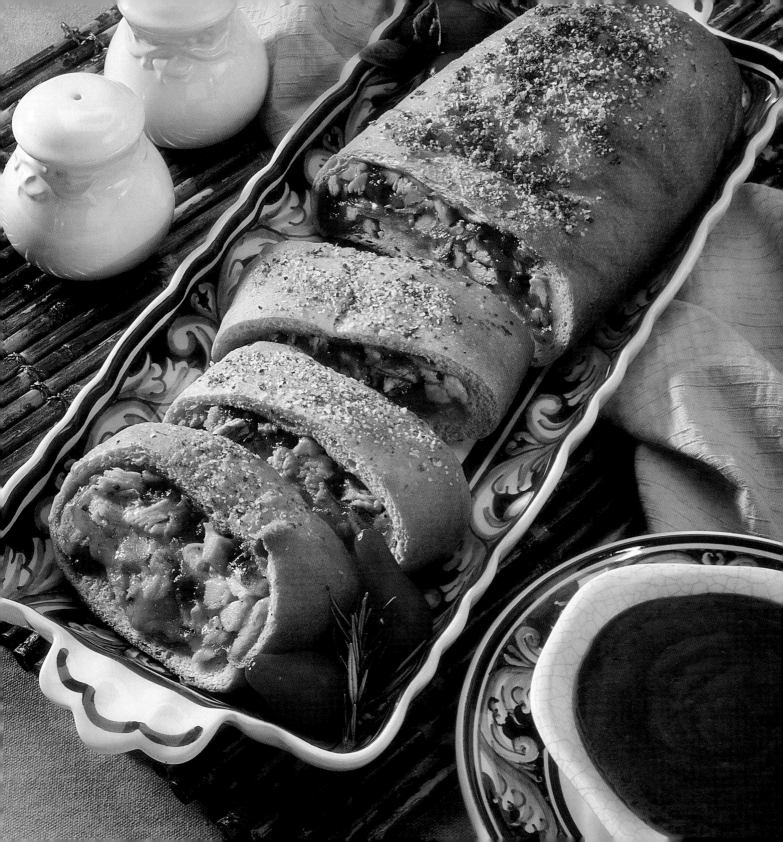

Grilled Panini Sandwiches

8 slices country Italian,
   sourdough or other
   firm-textured bread

8 slices SARGENTO® Deli Style
   Sliced Mozzarella Cheese

⅓ cup prepared pesto

4 large slices ripe tomato

2 tablespoons olive oil

1. Top each of 4 slices of bread with a slice of cheese. Spread pesto over cheese. Arrange tomatoes on top, then another slice of cheese. Close sandwiches with remaining 4 slices bread.

2. Brush olive oil lightly over both sides of sandwiches. Cook sandwiches over medium-low coals or in a preheated ridged grill pan over medium heat 3 to 4 minutes per side or until bread is toasted and cheese is melted.

Makes 4 servings

Prep Time: 5 minutes
Cook Time: 8 minutes

Italian Omelet

¼ cup chopped tomato

¼ cup (1 ounce) shredded part-
   skim mozzarella cheese

¼ teaspoon dried basil leaves

¼ teaspoon dried oregano
   leaves

1 teaspoon FLEISCHMANN'S®
   Original Margarine

1 cup EGG BEATERS® Healthy
   Real Egg Product

Chopped fresh parsley, for
   garnish

In small bowl, combine tomato, cheese, basil and oregano; set aside.

In 8-inch nonstick skillet, over medium heat, melt margarine. Pour Egg Beaters® into skillet. Cook, lifting edges to allow uncooked portion to flow underneath. When almost set, spoon tomato mixture over half of omelet. Fold other half over tomato mixture; cover and continue to cook for 1 to 2 minutes. Slide onto serving plate. Garnish with parsley.

Makes 2 servings

Prep Time: 10 minutes
Cook Time: 10 minutes

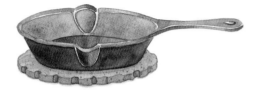

Grilled Panini Sandwich

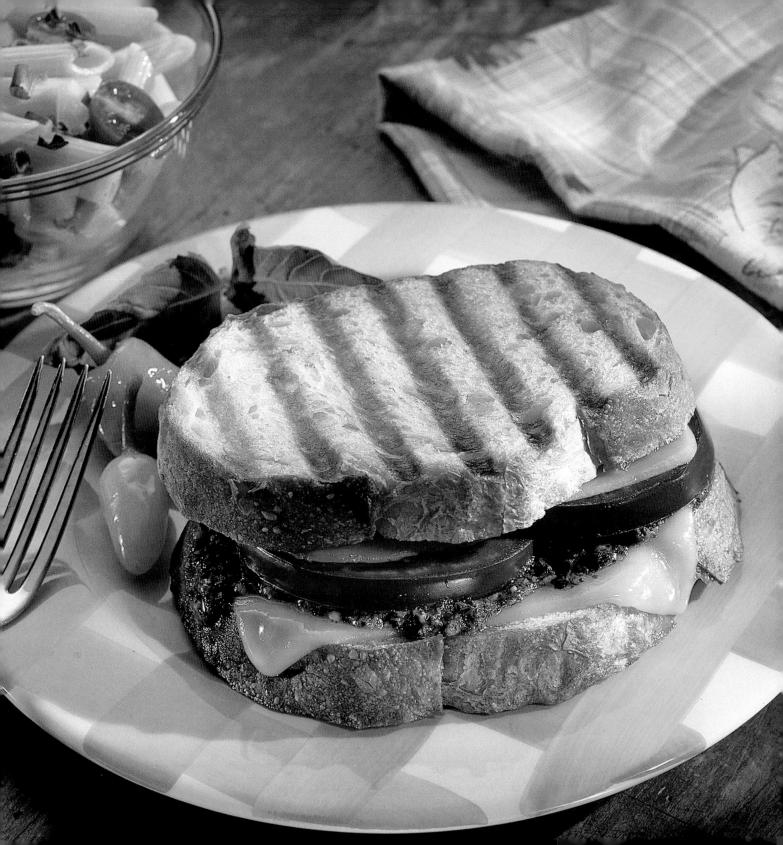

Personal Pizzas

- 1 pound BOB EVANS® Italian Roll Sausage
- 1 (8-ounce) can tomato sauce or pizza sauce
- ½ teaspoon garlic powder
- ½ teaspoon dried oregano leaves
- ¼ teaspoon dried basil leaves
- 8 English muffins *or* 1 pound loaf Italian bread, cut into 1-inch slices
- 3 cups (12 ounces) shredded Cheddar or mozzarella cheese or a combination
- 1 (4-ounce) can mushroom stems and pieces, drained
- 6 to 8 pimiento-stuffed green olives, sliced

Preheat oven to 425°F. Crumble sausage into medium skillet. Cook over medium heat until lightly browned, stirring occasionally. Drain on paper towels; set aside. Combine tomato sauce and seasonings in small bowl; spread evenly on muffins. Layer ⅔ of cheese on top of sauce. Layer sausage, mushrooms and olives evenly over cheese. Sprinkle with remaining cheese. Bake 15 to 20 minutes or until bubbly. Serve hot. Refrigerate leftovers.

Makes 8 servings

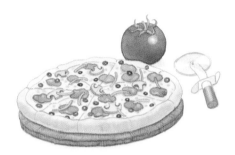

Classic Pepperoni Pizza

- 1 cup (½ of 15 ounce can) CONTADINA® Original Pizza Sauce
- 1 (12-inch) prepared, pre-baked pizza crust
- 1½ cups (6 ounces) shredded mozzarella cheese, divided
- 1½ ounces sliced pepperoni
- 1 tablespoon chopped fresh parsley

1. Spread pizza sauce onto crust to within 1 inch of edge.

2. Sprinkle with 1 cup cheese, pepperoni and remaining cheese.

3. Bake according to pizza crust package directions or until crust is crisp and cheese is melted. Sprinkle with parsley.

Makes 8 servings

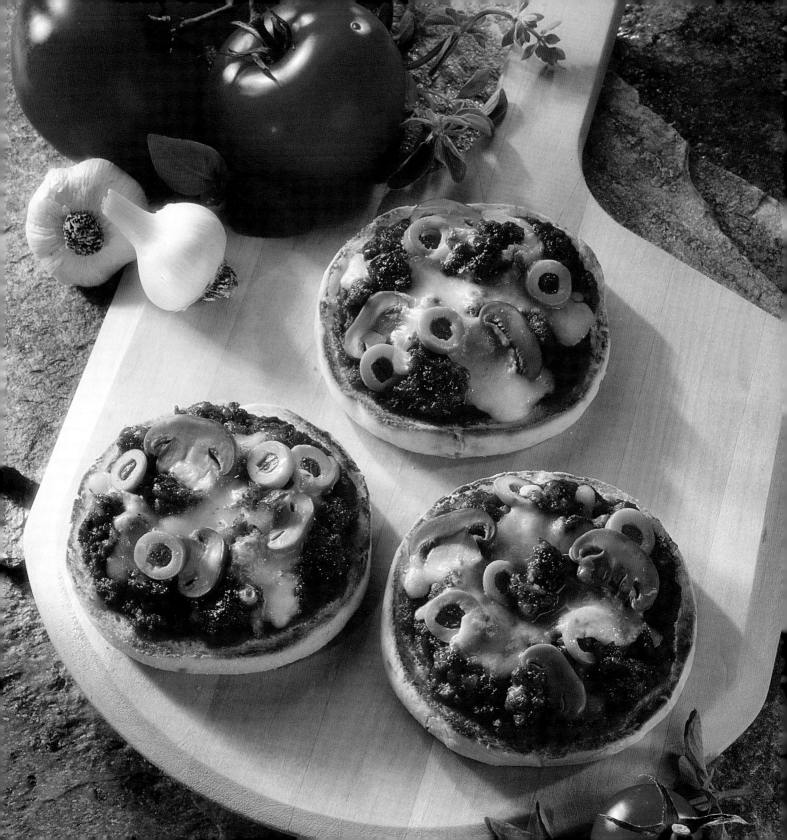

Italian Sausage and Rice Frittata

7 large eggs

¾ cup milk

½ teaspoon salt

½ pound mild or hot Italian sausage, casing removed and sausage broken into small pieces

1½ cups uncooked UNCLE BEN'S® Instant Brown Rice

1 can (14½ ounces) Italian-style stewed tomatoes

¼ teaspoon Italian herb seasoning

1½ cups (6 ounces) shredded Italian cheese blend, divided

1. Whisk together eggs, milk and salt in medium bowl. Set aside.

2. Preheat oven to 325°F. Cook sausage about 7 minutes in 11-inch ovenproof nonstick skillet over high heat until no longer pink.

3. Reduce heat to medium-low. Stir in rice, stewed tomatoes with their juices, breaking up any large pieces, and Italian seasoning. Sprinkle evenly with 1 cup cheese.

4. Pour egg mixture into skillet; stir gently to distribute egg. Cover and cook 15 minutes or until eggs are just set.

5. Remove from heat. Sprinkle remaining ½ cup cheese over frittata. Bake about 10 minutes more or until puffed and cheese is melted.

6. Remove skillet from oven. Cover and let stand 5 minutes. Cut into 6 wedges before serving.

Makes 6 servings

Cook's Tip: Choose a blend of shredded mozzarella and provolone for this frittata, or the blend of your choice.

Crispy Chicken Pizza Sandwiches

1 package (14 ounces) BUTTERBALL® Chicken Requests™ Italian Herb Crispy Baked Breasts

4 slices mozzarella cheese

4 Italian-style rolls, split

½ cup prepared pizza sauce

Red pepper flakes (optional)

Prepare chicken according to package directions. Place slice of cheese on top of each chicken piece during the last minute of heating. Spread rolls with pizza sauce. Place chicken on rolls; sprinkle with red pepper flakes.

Makes 4 sandwiches

Prep Time: 20 minutes

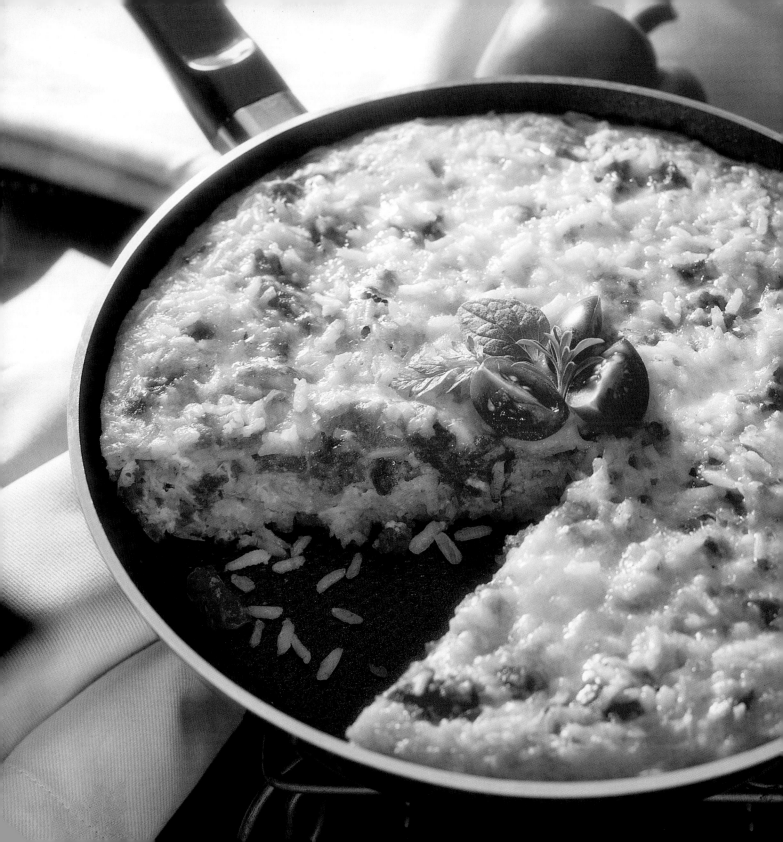

Hot Antipasto Subs

⅓ cup French's® Bold n' Spicy Brown Mustard

3 tablespoons mayonnaise

½ teaspoon dried oregano leaves

4 (6-inch) crusty Italian-style rolls, sliced lengthwise in half

1 jar (6 ounces) marinated artichoke hearts, drained and chopped

¼ cup chopped pitted cured olives

¼ cup sliced roasted red peppers, drained

¾ pound sliced deli meats and cheese such as salami, spiced ham and provolone cheese

1 cup arugula or spinach leaves, washed

1. Preheat oven to 400°F. Combine mustard, mayonnaise and oregano. Spread evenly on both sides of rolls.

2. Layer remaining ingredients on bottom of rolls, dividing evenly. Cover with top half, pressing firmly.

3. Wrap sandwiches in foil. Bake 10 minutes or until hot and cheese melts slightly.

Makes 4 servings

Prep Time: 20 minutes
Cook Time: 10 minutes

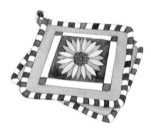

Hot Antipasto Sub

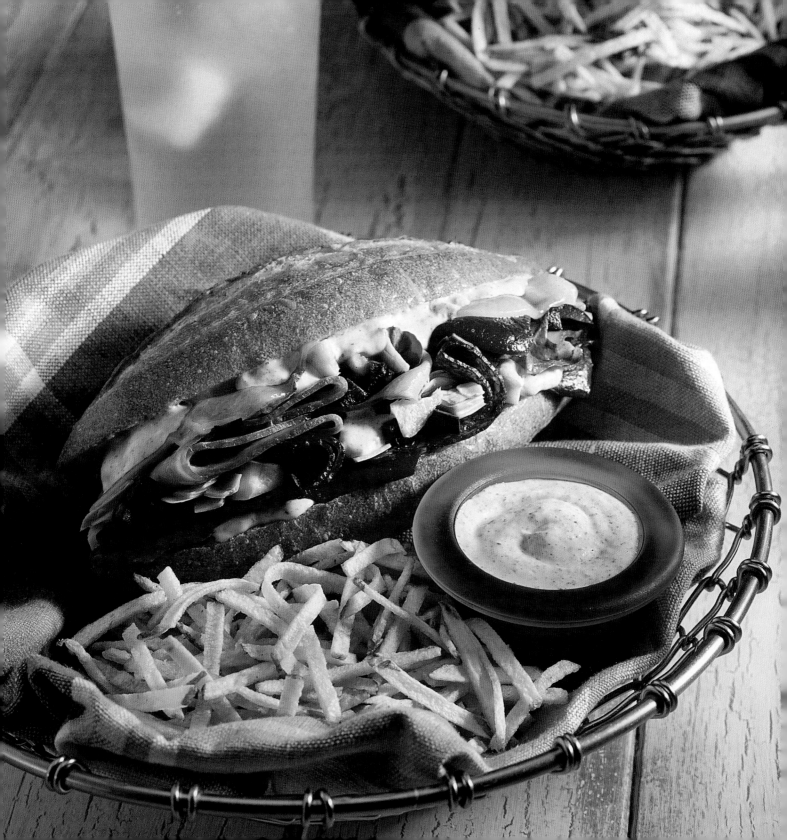

Plum Tomato Basil Pizza

1 cup (4 ounces) shredded mozzarella cheese

1 (10-ounce) package prepared pizza crust

4 ripe seeded Italian plum tomatoes, sliced

½ cup fresh basil leaves

1½ teaspoons TABASCO® brand Pepper Sauce

Olive oil

Preheat oven to 425°F. Sprinkle shredded mozzarella cheese evenly over pizza crust. Layer with tomatoes and basil. Drizzle with TABASCO® Sauce and olive oil. Bake on pizza pan or stone 15 minutes or until cheese is melted and crust is golden brown.

Makes 4 servings

BelGioioso® Caprese Sandwich

1 long (about 24 inches), slender baguette

1 clove garlic, cut in half

2 medium, fully-ripened tomatoes, thinly sliced and slices cut in half

24 fresh basil leaves

8 ounces BELGIOIOSO® Fresh Mozzarella, cut into ½-inch cubes

2 to 3 teaspoons extra virgin olive oil

2 teaspoons drained capers

Salt and freshly ground black pepper to taste

Make lengthwise cut down middle of baguette, starting on top of loaf and cut into, but not through, bottom. Gently open to make V-shaped cavity.

Rub cut sides of bread with garlic. Arrange tomato slices down each side of cavity followed by basil leaves.

In medium bowl, gently mix BelGioioso Fresh Mozzarella, oil, capers, salt and pepper. Spoon mixture into loaf between rows of tomato and basil. Cut sandwich crosswise into 6-inch lengths.

Makes 4 sandwiches

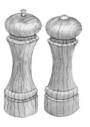

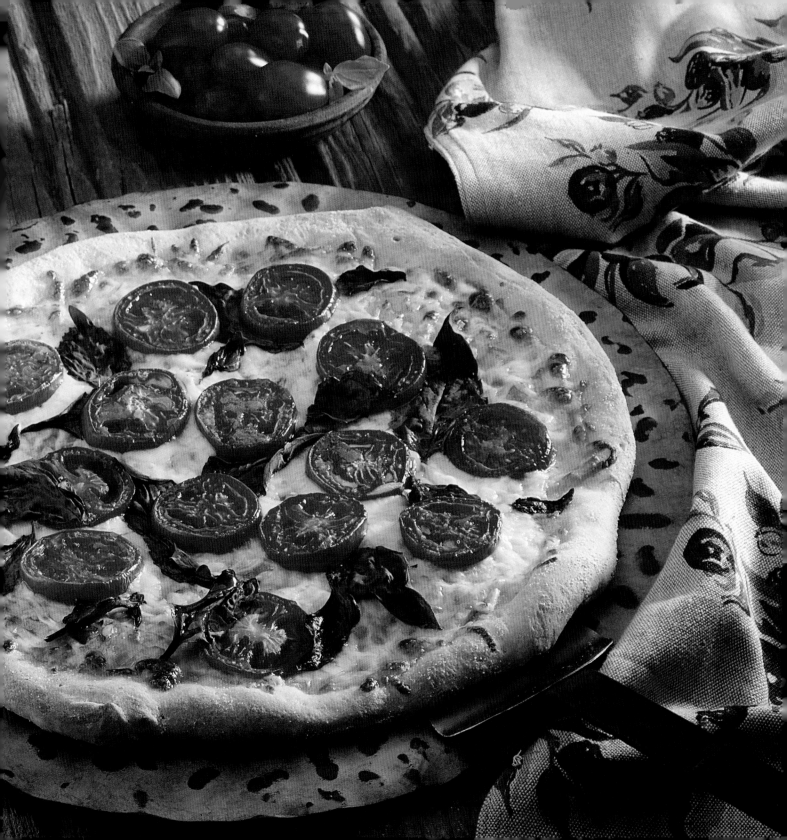

Calzone Italiano

Pizza dough for one 14-inch pizza

1 can (15 ounces) CONTADINA® Pizza Sauce, divided

3 ounces sliced pepperoni or ½ pound crumbled Italian sausage, cooked, drained

2 tablespoons chopped green bell pepper

1 cup (4 ounces) shredded mozzarella cheese

1 cup (8 ounces) ricotta cheese

1. Divide dough into 4 equal portions. Place on lightly floured, large, rimless cookie sheet. Press or roll out dough to 7-inch circles.

2. Spread 2 tablespoons pizza sauce onto half of each circle to within ½ inch of edge; top with ¼ each pepperoni, bell pepper and mozzarella cheese.

3. Spoon ¼ cup ricotta cheese onto remaining half of each circle; fold dough over. Press edges together tightly to seal. Cut slits into top of dough to allow steam to escape.

4. Bake in preheated 350°F oven for 20 to 25 minutes or until crusts are golden brown. Meanwhile, heat remaining pizza sauce; serve over calzones.

Makes 4 servings

Note: If desired, 1 large calzone may be made instead of 4 individual calzones. To prepare, shape dough into 1 (13-inch) circle. Spread ½ cup pizza sauce onto half of dough; proceed as above. Bake for 25 minutes.

Prep Time: 15 minutes
Cook Time: 25 minutes

Tuna and Pasta Frittata

1 tablespoon olive oil

2 cups cooked spaghetti

4 large eggs

¼ cup prepared pesto sauce

2 tablespoons milk

1 (3-ounce) pouch of STARKIST® Premium Albacore or Chunk Light Tuna

½ cup shredded mozzarella cheese

Preheat broiler. In medium ovenproof skillet, heat oil over medium-high heat; sauté spaghetti. In bowl, combine eggs, pesto sauce and milk; blend well. Add tuna; pour mixture over hot spaghetti. Cook over medium-low heat, stirring occasionally until eggs are almost completely set. Sprinkle cheese over cooked eggs; place under broiler until cheese is bubbly and golden. Serve hot or at room temperature.

Makes 2 to 4 servings

Prep Time: 8 minutes

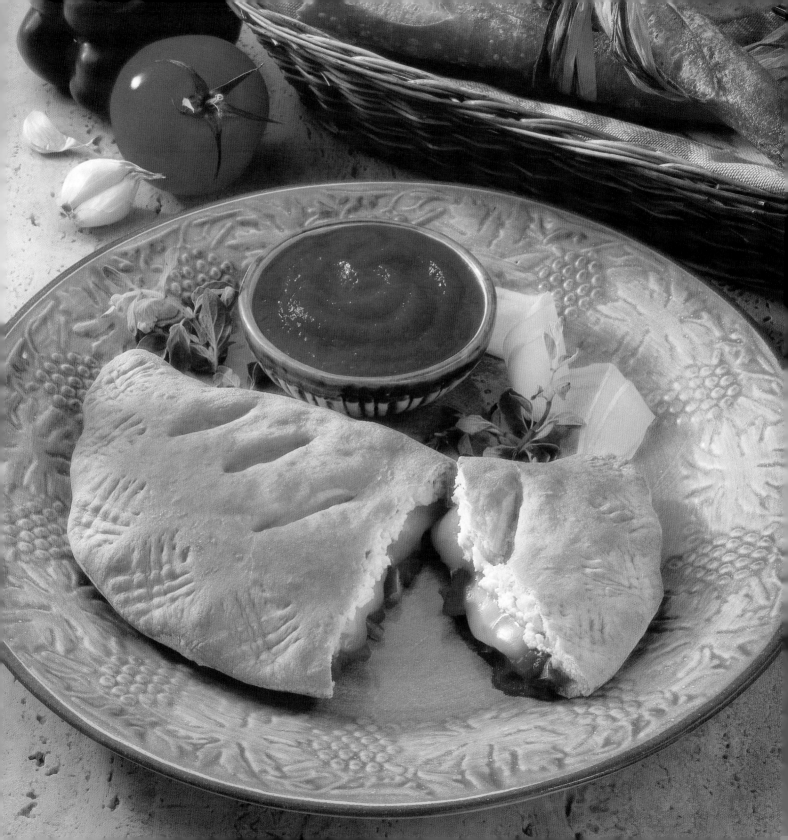

Open-Faced Italian Focaccia Sandwich

2 cups shredded cooked chicken

½ cup **HIDDEN VALLEY**® **The Original Ranch**® **Dressing**

¼ cup diagonally sliced green onions

1 piece focaccia bread, about ¾-inch thick, 10×7-inches

2 medium tomatoes, thinly sliced

4 cheese slices, such as provolone, Cheddar or Swiss

2 tablespoons grated Parmesan cheese (optional)

Stir together chicken, dressing and onions in a small mixing bowl. Arrange chicken mixture evenly on top of focaccia. Top with layer of tomatoes and cheese slices. Sprinkle with Parmesan cheese, if desired. Broil 2 minutes or until cheese is melted and bubbly. *Makes 4 servings*

Note: Purchase rotisserie chicken at your favorite store to add great taste and save preparation time.

Sausage, Peppers & Onion Pizza

½ pound bulk Italian sausage

1 medium red bell pepper, cut into strips

1 pre-baked pizza crust (14 inches)

1 cup spaghetti or pizza sauce

1½ cups shredded mozzarella cheese

1⅓ cups *French's*® **French Fried Onions**

1. Preheat oven to 450°F. Cook sausage in nonstick skillet over medium heat until browned, stirring frequently; drain. Add bell pepper and cook until crisp-tender, stirring occasionally.

2. Top pizza crust with sauce, sausage mixture and cheese. Bake 8 to 10 minutes or until cheese melts. Sprinkle with French Fried Onions; bake 2 minutes or until onions are golden. *Makes 8 servings*

Tip: You may substitute link sausage; remove meat from casing.

Prep Time: 10 minutes
Cook Time: 17 minutes

Open-Faced Italian Focaccia Sandwich

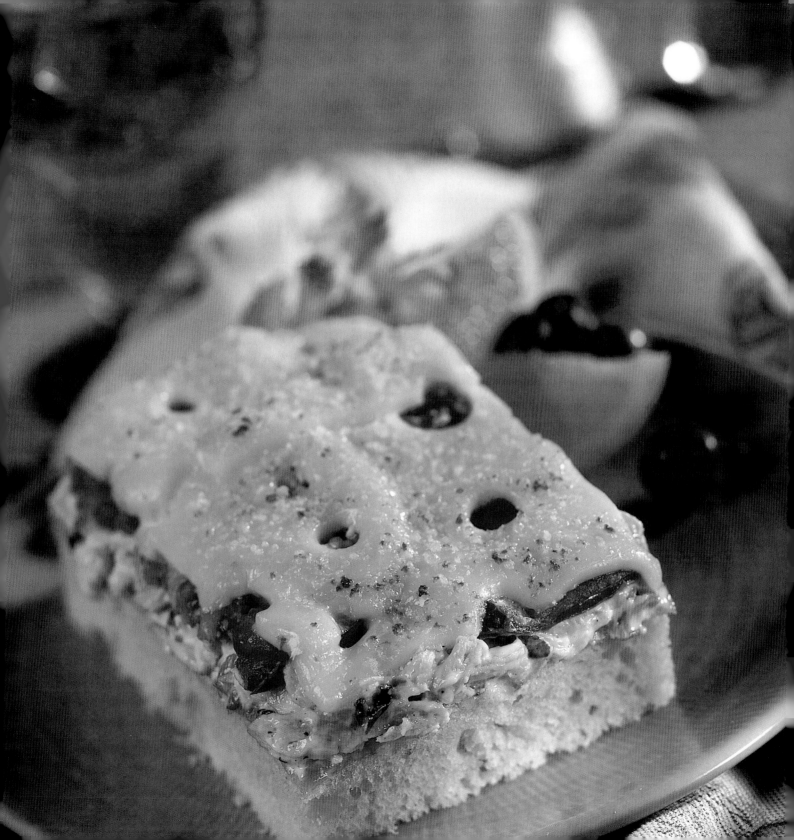

BelGioioso® Asiago and Sweet Pepper Sandwiches

2 tablespoons olive oil

1 red bell pepper, sliced into strips

1 yellow bell pepper, sliced into strips

1 medium onion, thinly sliced

1 teaspoon dried thyme

Hot pepper sauce

Salt and pepper to taste

4 ounces BELGIOIOSO® Asiago Cheese, thinly sliced

4 long sandwich buns, sliced open lengthwise

Heat olive oil in large skillet. Add red and yellow bell peppers and cook over medium heat about 6 minutes. Add onion and cook until vegetables are softened. Stir in thyme, hot pepper sauce, salt and pepper to taste.

Layer BelGioioso Asiago Cheese on bottom half of buns and top with vegetable mixture. Serve immediately. *Makes 4 servings*

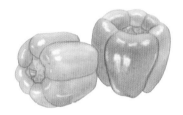

Herbed Mushroom Pizza

2 tablespoons olive oil

8 ounces sliced button or wild mushrooms, such as portobello or shiitake

1½ teaspoons minced garlic

½ teaspoon dried basil leaves

½ teaspoon dried thyme leaves

¼ teaspoon salt

¼ teaspoon black pepper

⅓ cup pizza or marinara sauce

1 bread-style pizza crust (12 inches)

1½ cups (6 ounces) shredded mozzarella cheese

1. Preheat oven to 450°F. Heat oil in large skillet over medium-high heat until hot. Add mushrooms and garlic; cook 4 minutes, stirring occasionally. Stir in basil, thyme, salt and pepper.

2. Spread pizza sauce evenly over crust. Top with mushroom mixture; sprinkle with cheese. Bake directly on oven rack 8 minutes or until crust is golden brown and cheese is melted. Slide cookie sheet under pizza to remove from oven. *Makes 4 servings*

Prep and Cook Time: 15 minutes

BelGioioso® Asiago and Sweet Pepper Sandwich

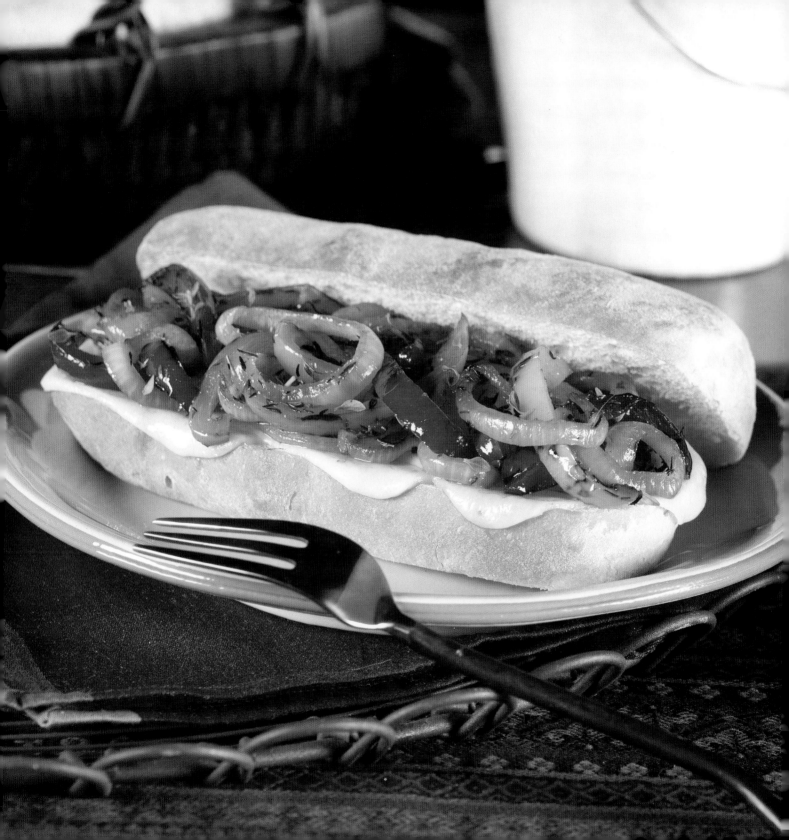

Zucchini Mushroom Frittata

1 ½ cups EGG BEATERS® Healthy
Real Egg Product

½ cup (2 ounces) shredded
reduced-fat Swiss cheese

¼ cup fat-free (skim) milk

½ teaspoon garlic powder

¼ teaspoon seasoned pepper

Nonstick cooking spray

1 medium zucchini, shredded
(1 cup)

1 medium tomato, chopped

1 (4-ounce) can sliced
mushrooms, drained

Tomato slices and fresh basil
leaves, for garnish

In medium bowl, combine Egg Beaters®, cheese, milk, garlic powder and seasoned pepper; set aside.

Spray 10-inch ovenproof nonstick skillet lightly with nonstick cooking spray. Over medium-high heat, sauté zucchini, tomato and mushrooms in skillet until tender. Pour egg mixture into skillet, stirring well. Cover; cook over low heat for 15 minutes or until cooked on bottom and almost set on top. Remove lid and place skillet under broiler for 2 to 3 minutes or until desired doneness. Slide onto serving platter; cut into wedges to serve. Garnish with tomato slices and basil.

Makes 6 servings

Prep Time: 20 minutes
Cook Time: 20 minutes

Quick and Easy Italian Sandwich

1 tablespoon olive or vegetable
oil

½ pound mild Italian sausage,
casing removed, sliced
½ inch thick

1 can (14.5 ounces)
CONTADINA® Recipe
Ready Diced Tomatoes
with Italian Herbs,
undrained

½ cup sliced green bell pepper

6 sandwich-size English
muffins, split, toasted

¼ cup (1 ounce) shredded
Parmesan cheese, divided

1. Heat oil in medium skillet. Add sausage; cook 3 to 4 minutes or until no longer pink in center, stirring occasionally. Drain.

2. Add undrained tomatoes and bell pepper; simmer, uncovered, 5 minutes, stirring occasionally.

3. Spread ½ cup meat mixture on each of 6 muffin halves; sprinkle with Parmesan cheese. Top with remaining muffin halves.

Makes 6 servings

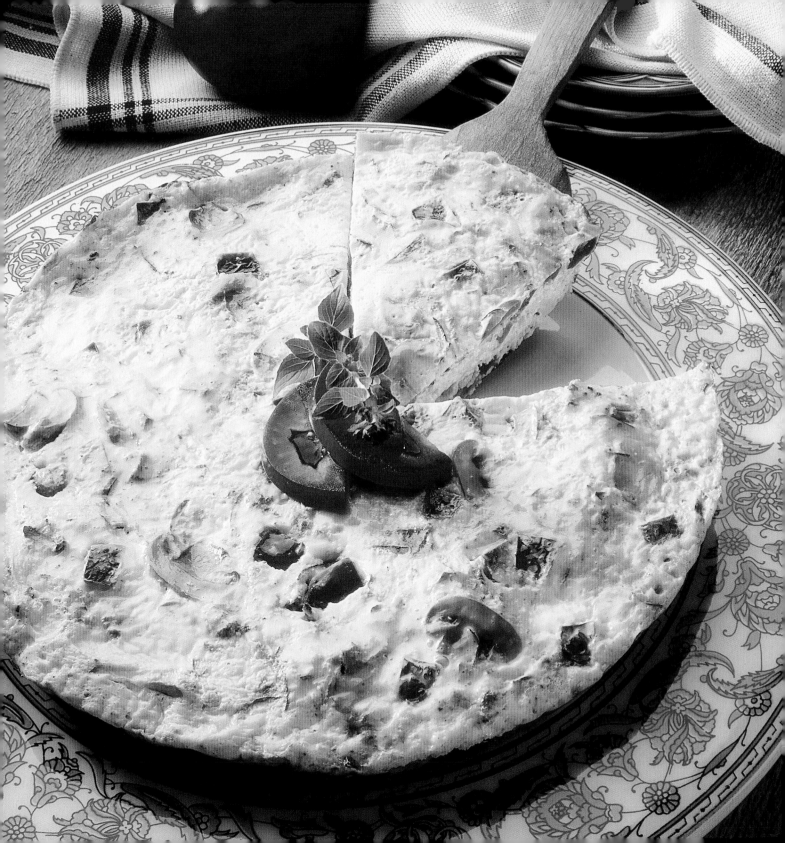

Chicken Parmesan Hero Sandwiches

4 boneless, skinless chicken breast halves (about 1¼ pounds)

1 egg, lightly beaten

¾ cup Italian seasoned dry bread crumbs

1 jar (1 pound 10 ounces) RAGÚ® Old World Style® Pasta Sauce

1 cup shredded mozzarella cheese (about 4 ounces)

4 long Italian rolls, halved lengthwise

1. Preheat oven to 400°F. Dip chicken in egg, then bread crumbs, coating well.

2. In 13×9-inch glass baking dish, arrange chicken. Bake uncovered 20 minutes.

3. Pour Ragú Pasta Sauce over chicken, then top with cheese. Bake an additional 10 minutes or until chicken is thoroughly cooked. To serve, arrange chicken and sauce on rolls. *Makes 4 servings*

Prep Time: 10 minutes
Cook Time: 30 minutes

Ranch Chicken Pizza

½ cup HIDDEN VALLEY® The Original Ranch® Dressing

1 package (3 ounces) cream cheese, softened

2 tablespoons tomato paste

1 cup chopped cooked chicken

1 (12-inch) prebaked pizza crust

½ cup roasted red pepper strips, rinsed and drained

1 can (2¼ ounces) sliced ripe olives, drained

¼ cup chopped green onions

1 cup (4 ounces) shredded mozzarella cheese

Preheat oven to 450°F. Beat dressing, cream cheese and tomato paste until smooth. Stir in chicken; spread mixture on pizza crust. Arrange red peppers, olives and onions on pizza; sprinkle with mozzarella cheese. Bake at 450°F. for 15 minutes or until hot and bubbly. *Makes 8 servings*

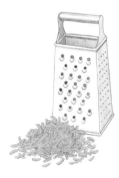

Chicken Parmesan Hero Sandwich

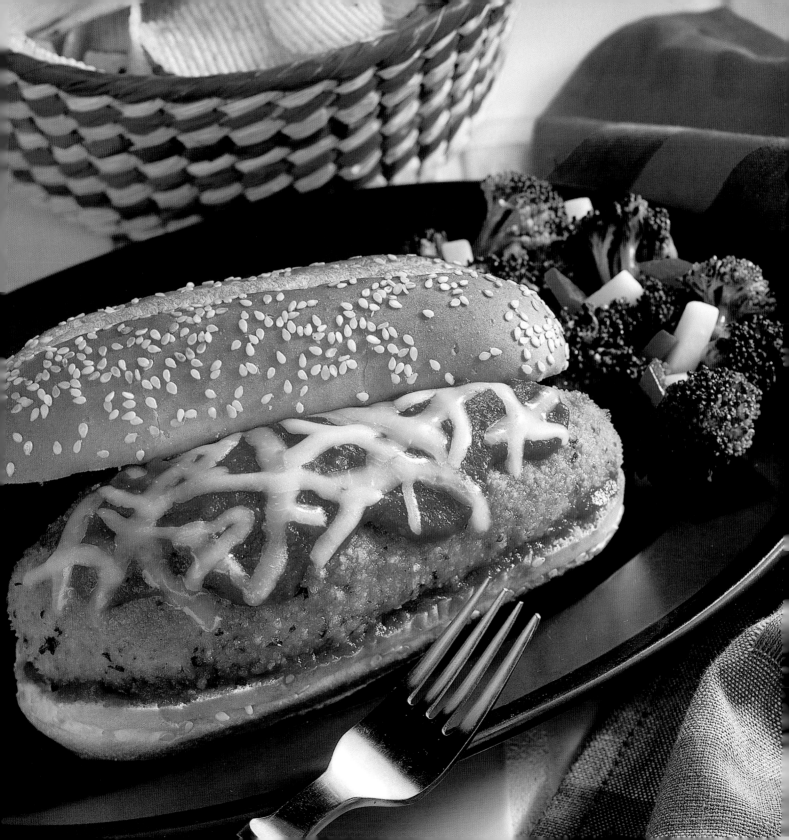

Stromboli

¼ cup French's® Bold n' Spicy Brown Mustard

2 tablespoons chopped fresh basil *or* 2 teaspoons dried basil leaves

1 tablespoon chopped green olives

1 pound frozen bread dough, thawed at room temperature

¼ pound sliced salami

¼ pound sliced provolone cheese

¼ pound sliced ham

⅛ pound thinly sliced pepperoni (2-inch diameter)

1 egg, beaten

1 teaspoon poppy or sesame seeds

1. Grease baking sheet. Stir mustard, basil and olives in small bowl; set aside.

2. Roll dough on floured surface to 16×10-inch rectangle.* Arrange salami on dough, overlapping slices, leaving 1-inch border around edges. Spread half of the mustard mixture thinly over salami. Arrange provolone and ham over salami. Spread with remaining mustard mixture. Top with pepperoni.

3. Fold one-third of dough toward center from long edge of rectangle. Fold second side toward center enclosing filling. Pinch long edge to seal. Pinch ends together and tuck under dough. Place on prepared baking sheet. Cover; let rise in warm place 15 minutes.

4. Preheat oven to 375°F. Cut shallow crosswise slits 3 inches apart on top of dough. Brush Stromboli lightly with beaten egg; sprinkle with poppy seeds. Bake 25 minutes or until browned. Remove to rack; cool slightly. Serve warm.

Makes 12 servings

If dough is too hard to roll, allow to rest on floured surface for 5 to 10 minutes.

Prep Time: 30 minutes
Cook Time: 25 minutes

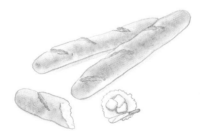

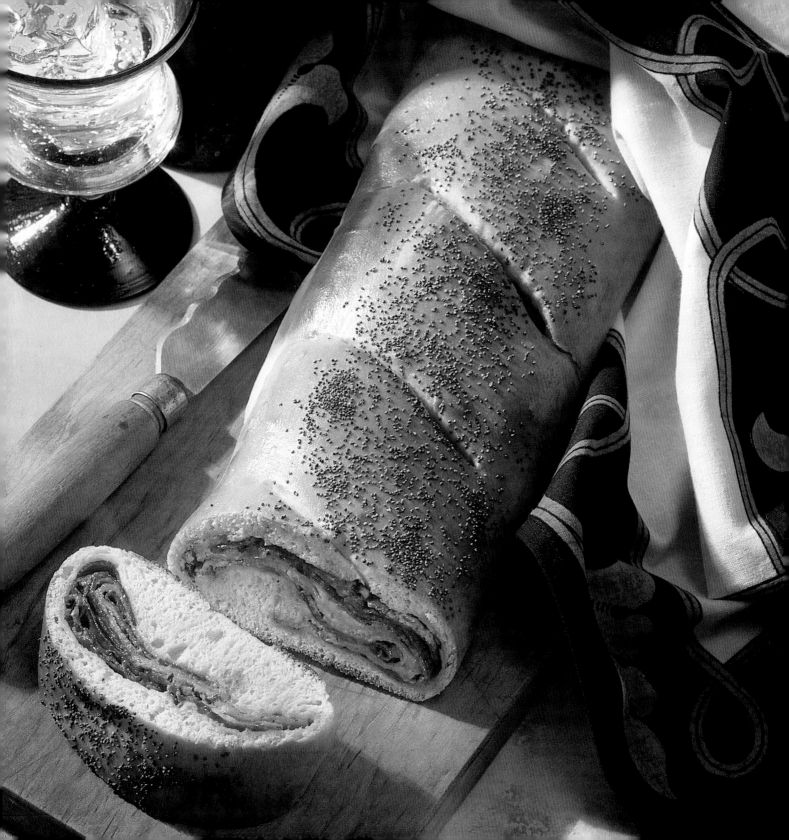

Vegetables & Sides

Italian Vegetables with Garlic Butter Rice

1 package UNCLE BEN'S
 NATURAL SELECT®
 Garlic & Butter Rice

1 yellow squash, sliced

1 zucchini, sliced

1 cup diced red bell pepper

1 cup sliced eggplant

⅓ cup balsamic vinaigrette

1 tablespoon chopped fresh
 rosemary

PREP: CLEAN: Wash hands. In large bowl, combine vegetables, vinaigrette and rosemary; set aside 15 minutes.

COOK: Meanwhile, prepare rice according to package directions; set aside. Sauté vegetables in marinade until crisp-tender.

SERVE: Serve vegetable mixture over rice.

CHILL: Refrigerate leftovers immediately.

Makes 4 servings

Prep Time: 5 minutes
Cook Time: 15 minutes

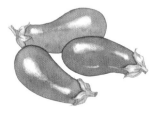

Italian Vegetables with Garlic Butter Rice

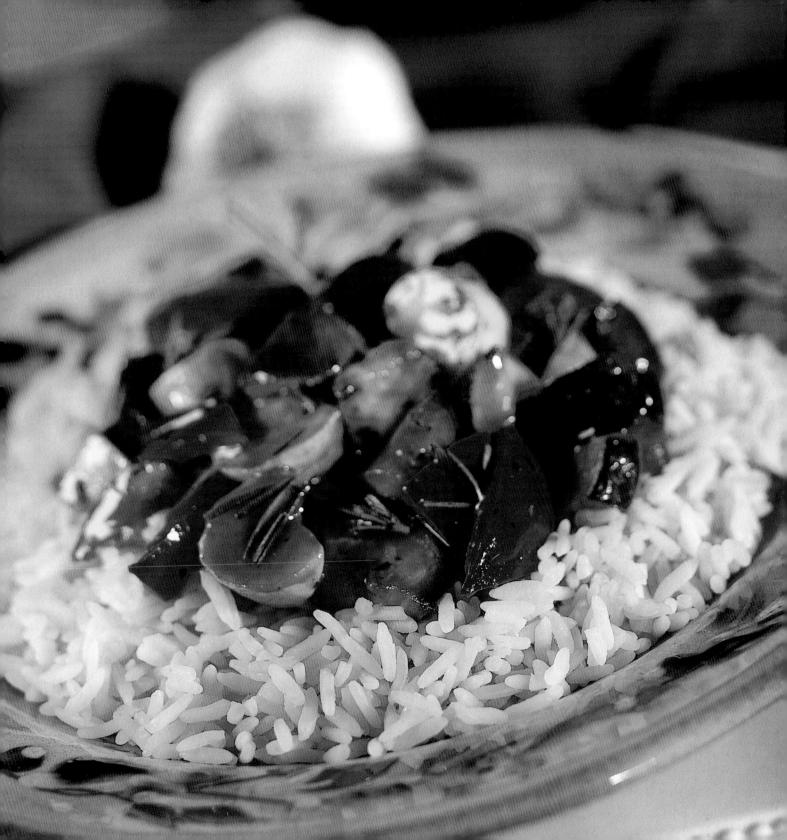

Baked Risotto with Asparagus, Spinach & Parmesan

1 tablespoon olive oil

1 cup finely chopped onion

1 cup arborio (risotto) rice

8 cups (8 to 10 ounces) spinach leaves, torn into pieces

2 cups chicken broth

¼ teaspoon salt

¼ teaspoon ground nutmeg

½ cup Parmesan cheese, divided

1½ cups diagonally sliced asparagus

1. Preheat oven to 400°F. Spray 13×9-inch baking dish with nonstick cooking spray.

2. Heat olive oil in large skillet over medium-high heat. Add onion; cook and stir 4 minutes or until tender. Add rice; stir to coat with oil.

3. Stir in spinach, a handful at a time, adding more as it wilts. Add broth, salt and nutmeg. Reduce heat and simmer 7 minutes. Stir in ¼ cup cheese.

4. Transfer to prepared baking dish. Cover tightly and bake 15 minutes.

5. Remove from oven and stir in asparagus; sprinkle with remaining ¼ cup cheese. Cover and bake 15 minutes more or until liquid is absorbed.

Makes 6 servings

Italian Broccoli with Tomatoes

4 cups broccoli florets

½ cup water

½ teaspoon dried Italian seasoning

½ teaspoon dried parsley flakes

¼ teaspoon salt (optional)

⅛ teaspoon black pepper

2 medium tomatoes, cut into wedges

½ cup shredded part-skim mozzarella cheese

MICROWAVE DIRECTIONS

Place broccoli and water in 2-quart microwavable casserole; cover. Microwave at HIGH (100% power) 5 to 8 minutes or until crisp-tender. Drain. Stir in Italian seasoning, parsley, salt, pepper and tomatoes. Microwave, uncovered, at HIGH (100% power) 2 to 4 minutes or until tomatoes are hot. Sprinkle with cheese. Microwave 1 minute or until cheese melts.

Makes 6 servings

Baked Risotto with Asparagus, Spinach & Parmesan

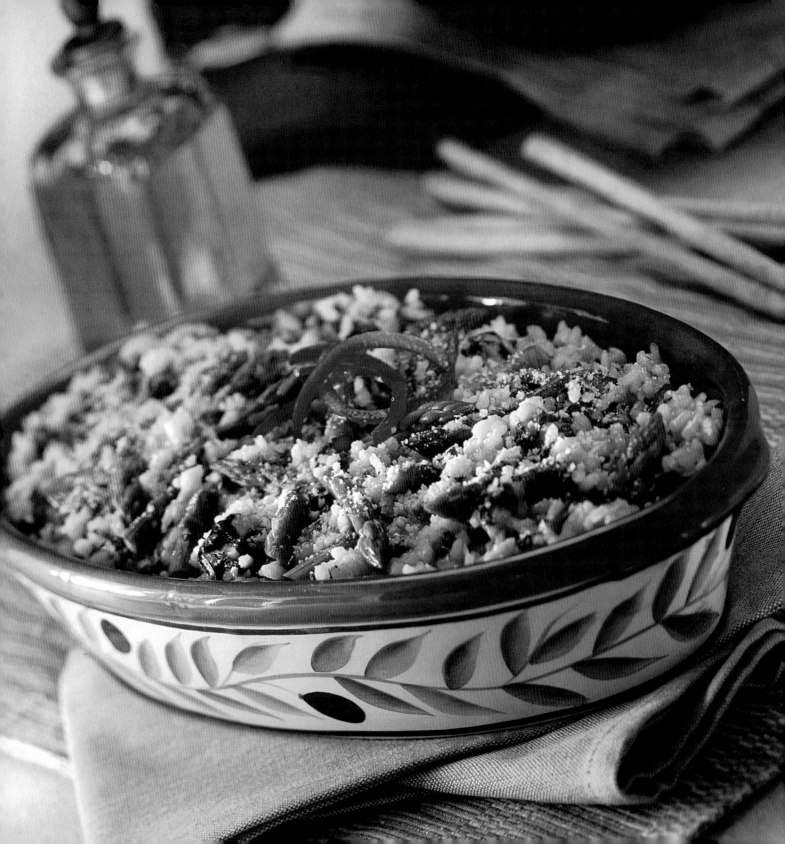

Creamy Spinach Italiano

1 cup ricotta cheese

¾ cup half-and-half or milk

2 packages (10 ounces each) frozen chopped spinach, thawed and squeezed dry

1⅓ cups *French's*® French Fried Onions, divided

½ cup chopped roasted red pepper

¼ cup chopped fresh basil

¼ cup grated Parmesan cheese

1 teaspoon garlic powder

¼ teaspoon salt

1. Preheat oven to 350°F. Whisk together ricotta cheese and half-and-half in large bowl until well combined. Stir in spinach, ⅔ *cup* French Fried Onions, red pepper, basil, Parmesan, garlic powder and salt. Pour mixture into greased deep-dish 9-inch pie plate.

2. Bake for 25 minutes or until heated through; stir. Sprinkle with remaining ⅔ *cup* onions. Bake for 5 minutes or until onions are golden.

Makes 4 servings

Prep Time: 10 minutes
Cook Time: 35 minutes

Peas Florentine Style

2 (10-ounce) packages frozen peas

¼ cup FILIPPO BERIO® Olive Oil

4 ounces Canadian bacon, cubed

1 clove garlic, minced

1 tablespoon chopped fresh Italian parsley

1 teaspoon sugar

Salt

Place peas in large colander or strainer; run under hot water until slightly thawed. Drain well. In medium skillet, heat olive oil over medium heat until hot. Add bacon and garlic; cook and stir 2 to 3 minutes or until garlic turns golden. Add peas and parsley; cook and stir over high heat 5 to 7 minutes or until heated through. Drain well. Stir in sugar; season to taste with salt.

Makes 5 servings

Creamy Spinach Italiano

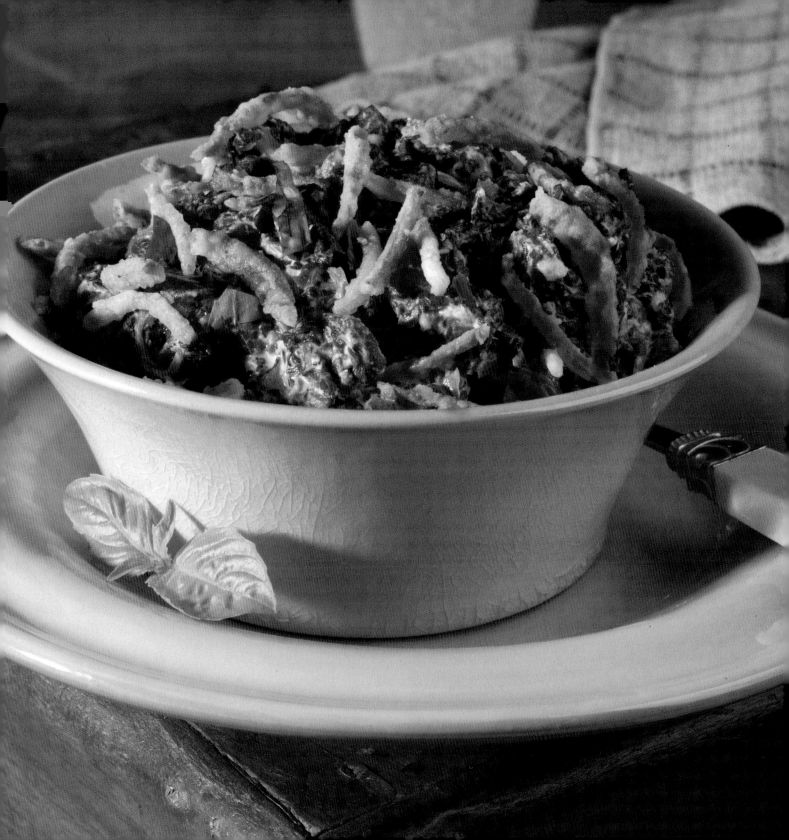

Garden-Style Risotto

1 can (14½ ounces) low-sodium
  chicken broth

1¾ cups water

2 garlic cloves, finely chopped

1 teaspoon dried basil leaves,
  crushed

½ teaspoon dried thyme leaves,
  crushed

1 cup arborio rice

2 cups packed DOLE®
  Fresh Spinach, torn

1 cup DOLE® Shredded Carrots

3 tablespoons grated
  Parmesan cheese

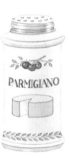

- Combine broth, water, garlic, basil and thyme in large saucepan. Bring to boil; meanwhile, prepare rice.

- Place rice in large, nonstick saucepan sprayed with vegetable cooking spray. Cook and stir rice over medium heat about 2 minutes or until rice is browned.

- Pour 1 cup boiling broth into saucepan with rice; cook, stirring constantly, until broth is almost absorbed (there should be some broth left).

- Add enough broth to barely cover rice; continue to cook, stirring constantly, until broth is almost absorbed. Repeat adding broth and cooking, stirring constantly, until broth is almost absorbed, about 15 minutes; add spinach and carrots with the last addition of broth.

- Cook 3 to 5 minutes more, stirring constantly, or until broth is almost absorbed and rice and vegetables are tender. Do not overcook. (Risotto will be saucey and have a creamy texture.) Stir in Parmesan cheese. Serve warm.

Makes 6 servings

Garden Pilaf: Substitute 1 cup uncooked long grain white rice for arborio rice and reduce water from 1¾ cups to ½ cup. Prepare broth as directed above with ½ cup water; meanwhile, brown rice as directed above. Carefully add browned rice into boiling broth. Reduce heat to low; cover and cook 15 minutes. Stir in vegetables; cover and cook 4 to 5 minutes longer or until rice and vegetables are tender. Stir in Parmesan cheese.

Prep Tme: 5 minutes
Cook Time: 25 minutes

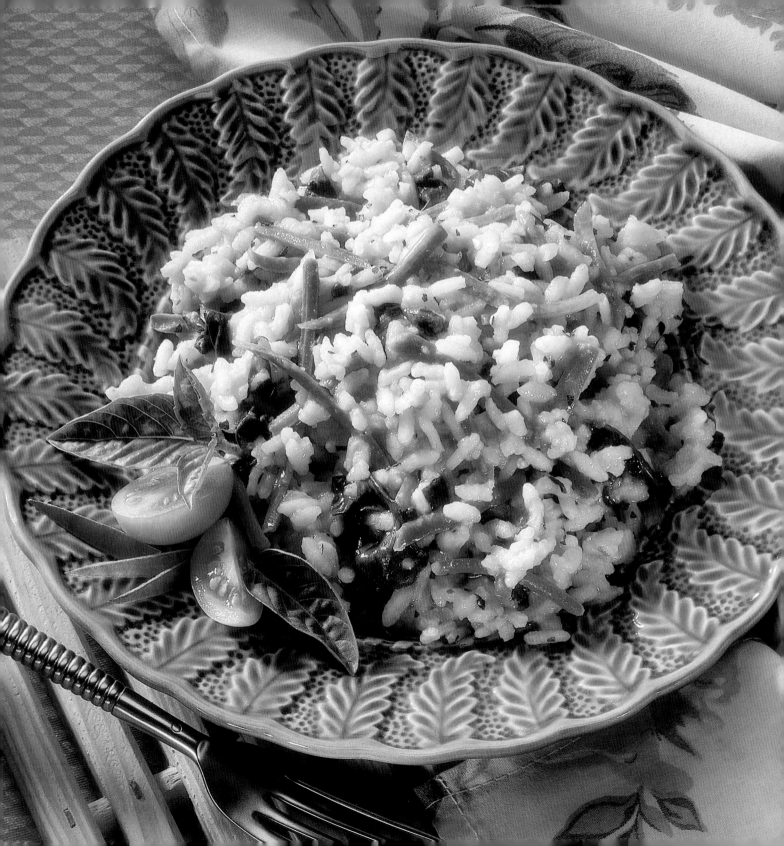

Zucchini Tomato Bake

1 pound eggplant, coarsely chopped

2 cups zucchini slices

2 cups mushrooms slices

3 sheets (18×12 inches) heavy-duty foil, lightly sprayed with nonstick cooking spray

2 teaspoons olive oil

½ cup chopped onion

½ cup chopped fresh fennel (optional)

2 cloves garlic, minced

1 can (14½ ounces) no-salt-added whole tomatoes, undrained

1 tablespoon tomato paste

2 teaspoons dried basil leaves

1 teaspoon sugar

1. Preheat oven to 400°F. Divide eggplant, zucchini and mushrooms into 3 portions. Arrange each portion on foil sheet.

2. Heat oil in small skillet over medium heat. Add onion, fennel, if desired, and garlic. Cook and stir 3 to 4 minutes or until onion is tender. Add tomatoes, tomato paste, basil and sugar. Cook and stir about 4 minutes or until sauce thickens.

3. Pour sauce over eggplant mixture. Double fold sides and end of foil to seal packets, leaving head space for heat circulation. Place on baking sheet.

4. Bake 30 minutes. Remove from oven. Carefully open one end of each packet to allow steam to escape. Open and transfer contents to serving dish.

Makes 6 servings

Green Beans with Pine Nuts

1 pound green beans, ends removed

2 tablespoons butter or margarine

2 tablespoons pine nuts

Salt

Pepper

Cook beans in 1 inch water in covered 3-quart pan 4 to 8 minutes or until crisp-tender; drain. Melt butter in large skillet over medium heat. Add pine nuts; cook, stirring frequently, until golden. Add beans; stir gently to coat beans with butter. Season with salt and pepper to taste. *Makes 4 servings*

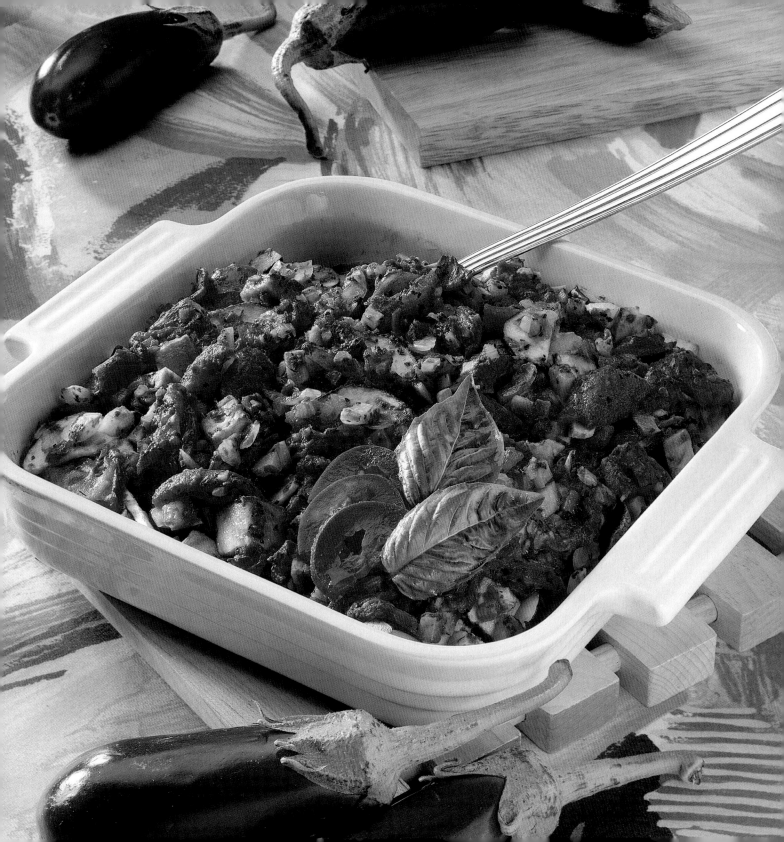

Risotto-Style Primavera

1 tablespoon FILIPPO BERIO®
   Olive Oil

1 small zucchini, sliced

1 medium onion, sliced

½ red bell pepper, seeded and
   cut into thin strips

3 mushrooms, sliced

½ cup uncooked long grain rice

¼ cup dry white wine

1 cup chicken broth

1¾ cups water, divided

2 tablespoons grated
   Parmesan cheese

Salt and freshly ground black
   pepper

In large saucepan or skillet, heat olive oil over medium heat until hot. Add zucchini, onion, bell pepper and mushrooms. Cook and stir 5 to 7 minutes or until zucchini is tender-crisp. Remove vegetables; set aside. Add rice and wine; stir until wine is absorbed. Add chicken broth. Cook, uncovered, stirring frequently, until absorbed. Add 1 cup water. Cook, uncovered, stirring frequently, until absorbed. Add remaining ¾ cup water. Cook, uncovered, stirring frequently, until absorbed. (Total cook time will be about 25 minutes until rice is tender and mixture is creamy.) Stir in vegetables and Parmesan cheese. Season to taste with salt and black pepper. *Makes 4 servings*

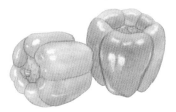

Herbed Green Beans

1 pound fresh green beans,
   ends removed

1 teaspoon extra-virgin olive oil

2 tablespoons chopped fresh
   basil *or* 2 teaspoons dried
   basil leaves

1. Steam green beans 5 minutes or until crisp-tender. Rinse under cold running water; drain and set aside.

2. Just before serving, heat oil over medium-low heat in large nonstick skillet. Add basil; cook and stir 1 minute, then add green beans. Cook until heated through. Garnish with additional fresh basil, if desired. Serve immediately.

Makes 6 servings

Tip: When buying green beans, look for vivid green, crisp beans without scars. Pods should be well shaped and slim with small seeds. Buy beans of uniform size to ensure even cooking and avoid bruised or large beans.

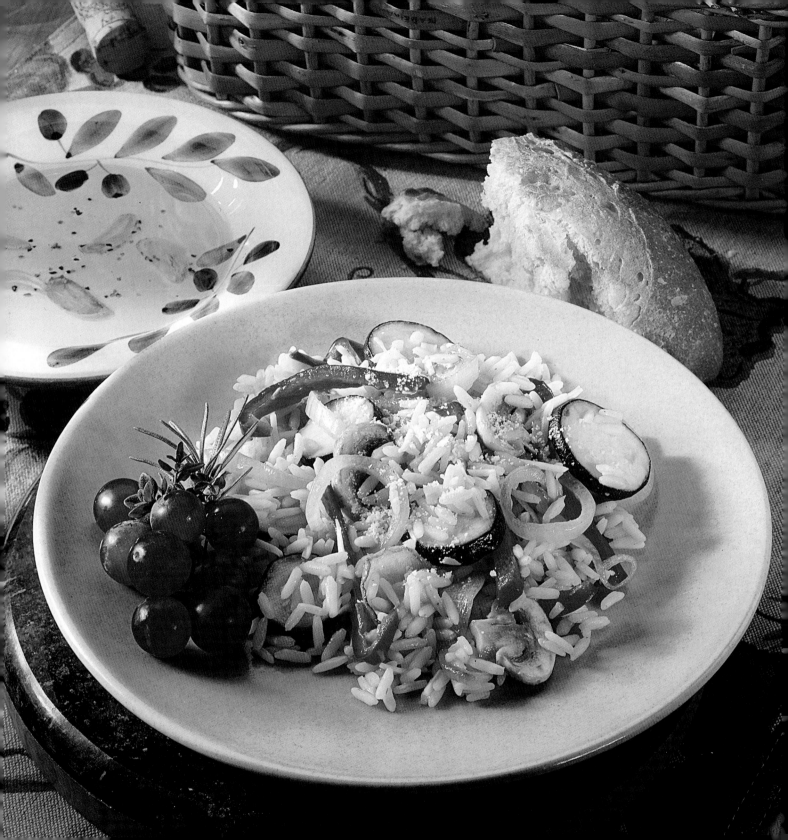

Cannellini Parmesan Casserole

2 tablespoons olive oil

1 cup chopped onion

2 teaspoons minced garlic

1 teaspoon dried oregano leaves

¼ teaspoon black pepper

2 cans (14½ ounces each) onion- and garlic-flavored diced tomatoes, undrained

1 jar (14 ounces) roasted red peppers, drained and cut into ½-inch squares

2 cans (19 ounces each) white cannellini beans or Great Northern beans, rinsed and drained

1 teaspoon dried basil leaves *or* 1 tablespoon chopped fresh basil

¾ cup (3 ounces) grated Parmesan cheese

1. Heat oil in Dutch oven over medium heat until hot. Add onion, garlic, oregano and pepper; cook and stir 5 minutes or until onion is tender.

2. Increase heat to high. Add tomatoes with juice and red peppers; cover and bring to a boil.

3. Reduce heat to medium. Stir in beans; cover and simmer 5 minutes, stirring occasionally. Stir in basil and sprinkle with cheese.

Makes 6 servings

Prep and Cook Time: 20 minutes

 Cannellini beans are cultivated large, white kidney beans used extensively in Italian cooking, particularly in soups and salads. They are available in both dry and canned forms. Great Northern beans are often substituted when cannellini beans prove difficult to find.

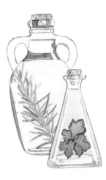

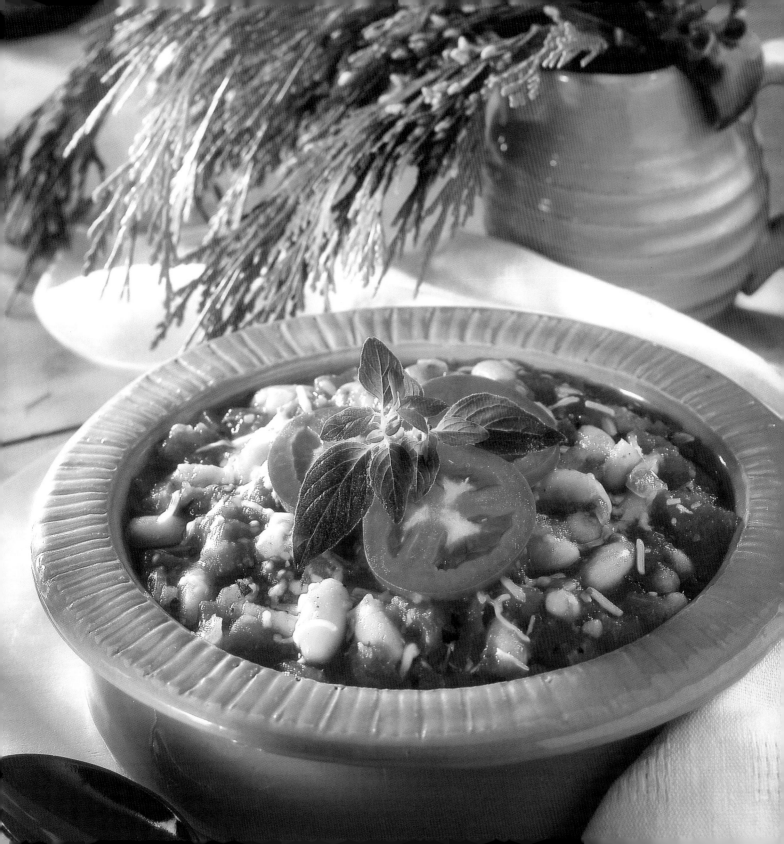

Lemon and Fennel Marinated Vegetables

1 cup water

2 medium carrots, diagonally sliced ½ inch thick

1 cup small whole fresh mushrooms

1 small red or green bell pepper, cut into ¾-inch pieces

3 tablespoons lemon juice

1 tablespoon sugar

1 tablespoon olive oil

1 clove garlic, minced

½ teaspoon fennel seeds, crushed

½ teaspoon dried basil leaves, crushed

¼ teaspoon black pepper

Bring water to a boil over high heat in small saucepan. Add carrots. Return to a boil. Reduce heat to medium-low. Cover and simmer about 5 minutes or until carrots are crisp-tender. Drain and cool.

Place carrots, mushrooms and bell pepper in large resealable plastic food storage bag. Combine lemon juice, sugar, oil, garlic, fennel seeds, basil and black pepper in small bowl. Pour over vegetables. Close bag securely; turn to coat. Marinate in refrigerator 8 to 24 hours, turning occasionally.

Drain vegetables; discard marinade. Place vegetables in serving dish.

Makes 4 servings

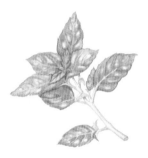

Golden Mushroom Risotto

1 boil-in-bag rice package

3 cups (8 ounces) sliced mushrooms

1 can (10¾ ounces) condensed golden mushroom soup

½ cup grated Parmesan cheese

1⅓ cups *French's®* French Fried Onions, divided

2 tablespoons chopped parsley

1. Cook rice according to package directions; drain and set aside.

2. Heat 1 *tablespoon oil* in medium saucepan over medium-high heat until hot. Sauté mushrooms until golden brown. Stir in hot rice, soup, ¾ *cup water*, cheese and ⅔ *cup* French Fried Onions. Cook until heated through; stirring often.

3. Sprinkle with remaining ⅔ *cup* onions and parsley before serving.

Makes 6 servings

Prep Time: 10 minutes
Cook Time: 20 minutes

Lemon and Fennel Marinated Vegetables

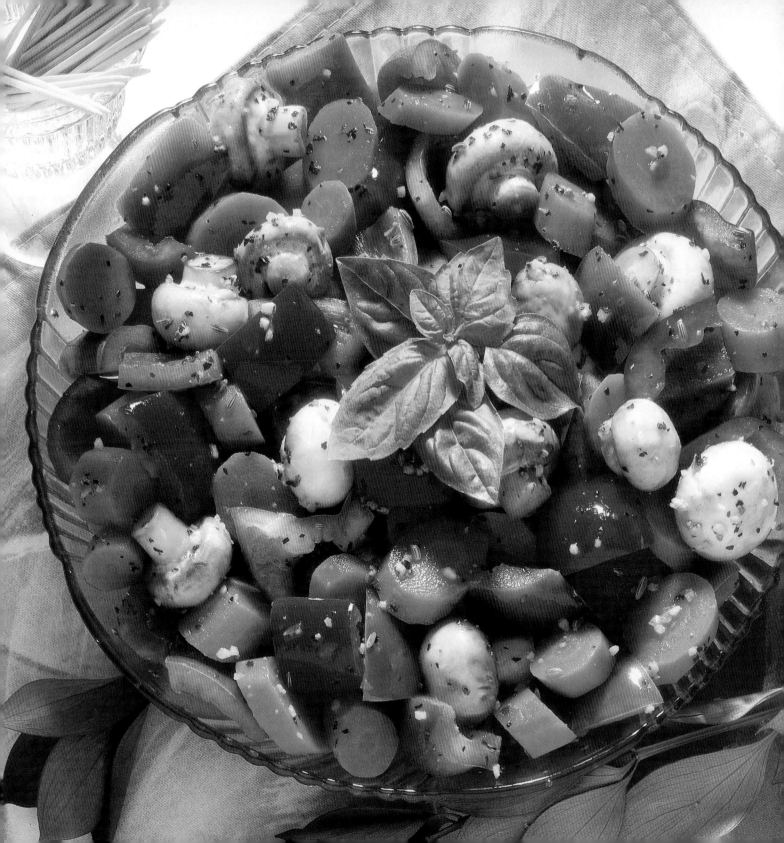

Sausage & Red Pepper Risotto

4½ cups chicken broth

8 ounces sweet Italian sausage links, removed from casing

1 tablespoon BERTOLLI® Olive Oil

1 large onion, chopped

1 medium red bell pepper, chopped

1 clove garlic, finely chopped

1½ cups arborio or regular rice

⅓ cup dry white wine or chicken broth

⅛ teaspoon dried oregano leaves, crushed

1 cup RAGÚ® Light Pasta Sauce

¼ cup grated Parmesan cheese

⅛ teaspoon ground black pepper

In 2-quart saucepan, heat chicken broth; set aside.

In heavy-duty 3-quart saucepan, brown sausage over medium-high heat 4 minutes or until sausage is no longer pink; remove sausage. In same 3-quart saucepan, add oil and cook onion over medium heat, stirring occasionally, 3 minutes. Stir in bell pepper and garlic and cook 1 minute. Add rice and cook, stirring occasionally, 1 minute. Slowly add 1 cup broth, wine and oregano and cook, stirring constantly, until liquid is absorbed. Continue adding 2 cups broth, 1 cup at a time, stirring frequently, until liquid is absorbed.

Meanwhile, stir Ragú Light Pasta Sauce into remaining 1½ cups broth; heat through. Continue adding broth mixture, 1 cup at a time, stirring frequently, until rice is slightly creamy and just tender. Return sausage to saucepan and stir in cheese and black pepper. Serve immediately.

Makes 4 main-dish or 8 side-dish servings

BelGioioso® Parmesan Polenta

Nonstick vegetable oil spray

4 cups canned vegetable broth

1½ cups yellow cornmeal

¾ cup grated BELGIOIOSO® Parmesan Cheese (about 2 ounces)

Preheat oven to 375°F. Spray 8×8×2-inch glass baking dish with vegetable oil spray. Bring vegetable broth to a boil in medium heavy saucepan over medium heat. Gradually whisk in cornmeal. Continue to whisk until mixture is very thick, about 3 minutes. Mix in BelGioioso Parmesan Cheese and pour mixture into prepared dish. Bake polenta until top begins to brown, about 30 minutes. Serve hot.

Makes 4 to 6 servings

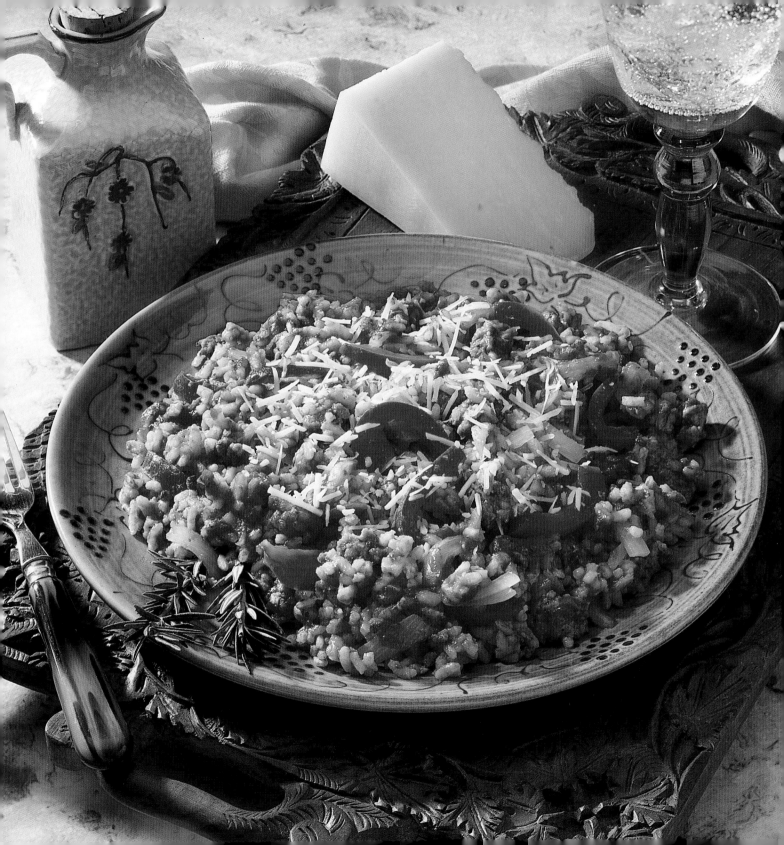

Oven-Roasted Peppers and Onions

Olive oil cooking spray

2 medium green bell peppers

2 medium red bell peppers

2 medium yellow bell peppers

4 small onions

1 teaspoon Italian herb seasoning

½ teaspoon dried basil leaves

¼ teaspoon ground cumin

1. Preheat oven to 375°F. Spray 15×10-inch jelly-roll pan with cooking spray. Cut bell peppers into 1½-inch pieces. Cut onions into quarters. Place vegetables on prepared pan. Spray vegetables with cooking spray. Bake 20 minutes; stir. Sprinkle with Italian seasoning, basil and cumin.

2. *Increase oven temperature to 425°F. Bake 20 minutes or until edges are darkened and vegetables are crisp-tender.* *Makes 6 servings*

Baked Spinach Risotto

1 tablespoon olive oil

1 green bell pepper, chopped

1 medium onion, chopped

2 cloves garlic, minced

1 cup arborio rice

3 cups chopped fresh spinach leaves

1 (14½-ounce) can chicken broth

½ cup grated Parmesan cheese, divided

1 tablespoon TABASCO® brand Green Pepper Sauce

1 teaspoon salt

Preheat oven to 400°F. Grease 1½-quart casserole. Heat oil in 10-inch skillet over medium heat. Add green bell pepper, onion and garlic; cook 5 minutes. Add rice; stir to coat well. Stir in spinach, chicken broth, ¼ cup Parmesan cheese, TABASCO® Green Pepper Sauce and salt. Spoon mixture into prepared baking dish. Sprinkle with remaining ¼ cup Parmesan cheese. Bake 35 to 40 minutes or until rice is tender. *Makes 4 servings*

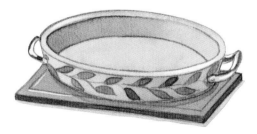

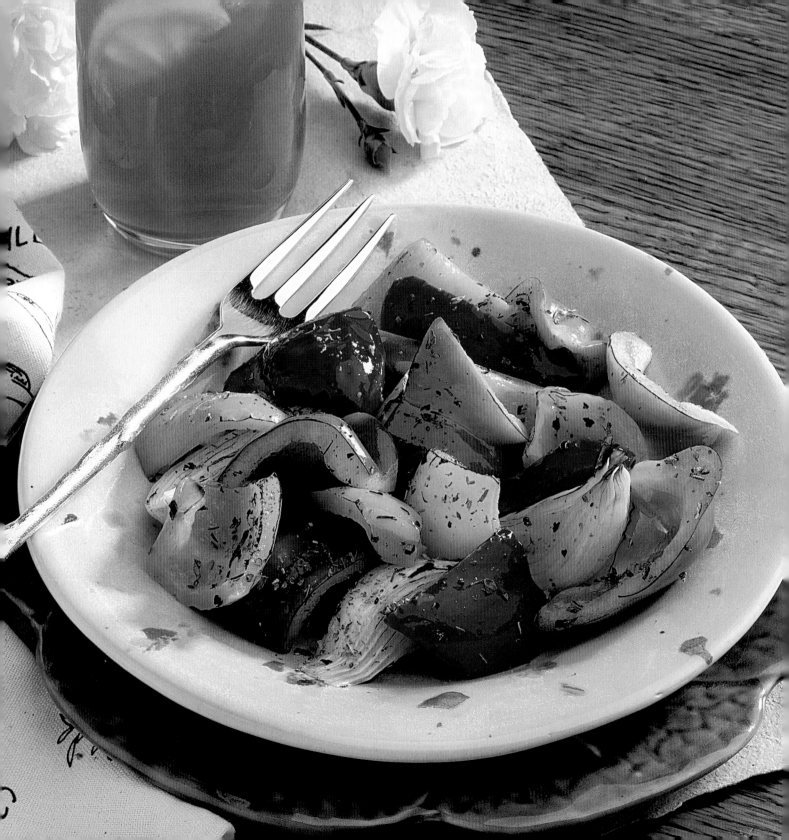

Fennel with Parmesan Bread Crumbs

2 large fennel bulbs

½ cup dry bread crumbs

¼ cup lemon juice

1 tablespoon freshly grated Parmesan cheese

1 tablespoon capers

2 teaspoons olive oil

⅛ teaspoon black pepper

½ cup reduced-sodium chicken broth

1. Preheat oven to 375°F. Spray 9-inch square baking dish with nonstick cooking spray; set aside.

2. Remove outer leaves and wide base from fennel bulbs. Slice bulbs crosswise.

3. Combine fennel and ¼ cup water in medium nonstick skillet with tight-fitting lid. Bring to a boil over high heat; reduce heat to medium. Cover and steam 4 minutes or until fennel is crisp-tender. Cool slightly; arrange in prepared baking pan.

4. Combine bread crumbs, lemon juice, Parmesan, capers, oil and black pepper in small bowl. Sprinkle bread crumb mixture over fennel; pour broth over top.

5. Bake, uncovered, 20 to 25 minutes or until golden brown. Garnish with minced fennel leaves and red bell pepper strips, if desired.

Makes 4 servings

Vegetables Italiano

2 tablespoons olive oil

1 cup sliced peeled carrots

¾ cup halved onion slices

2 cloves garlic, minced

1 can (14.5 ounces) CONTADINA® Stewed Tomatoes, undrained

3 cups sliced zucchini

1 cup fresh mushrooms, halved

¼ teaspoon salt, or to taste

⅛ teaspoon ground black pepper

1. Heat oil in large skillet. Add carrots, onion and garlic; sauté for 3 minutes.

2. Stir in undrained tomatoes, zucchini, mushrooms, salt and pepper.

3. Bring to a boil. Reduce heat to low; simmer, uncovered, for 5 to 6 minutes or until vegetables are crisp-tender. Serve over pasta, if desired.

Makes 4 side-dish servings

Prep Time: 8 minutes
Cook Time: 10 minutes

Fennel with Parmesan Bread Crumbs

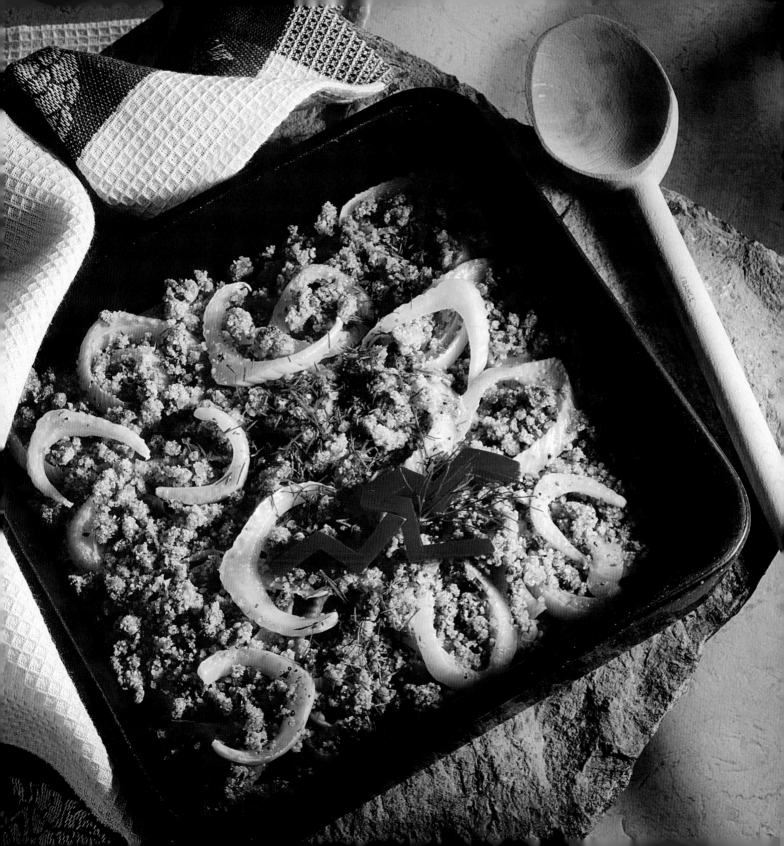

Polenta with Fresh Tomato-Bean Salsa

½ (16-ounce) package
    prepared polenta

Nonstick cooking spray

1⅓ cups chopped plum tomatoes

⅔ cup canned black beans or
    red kidney beans, rinsed
    and drained

2 tablespoons chopped fresh
    basil leaves

¼ teaspoon black pepper

2 tablespoons grated
    Parmesan cheese

1. Preheat oven to 450°F. Cut polenta into ¼-inch-thick slices. Lightly spray shallow baking pan with cooking spray. Place polenta slices in a single layer in baking pan. Lightly spray top of polenta with cooking spray. Bake 15 to 20 minutes or until edges are slightly brown.

2. Meanwhile, stir together tomatoes, beans, basil and pepper. Let stand at room temperature 15 minutes to blend flavors.

3. Arrange polenta on serving plates. Spoon tomato mixture on top. Sprinkle with cheese. *Makes 2 servings*

Tip: Salsa may be cooked, if desired. Cook and stir tomatoes and beans in large skillet over medium heat until hot. Stir in basil and pepper. Serve as directed.

Tomato Risotto Pronto

1 can (14½ ounces)
    DEL MONTE® Diced
    Tomatoes with Basil, Garlic
    & Oregano

2 large mushrooms, sliced

1 tablespoon olive oil

1 cup uncooked long grain
    white rice

1 clove garlic, minced

⅛ to ¼ teaspoon pepper

1¼ cups chicken broth

¼ cup grated Parmesan cheese

1. Drain tomatoes reserving liquid; pour liquid into measuring cup. Add water to measure 1⅔ cups.

2. Brown mushrooms in oil in large saucepan. Add rice, garlic and pepper; cook 2 minutes. Add reserved liquid and tomatoes; bring to boil.

3. Cover and cook over low heat 18 minutes. Remove cover; increase heat to medium.

4. Gradually stir in ½ cup broth. When liquid is gone, gradually add another ½ cup broth, adding remaining ¼ cup broth when liquid is gone. Add cheese. Rice should be tender-firm but creamy. Serve immediately.
Makes 4 to 6 servings

Prep Time: 8 minutes
Cook Time: 32 minutes

Polenta with Fresh Tomato-Bean Salsa

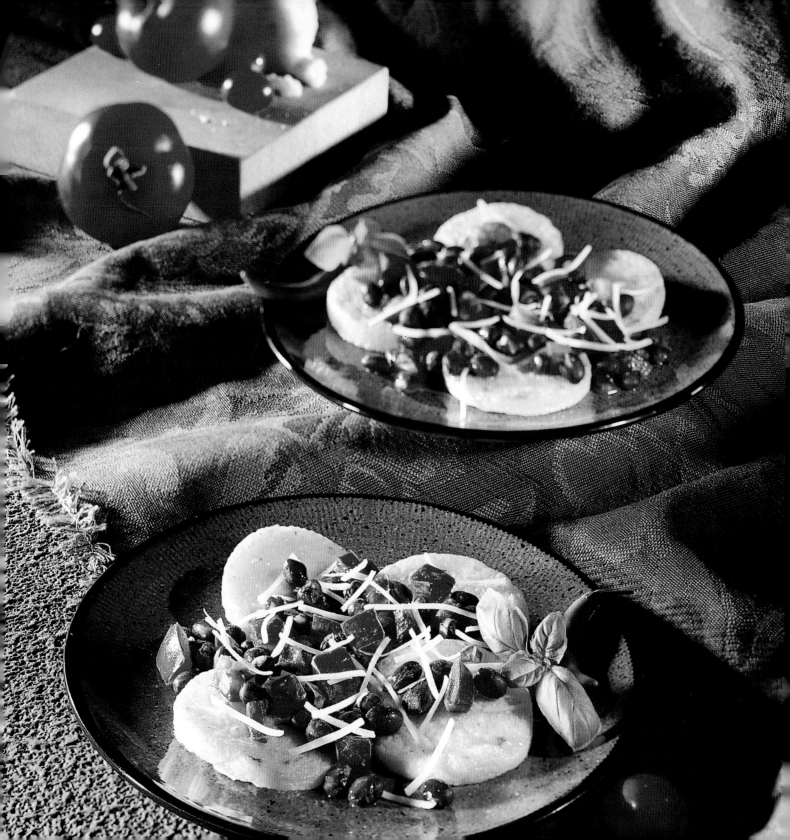

Seafood Risotto

1 package (5.2 ounces) rice in
   creamy sauce (Risotto
   Milanese flavor)

1 package (14 to 16 ounces)
   frozen fully cooked shrimp

1 box (10 ounces) BIRDS EYE®
   frozen Mixed Vegetables

2 teaspoons grated Parmesan
   cheese

- In 4-quart saucepan, prepare rice according to package directions. Add frozen shrimp and vegetables during last 10 minutes of cooking.

- Sprinkle with cheese.

Makes 4 servings

Serving Suggestion: Serve with garlic bread and a tossed green salad.

Prep Time: 5 minutes
Cook Time: 15 minutes

Parmesano Zucchini

2 tablespoons olive oil

2 medium zucchini, cut into
   julienne strips

1 small red onion, thinly sliced

6 ounces sliced fresh
   mushrooms (about 2 cups)

¼ cup chopped fresh basil
   leaves

½ teaspoon LAWRY'S® Garlic
   Powder with Parsley

½ teaspoon LAWRY'S®
   Seasoned Salt

⅓ cup freshly grated Parmesan
   cheese

In medium skillet, heat oil. Add all remaining ingredients except cheese and cook over medium-high heat 3 minutes or until zucchini is tender. Sprinkle with Parmesan cheese just before serving.

Makes 4 servings

tip   *Choose zucchini that are heavy for their size, firm and well shaped. They should have a bright color and be free of cuts and any soft spots. Before using, rinse zucchini under cold running water, scrubbing lightly with a vegetable brush, and trim off both ends.*

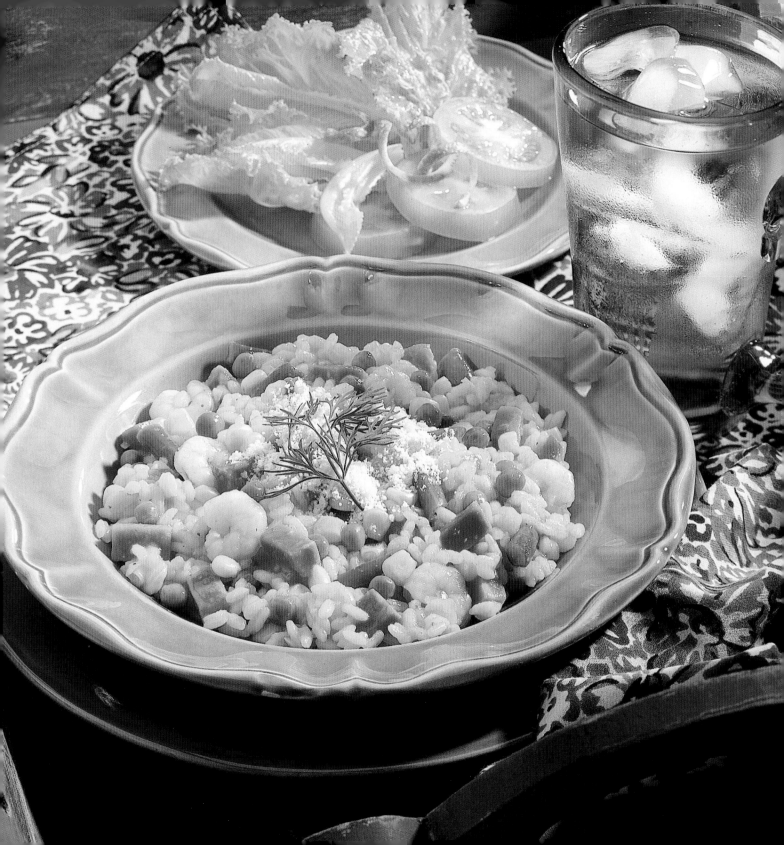

Easy Polenta Marinara

1 can (about 14 ounces) reduced-sodium chicken broth

1 cup yellow cornmeal

3 tablespoons grated Parmesan cheese

1½ cups prepared marinara sauce

½ cup (2 ounces) shredded mozzarella cheese

Fresh basil leaves for garnish (optional)

1. Preheat oven to 375°F. Grease 9-inch square baking dish; set aside.

2. Combine broth and 1 cup water in medium saucepan. Whisk cornmeal into liquid. Bring to a boil over medium-high heat, stirring to prevent lumps.

3. Reduce heat to medium-low; cook about 7 minutes or until mixture is very thick, stirring constantly. Stir in Parmesan cheese; season with salt and pepper to taste.

4. Pour hot polenta into prepared dish, spreading evenly with spatula. Pour marinara sauce over polenta; sprinkle with mozzarella cheese. Bake 10 minutes or until cheese is melted and sauce is heated through.

Makes 6 servings

Creamy Italian-Style Rice

1 tablespoon margarine or butter

1 small onion, finely chopped

1 teaspoon dried Italian seasoning

3⅓ cups water

1½ cups uncooked regular or converted rice

1 package (10 ounces) frozen mixed vegetables, thawed

1 jar (1 pound) RAGÚ® Cheese Creations!® Four Cheese Sauce

1. In 2½-quart saucepan, melt margarine over medium-high heat and cook onion with Italian seasoning, stirring occasionally, 2 minutes or until onion is tender. Stir in water and bring to a boil over high heat. Stir in rice. Reduce heat to low and simmer covered 15 minutes.

2. Stir in mixed vegetables and Ragú Cheese Creations! Sauce and cook 5 minutes. Remove from heat and let stand covered, stirring occasionally, 5 minutes or until liquid is absorbed.

3. Season, if desired, with salt and ground black pepper and garnish with grated Parmesan cheese.

Makes 6 servings

Prep Time: 10 minutes
Cook Time: 30 minutes

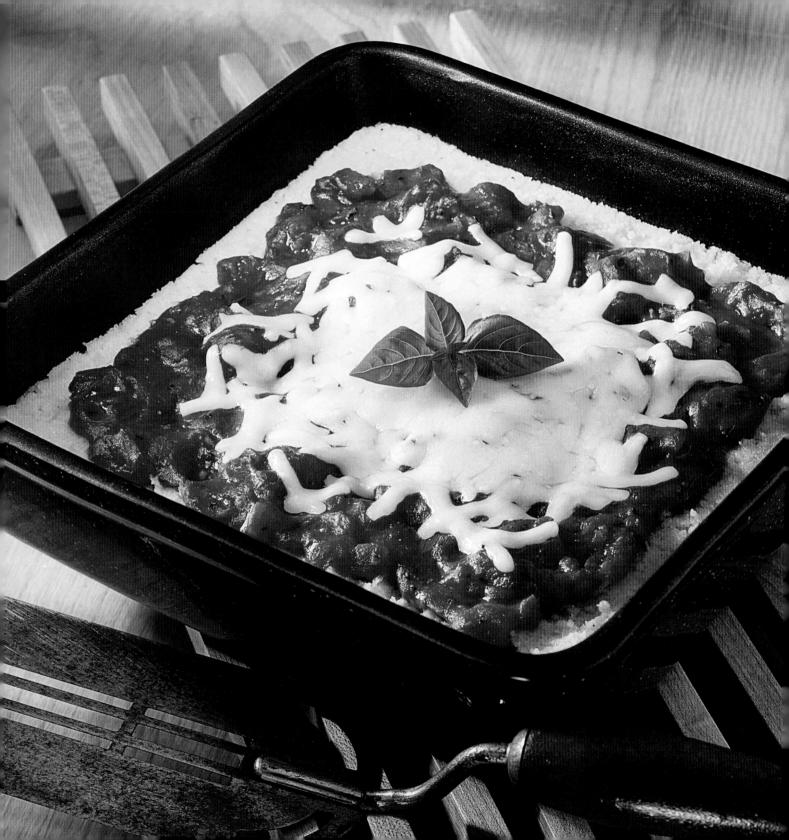

Peasant Risotto

1 teaspoon olive oil

3 ounces chopped low-fat turkey-ham

2 cloves garlic, minced

1 cup arborio or white short-grain rice

1 can (15 ounces) Great Northern beans, rinsed and drained

¼ cup chopped green onions with tops

½ teaspoon dried sage leaves

2 cans (14 ounces each) reduced-sodium chicken broth, heated

1½ cups Swiss chard, rinsed, stems removed and shredded

¼ cup freshly grated Parmesan cheese

1. Heat oil in large saucepan over medium heat. Add turkey-ham and garlic. Cook and stir until garlic is browned. Add rice, beans, green onions and sage; mix well. Add warm broth; bring to a boil. Reduce heat to low. Cook about 25 minutes or until rice is creamy, stirring frequently.

2. Add Swiss chard and Parmesan; mix well. Cover; remove from heat. Let stand, covered, 2 minutes or until Swiss chard is wilted. Serve immediately.

Makes 4 servings

 tip Swiss chard is a member of the beet family. It has large, crinkly green leaves and silvery stalks. It should be stored in a plastic bag in the refrigerator for up to three days.

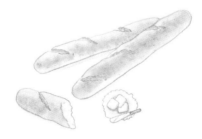

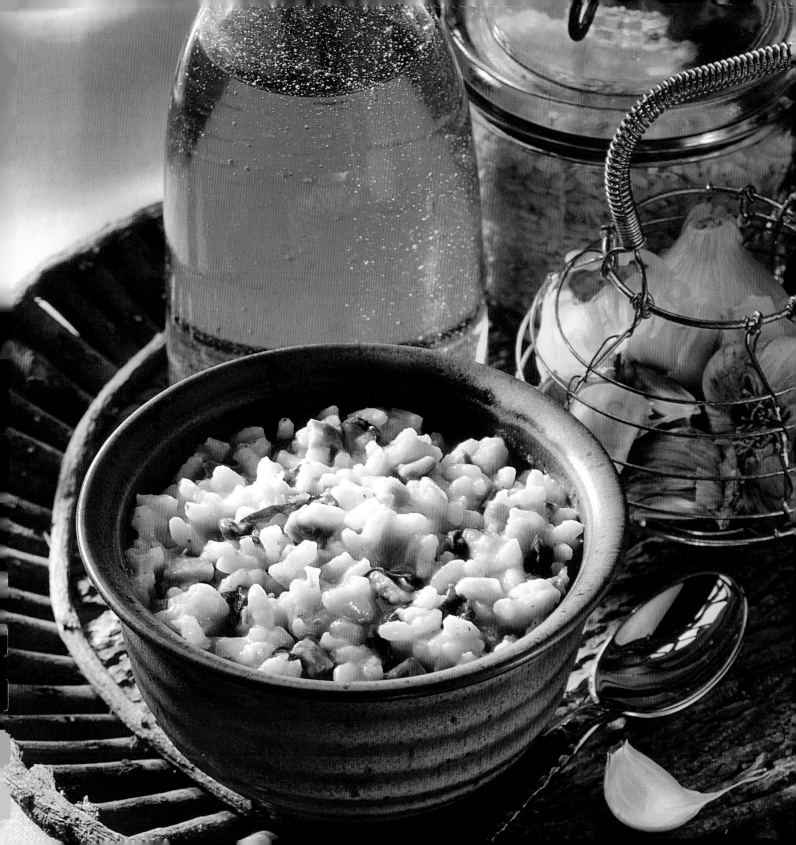

Desserts

Polenta Apricot Pudding Cake

¼ **cup chopped dried
  apricots**

2 **cups orange juice**

1 **cup part-skim ricotta
  cheese**

3 **tablespoons honey**

¾ **cup sugar**

½ **cup cornmeal**

½ **cup all-purpose flour**

¼ **teaspoon grated nutmeg**

¼ **cup slivered almonds**

  Powdered sugar (optional)

1. Preheat oven to 300°F. Soak apricots in ¼ cup water in small bowl 15 minutes. Drain and discard water. Pat apricots dry with paper towels.

2. Combine orange juice, ricotta cheese and honey in medium bowl. Mix on medium speed of electric mixer 5 minutes or until smooth. Combine sugar, cornmeal, flour and nutmeg in small bowl. Gradually add sugar mixture to orange juice mixture; blend well. Slowly stir in apricots.

3. Spray 10-inch nonstick springform pan with nonstick cooking spray. Pour batter into prepared pan. Sprinkle with almonds. Bake 60 to 70 minutes or until center is firm and cake is golden brown. Garnish with powdered sugar, if desired. Serve warm. *Makes 8 servings*

Polenta Apricot Pudding Cake

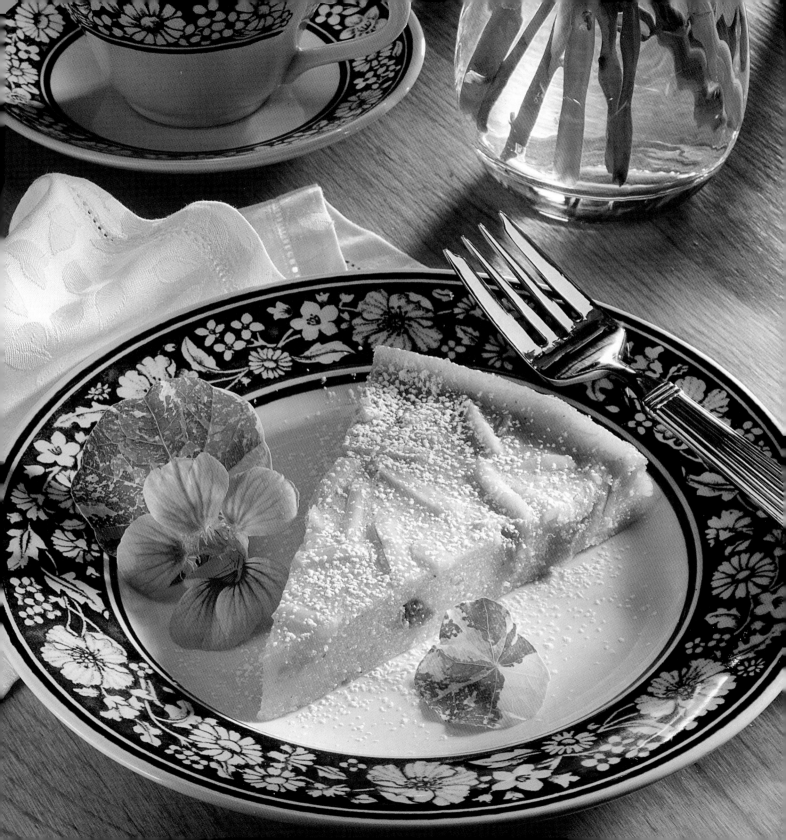

Tiramisu

2 tablespoons instant coffee crystals

½ cup hot water

2 (3-ounce) packages ladyfingers (24), cut crosswise into quarters

1 (14-ounce) can EAGLE® BRAND Sweetened Condensed Milk (NOT evaporated milk), divided

8 ounces mascarpone or cream cheese, softened

2 cups (1 pint) whipping cream, divided

1 teaspoon vanilla extract

1 cup (6 ounces) miniature semi-sweet chocolate chips, divided

Grated semi-sweet chocolate and/or strawberries, if desired

1. In small mixing bowl, dissolve coffee crystals in water; set aside 1 tablespoon coffee mixture. Brush remaining coffee mixture on cut sides of ladyfingers; set aside.

2. In large mixing bowl, gradually beat ¾ cup Eagle Brand and mascarpone. Add 1¼ cups whipping cream, vanilla and reserved 1 tablespoon coffee mixture; beat until soft peaks form. Fold in half the chips.

3. In heavy saucepan over low heat, melt remaining chips with remaining Eagle Brand.

4. Using 8 tall dessert glasses or parfait glasses, layer mascarpone mixture, chocolate mixture and ladyfinger pieces, beginning and ending with mascarpone mixture. Cover and chill at least 4 hours.

5. In medium mixing bowl, beat remaining ¾ cup whipping cream until soft peaks form. To serve, spoon whipped cream over dessert. Garnish as desired. Store covered in refrigerator.

Makes 8 servings

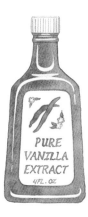

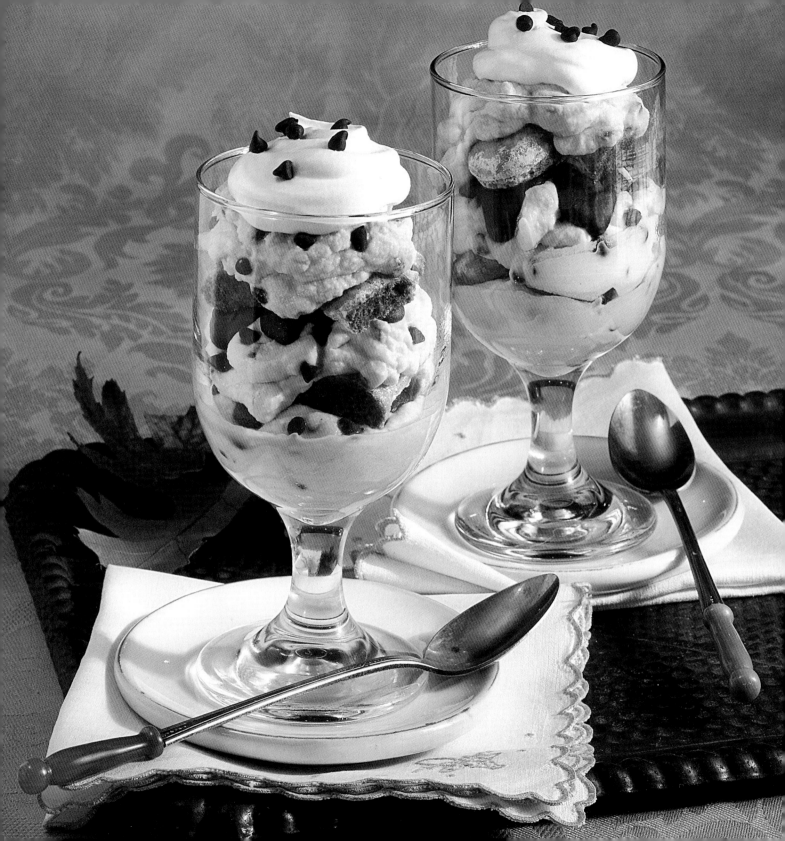

Chocolate Almond Biscotti

1 package DUNCAN HINES®
Moist Deluxe® Dark
Chocolate Cake Mix

1 cup all-purpose flour

½ cup butter or margarine,
melted

2 eggs

1 teaspoon almond extract

½ cup chopped almonds

White chocolate, melted
(optional)

1. Preheat oven to 350°F. Line 2 baking sheets with parchment paper.

2. Combine cake mix, flour, butter, eggs and almond extract in large bowl. Beat at low speed with electric mixer until well blended; stir in almonds. Divide dough in half. Shape each half into 12×2-inch log; place logs on prepared baking sheets. (Bake logs separately.)

3. Bake at 350°F for 30 to 35 minutes or until toothpick inserted in centers comes out clean. Remove logs from oven; cool on baking sheets 15 minutes. Using serrated knife, cut logs into ½-inch slices. Arrange slices on baking sheets. Bake biscotti 10 minutes. Remove to cooling racks; cool completely.

4. Dip one end of each biscotti in melted white chocolate, if desired. Allow white chocolate to set at room temperature before storing biscotti in airtight container. *Makes about 2½ dozen cookies*

Italian Chocolate Pie alla Lucia

4 tablespoons pine nuts

3 tablespoons brown sugar

1 tablespoon grated orange
peel

1 unbaked (9-inch) pie crust

4 ounces bittersweet chocolate,
coarsely chopped

3 tablespoons unsalted butter

1 can (5 ounces) evaporated
milk

3 eggs

3 tablespoons hazelnut liqueur

1 teaspoon vanilla

1. Toast pine nuts in dry nonstick skillet over medium heat, stirring constantly until golden brown and aromatic. Remove from heat and finely chop; cool. Combine pine nuts, brown sugar and orange peel in small bowl. Sprinkle in bottom of prepared pie crust and gently press into place with fingertips or back of spoon.

2. Preheat oven to 325°F. Melt chocolate and butter in small saucepan over low heat; stir until well blended. Let cool to room temperature.

3. Combine chocolate mixture with evaporated milk in medium bowl with electric mixer at medium speed. Add eggs, one at a time, beating well after each addition. Stir in hazelnut liqueur and vanilla. Pour into pie shell over pine nuts.

4. Bake on middle rack of oven 30 to 40 minutes or until filling is set.

5. Remove from oven and cool. Refrigerate until ready to serve. Serve with whipped cream and chocolate curls. *Makes 8 servings*

Chocolate Almond Biscotti

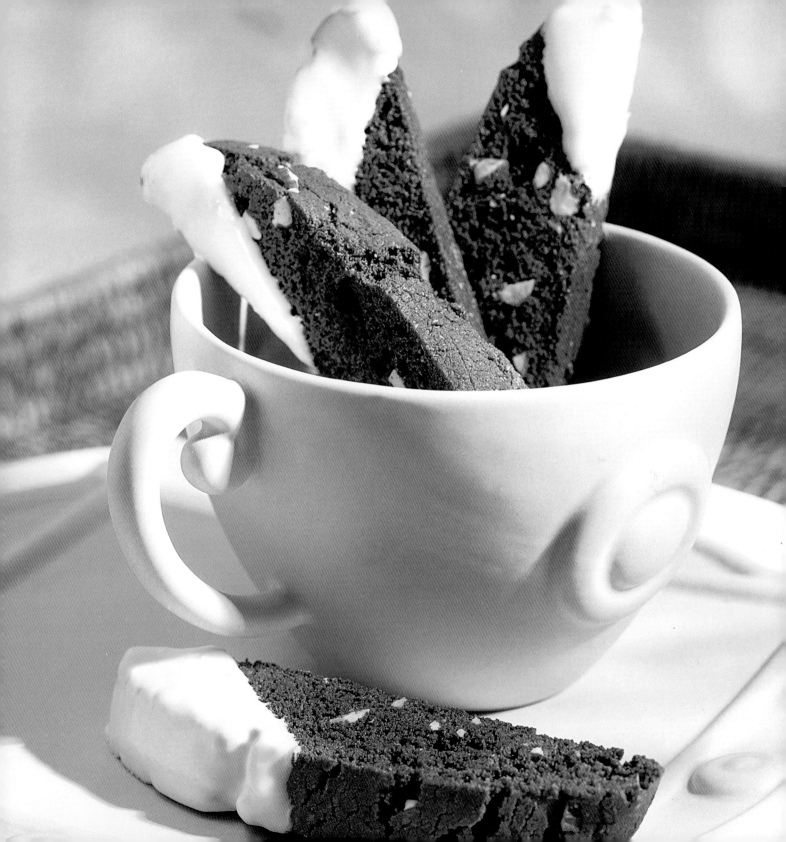

Summertime Fruit Medley

2 large ripe peaches, peeled and sliced

2 large ripe nectarines, sliced

1 large mango, peeled and cut into 1-inch chunks

1 cup blueberries

2 cups orange juice

¼ cup amaretto *or* ½ teaspoon almond extract

2 tablespoons sugar

1. Combine peaches, nectarines, mango and blueberries in large bowl.

2. Whisk orange juice, amaretto and sugar in small bowl until sugar is dissolved. Pour over fruit mixture; toss. Marinate 1 hour at room temperature, gently stirring occasionally. Garnish with mint, if desired.   *Makes 8 servings*

Fruit & Nut Biscotti Toasts

2 cups all-purpose flour

¾ cup sugar

½ cup cornmeal

½ cup finely chopped toasted walnuts

1½ teaspoon baking powder

½ teaspoon baking soda

¾ cup I CAN'T BELIEVE IT'S NOT BUTTER!® Spread, melted and cooled

3 eggs

1½ teaspoons vanilla extract

½ cup finely chopped citron (optional)

¼ cup dried cranberries or raisins

Preheat oven to 325°F.

In large bowl, combine flour, sugar, cornmeal, walnuts, baking powder and baking soda; set aside.

In small bowl, with wire whisk, beat I Can't Believe It's Not Butter! Spread, eggs and vanilla. Add to flour mixture, stirring until mixture forms a dough. Stir in citron and cranberries. Chill 1 hour.

On lightly floured surface, knead dough. Divide in half. On greased baking sheet, with floured hands, shape dough into two flat logs, about 14×1½-inches each. Bake 30 minutes or until firm. On wire rack, cool 10 minutes.

On cutting board, cut logs into ½-inch-thick diagonal slices. On baking sheet, arrange cookies cut side down. Bake an additional 20 minutes, turning over once. On wire rack, cool completely. Store in airtight container.

Makes about 2½ dozen toasts

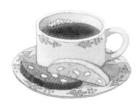

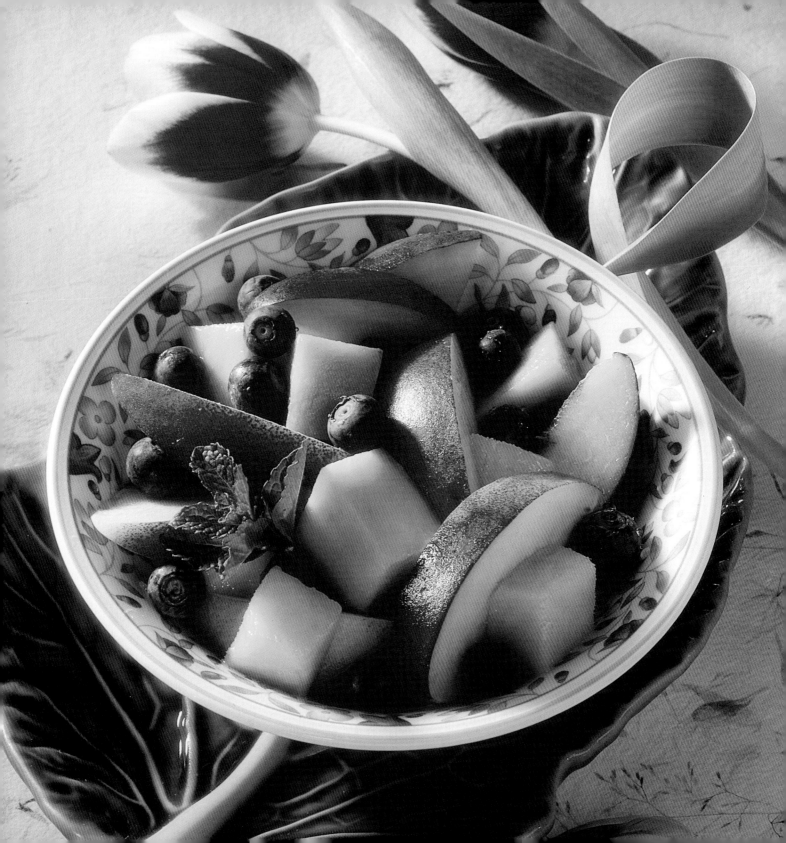

Quick Tiramisu

1 package (18 ounces) NESTLÉ® TOLL HOUSE® Refrigerated Sugar Cookie Bar Dough

1 package (8 ounces) ⅓ less fat cream cheese

½ cup granulated sugar

¾ teaspoon TASTER'S CHOICE® 100% Pure Instant Coffee dissolved in ¾ cup cold water, *divided*

1 container (8 ounces) frozen nondairy whipped topping, thawed

1 tablespoon NESTLÉ® TOLL HOUSE® Baking Cocoa

PREHEAT oven to 325°F.

DIVIDE cookie dough into 20 pieces. Shape into 2½×1-inch oblong shapes. Place on ungreased baking sheets.

BAKE for 10 to 12 minutes or until light golden brown around edges. Cool on baking sheets for 1 minute; remove to wire racks to cool completely.

BEAT cream cheese and sugar in large mixer bowl until smooth. Beat in ¼ *cup* Taster's Choice. Fold in whipped topping. Layer 6 cookies in 8-inch-square baking dish. Sprinkle each cookie with 1 *teaspoon* Taster's Choice. Spread *one-third* cream cheese mixture over cookies. Repeat layers 2 more times with 12 cookies, *remaining* coffee and *remaining* cream cheese mixture. Cover; refrigerate for 2 to 3 hours. Crumble *remaining* cookies over top. Sift cocoa over cookies. Cut into squares. *Makes 6 to 8 servings*

Caffè en Forchetta

2 cups reduced-fat (2%) milk

1 cup egg substitute

½ cup sugar

2 tablespoons mocha-flavored instant coffee

Grated chocolate or 6 chocolate-covered coffee beans (optional)

1. Preheat oven to 325°F.

2. Combine all ingredients in medium bowl except grated chocolate. Whisk until instant coffee has dissolved and mixture is foamy. Pour into six individual custard cups. Place cups in 13×9-inch baking pan. Fill with hot water halfway up side of cups.

3. Bake 55 to 60 minutes or until knife inserted halfway between center and edge comes out clean. Serve warm or at room temperature. Garnish with grated chocolate or chocolate-covered coffee beans, if desired. *Makes 6 servings*

Note: Enjoy your dinner coffee a whole new way. Translated from Italian, Caffè en Forchetta literally means "coffee on a fork." However, a spoon is recommended when serving this wonderfully creamy dessert.

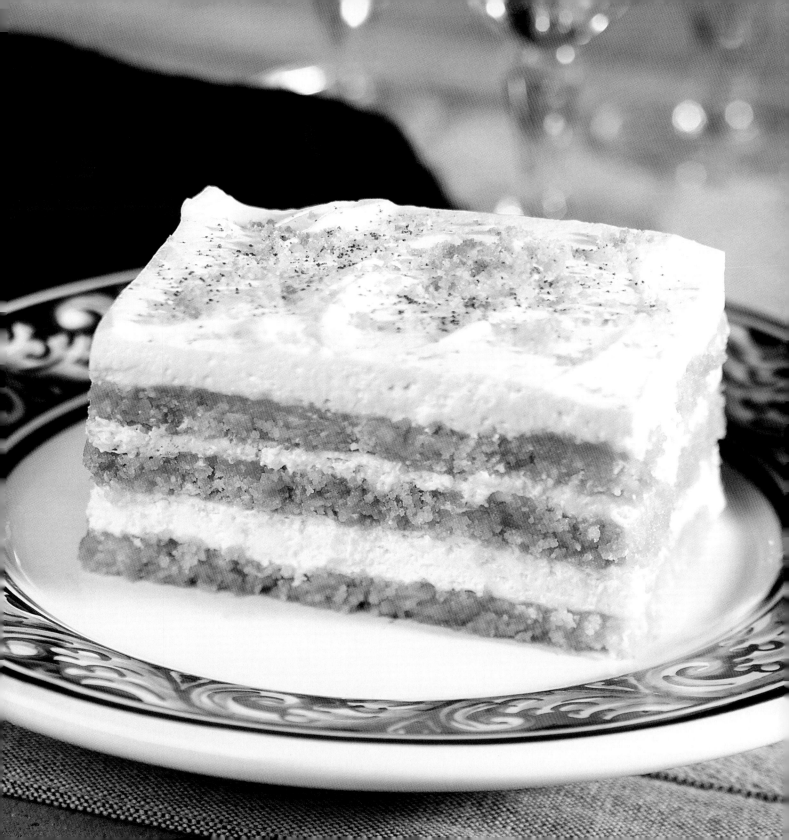

Apricot Biscotti

3 cups all-purpose flour

1½ teaspoons baking soda

½ teaspoon salt

⅔ cup sugar

3 eggs

1 teaspoon vanilla

½ cup chopped dried apricots*

⅓ cup sliced almonds, chopped

1 tablespoon reduced-fat (2%) milk

Other chopped dried fruits, such as dried cherries, cranberries or blueberries, can be substituted.

1. Preheat oven to 350°F. Lightly coat cookie sheet with nonstick cooking spray; set aside.

2. Combine flour, baking soda and salt in medium bowl; set aside.

3. Beat sugar, eggs and vanilla in large bowl with electric mixer at medium speed until combined. Add flour mixture; beat well.

4. Stir in apricots and almonds. Turn dough out onto lightly floured work surface. Knead 4 to 6 times. Shape dough into 20-inch log; place on prepared cookie sheet. Brush dough with milk.

5. Bake 30 minutes or until firm. Remove from oven; cool 10 minutes. Diagonally slice into 30 biscotti. Place slices on cookie sheet. Bake 10 minutes; turn and bake additional 10 minutes. Cool on wire racks. Store in airtight container.

Makes 2½ dozen biscotti

Rustic Honey Polenta Cake

2½ cups all-purpose flour

1 cup yellow cornmeal

2 tablespoons baking powder

1 teaspoon salt

1 cup (2 sticks) butter or margarine, melted

1¾ cups milk

¾ cup honey

2 eggs, slightly beaten

Honey-Orange Syrup (recipe follows)

Sweetened whipped cream and orange segments for garnish (optional)

In large bowl, combine flour, cornmeal, baking powder and salt; mix well. In small bowl, combine melted butter, milk, honey and eggs; mix well. Stir into flour mixture, mixing until just blended. Pour into lightly greased 13×9-inch baking pan.

Bake at 325°F for 25 to 30 minutes, or until toothpick comes out clean. Meanwhile prepare Honey-Orange Syrup. When cake is done, remove from oven to wire rack. Pour hot syrup evenly over top of cake, spreading if necessary to cover entire surface. Cool completely. Garnish with a dollop of whipped cream and orange segments, if desired.

Makes 12 servings

Honey-Orange Syrup: In small saucepan, whisk together ½ cup honey, 3 tablespoons orange juice concentrate and 1 tablespoon freshly grated orange peel. Heat over medium-high heat until mixture begins to boil; remove from heat.

Favorite recipe from **National Honey Board**

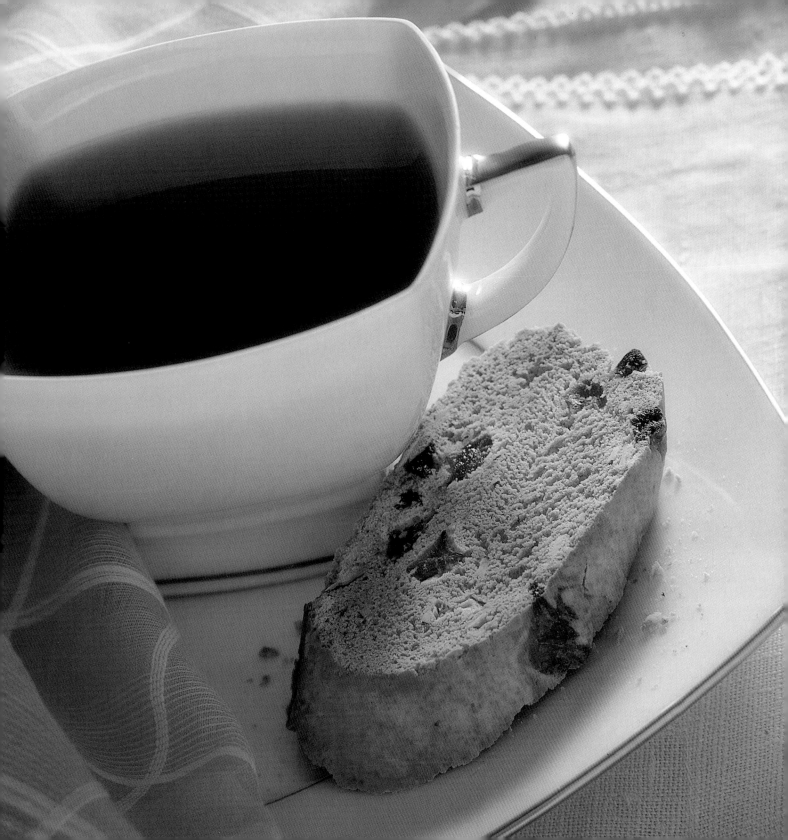

Chocolate-Amaretto Ice

¾ cup sugar

½ cup HERSHEY'S Cocoa

2 cups (1 pint) light cream or half-and-half

2 tablespoons amaretto (almond flavored liqueur)

Sliced almonds (optional)

1. Stir together sugar and cocoa in small saucepan; gradually stir in light cream. Cook over low heat, stirring constantly, until sugar dissolves and mixture is smooth and hot. Do not boil.

2. Remove from heat; stir in liqueur. Pour into 8-inch square pan. Cover; freeze until firm, stirring several times before mixture freezes. Scoop into dessert dishes. Serve frozen. Garnish with sliced almonds, if desired.

Makes 4 servings

Macédoine

Finely grated peel and juice of 1 lemon

Finely grated peel and juice of 1 lime

8 cups diced assorted seasonal fruits*

1 cup sweet spumante wine or freshly squeezed orange juice

¼ cup sugar

¼ cup coarsely chopped walnuts or almonds, toasted (optional)

Apples, pears and bananas are essential fruits in a traditional Macédoine. Add as many seasonally ripe fruits to them as you can— variety is the key. As you select fruits, try to achieve a diversity of textures, being sure to avoid mushy, overripe fruit.

1. Combine lemon juice and lime juice; place in large bowl. Place assorted fruits in bowl with citrus juice mixture; toss to coat.

2. Combine wine, sugar and citrus peels in small bowl, stirring until sugar is dissolved. Pour over fruit mixture; toss gently. Cover; refrigerate 1 hour.

3. Sprinkle walnuts on fruit mixture just before serving, if desired.

Makes 8 servings

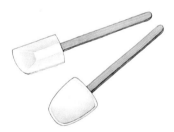

Acknowledgments

The publisher would like to thank the companies and organizations listed below for the use of their recipes and photographs in this publication.

Barilla America, Inc.
BelGioioso® Cheese, Inc.
Birds Eye®
Bob Evans®
Butterball® Turkey Company
Del Monte Corporation
Dole Food Company, Inc.
Duncan Hines® and Moist Deluxe® are registered trademarks of Aurora Foods Inc.
Eagle Brand®
Egg Beaters®
Filippo Berio® Olive Oil
The Golden Grain Company®
Hebrew National®
Hershey Foods Corporation
The Hidden Valley® Food Products Company
Holland House® is a registered trademark of Mott's, Inc.
Lawry's® Foods
McIlhenny Company (TABASCO® brand Pepper Sauce)
National Honey Board
National Pork Board
Nestlé USA
Perdue Farms Incorporated
Reckitt Benckiser Inc.
Sargento® Foods Inc.
The J.M. Smucker Company
Sonoma® Dried Tomatoes
StarKist® Seafood Company
Tyson Foods, Inc.
Uncle Ben's Inc.
Unilever Bestfoods North America
Veg•All®

Index

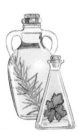

Metric Conversion Chart

VOLUME MEASUREMENTS (dry)

1/8 teaspoon = 0.5 mL
1/4 teaspoon = 1 mL
1/2 teaspoon = 2 mL
3/4 teaspoon = 4 mL
1 teaspoon = 5 mL
1 tablespoon = 15 mL
2 tablespoons = 30 mL
1/4 cup = 60 mL
1/3 cup = 75 mL
1/2 cup = 125 mL
2/3 cup = 150 mL
3/4 cup = 175 mL
1 cup = 250 mL
2 cups = 1 pint = 500 mL
3 cups = 750 mL
4 cups = 1 quart = 1 L

VOLUME MEASUREMENTS (fluid)

1 fluid ounce (2 tablespoons) = 30 mL
4 fluid ounces (1/2 cup) = 125 mL
8 fluid ounces (1 cup) = 250 mL
12 fluid ounces (1 1/2 cups) = 375 mL
16 fluid ounces (2 cups) = 500 mL

WEIGHTS (mass)

1/2 ounce = 15 g
1 ounce = 30 g
3 ounces = 90 g
4 ounces = 120 g
8 ounces = 225 g
10 ounces = 285 g
12 ounces = 360 g
16 ounces = 1 pound = 450 g

DIMENSIONS

1/16 inch = 2 mm
1/8 inch = 3 mm
1/4 inch = 6 mm
1/2 inch = 1.5 cm
3/4 inch = 2 cm
1 inch = 2.5 cm

OVEN TEMPERATURES

250°F = 120°C
275°F = 140°C
300°F = 150°C
325°F = 160°C
350°F = 180°C
375°F = 190°C
400°F = 200°C
425°F = 220°C
450°F = 230°C

BAKING PAN SIZES

Utensil	Size in Inches/Quarts	Metric Volume	Size in Centimeters
Baking or Cake Pan (square or rectangular)	8×8×2	2 L	20×20×5
	9×9×2	2.5 L	23×23×5
	12×8×2	3 L	30×20×5
	13×9×2	3.5 L	33×23×5
Loaf Pan	8×4×3	1.5 L	20×10×7
	9×5×3	2 L	23×13×7
Round Layer Cake Pan	8×1½	1.2 L	20×4
	9×1½	1.5 L	23×4
Pie Plate	8×1¼	750 mL	20×3
	9×1¼	1 L	23×3
Baking Dish or Casserole	1 quart	1 L	—
	1½ quart	1.5 L	—
	2 quart	2 L	—